the
ETHICS
of
Touch

The Hands-on Practitioner's Guide
To Creating a Professional, Safe and Enduring Practice

Ben E. Benjamin, Ph.D., and Cherie Sohnen-Moe

 SMA Inc., Tuscon, Arizona, USA

3906 W. Ina Road #200-347
Tucson, AZ 85741-2295
520-743-3936 800-786-4774
www.sohnen-moe.com

Publisher's Cataloging-in-Publication
(Provided by Quality Books, Inc.)

Benjamin, Ben E., 1944-
    The ethics of touch : the hands-on practioner's
guide to creating a professional, safe and eduring
practice / by Ben E. Benjamin and Cherie Sohnen-Moe.
    p. cm.
    Includes bibliographical references and index.
    LCCN 2002096403
    ISBN 1-880908-40-6

    1. Touch—Theraputic use—Moral and ethical aspects.
2. Allied health personnel—Professional ethics.
I. Sohnen-Moe, Cherie. II. Title.

RZ999.B465 2003   174'.29582
                    QBI03-200040

Cover design and illustrations: Umanga deSilva and James Moe
Editors: Joelle Andre, James Moe and Melissa B. Mower
Printed in the United States of America
First Edition, 2003

Preface

Ethics is an exciting, vital field of study for all professionals. Life is more fulfilling and satisfying if we live with honor and integrity in all our relationships and business dealings, yet much confusion exists among practitioners about what is and what is not ethical behavior. This confusion can be even more complex for somatic practitioners. This book helps to clarify an often vague, amorphous topic. Applying a professional code of ethics to practical behavior is not always easy. It is our desire to assist practitioners in developing an ethical foundation beyond reproach.

We created this ethics book because of the lack of resource materials written specifically for somatic practitioners. Most massage therapists, bodyworkers, chiropractors, acupuncturists, physical therapists and other somatic practitioners do not receive adequate ethics training. It is our mission to support hands-on professionals in expanding their knowledge about the field of ethics, better managing boundaries, and running ethical practices. We want to reach students as well as seasoned practitioners.

The Ethics of Touch was also written to facilitate exploration. Throughout this book you will find thought-provoking examples, models and exercises that make this information personally relevant.

We first develop a theoretical foundation and define key terms. Then we present methods for resolving ethical dilemmas and provide information on critical topics. We also incorporate specific methods and techniques for maintaining healthy boundaries, enhancing communication, fostering a sense of safety and managing your practice.

We encourage you to read each chapter and evaluate how to put these behaviors and skills into practice. Some of these issues may not be critical at your current setting, yet we have found that most practitioners face these issues at some point in their careers. If you seriously think about these issues ahead of time, you are prepared when they arise. The information, models and suggestions are meant as a starting point for you to customize and apply them to the unique aspects of your practice.

Terminology
What's In A Name?

This book is directed at health care professionals who touch the body as a primary method of delivering care. For consistency, and when speaking of all providers, we have chosen to use the words practitioner, health care provider, somatic practitioner, hands-on practitioner, and manual practitioner instead of specific titles such as massage therapist, bodyworker, acupuncturist, yoga instructor, chiropractor, Feldenkrais practitioner, physical therapist, Rolf© practitioner, polarity therapist, Shiatsu practitioner or Alexander teacher. Some of the scenarios do refer to specific professions yet are relevant to almost every field. Also, the terms bodywork, body therapy, touch therapy, somatic therapy, manual therapies, treatment and session are all interchangeable. We hope the information in this book is used by all professionals in the health care field, as the same concepts and basic information applies equally to all these professions.

Patient or Client?

We use the word "client" instead of "patient" throughout this book. We have done this purposefully because in our culture the word patient has come to indicate a person who is somewhat helpless and passive in relation to the health care provider.

The dictionary defines the word patient as follows: "from the Latin of *pati*, to suffer, bearing or enduring pain; a person under the care of a doctor; a person or thing that receives impressions from external agents; one who or that which is passively affected." We view the client as the employer of the practitioner who has been engaged to assist the client. This creates a context which places the client in charge, or at least in partnership, creating the best care possible. This attitude serves the best interests of the client/ practitioner relationship.

Him or Her?

Throughout history the male gender has been used exclusively to denote the generic pronoun when referring to women as well as men. As our culture and language has evolved, we have struggled to find the appropriate way to refer to all persons equally. Unfortunately, in English at least, a gender neutral pronoun does not exist and thus there is no way to easily accomplish this except by using the clumsy terms s/he, his or her, and himself/herself. We chose to alternate the use of the female and male pronouns throughout the book, but we intend for the principles illustrated by the examples to apply to both genders.

How to Use This book

The Ethics of Touch is intended for use both by hands-on healthcare practitioners in training and by professionals in the field. To fully assimilate the material in this book, it is best to read and study one chapter or even one section at a time. Although each chapter is self-contained, we suggest reading chapters One and Two first to gain an understanding of the core concepts that are carried throughout the book.

Many of the chapters include useful exercises, and at the end of each chapter are thought-provoking activities and questions for personal exploration. While you can do these on your own, they are much more valuable if you discuss them with peers and colleagues.

Continuing Education Units

You can obtain Continuing Education Units (CEUs) for each chapter. Our courses are recognized by many organizations, and we are category A providers for the National Certification Board for Therapeutic Massage and Bodywork.

If you are interested in using this material for CEUs, please call 800-786-4774 or visit our web site, www.TheEthicsOfTouch.com. If you have any questions regarding CEUs, please contact us, your professional organization or your state licensing board.

About the Authors

BEN BENJAMIN holds a PH.D. in Education and Sports Medicine. He is the founder and president of the Muscular Therapy Institute in Cambridge, Massachusetts, and has been in private practice for 40 years. He is the author of the widely-used books *Listen To Your Pain, Are You Tense?* and *Exercise Without Injury*. He has also written many professional articles on working with pain and injury problems and has been a regular columnist for the AMTA *Massage Therapy Journal* since 1986.

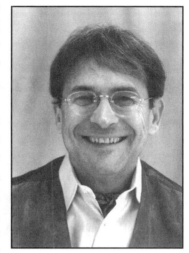

Dr. Benjamin was the initiator and chairperson of the AMTA Council of Schools Professional and Sexual Ethics Task Force for four years and is considered an authority on ethics and boundaries in the body therapy field. He was one of the first to write extensively about boundaries, ethical issues and sexual abuse in alternative health care, and since the early 1990s has published many articles on these topics in professional journals. Among the workshops he teaches throughout North America are Creating Healthy Boundaries in Health Care Settings, Working with Survivors of Trauma and Abuse, Assertiveness and Effective Communication, and Sexuality and Dual Relationships.

CHERIE SOHNEN-MOE is an author, business coach, international workshop leader and successful business owner since 1978. Before shifting her focus to education and coaching, she was in private practice for many years as a massage practitioner and holistic health educator. Cherie is the president of Sohnen-Moe Associates, Inc. Her company publishes business and practice mangement books in addition to distributing professional development products created by others. She holds a degree in psychology from UCLA and has extensive experience in the areas of business management, marketing, communication, training and creative problem solving.

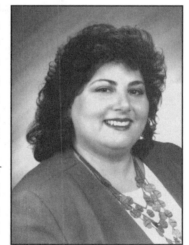

Ms. Sohnen-Moe is the author of *Present Yourself Powerfully* and *Business Mastery*; the latter is a required text in 400+ schools. She has written more than 100 articles that have been published in over 15 national and international magazines. Her most popular workshops are Marketing from Your Heart, The Four Keys to Publicity, The Ethics of Touch, Therapeutic Communications, Take Your Practice to the Next Level, Present Yourself Powerfully and Creative Teaching Techniques.

Contributing Authors

This book has been a work in progress for a decade. We had both been focusing our attention and expertise on different aspects of ethical behavior and realized that combining our backgrounds, education and experience would create a dynamic, useful resource.

In the process of research and writing, we sought the assistance of experts in a variety of fields to give breadth and depth to this book. Many people contributed ideas and stories, and several wrote major sections. Along with our original writing, we blended the contributed materials to fit the style, tone and focus of this book. We are grateful for all the support from our colleagues and their permission to adapt and expand their writings. We are true believers in collaboration and this book is the synergistic result of many creative minds.

DOUGLAS BOLTON, PH.D., is a clinical psychologist and certified school psychologist. He graduated from the University of Vermont and is currently working in a therapeutic school for students with severe emotional and behavioral problems. Robert and Douglas Bolton are the primary authors of the Dynamics of Effective Communication chapter.

ROBERT BOLTON, PH.D., is the co-founder of Ridge Associates, Inc., a consulting firm that serves Fortune 500 companies. He has designed training programs for the New York State Department of Mental Hygiene and co-founded a psychiatric outpatient clinic. He is the author of *People Skills: How to Assert Yourself, Listen to Others and Resolve Conflicts* and *People Styles at Work.*

NANCY BRIDGES, M.S.W., is a supervisor in the Dept. of Psychiatry at the Cambridge Health Alliance, an instructor at the Harvard Medical School and lecturer at Smith College School for Social Work. She has written numerous articles and presents widely on the therapeutic process and relationship. She is the primary author of the Supervision Chapter.

DAPHNE CHELLOS, M.A., is a psychotherapist, sex therapist and former massage therapist with 20 years of experience in teaching sexuality, ethics and communication. She holds a master's in counseling and directs the outreach program at the Naropa Institute in Colorado. Ms. Chellos is the primary author of the chapter on Sex, Touch and Intimacy.

REBECCA GWYNNE, B.A., L.M.T., is a Reiki Master/Teacher and has been practicing Reiki for 10 years and massage for nearly seven years. Ms. Gwynne works at Sohnen-Moe Associates, Inc. and contributed to the energy information in the Boundaries chapter.

LINDA MABUS JORGENSON, M.A., J.D., has considerable legal experience in the area of sexual exploitation by professionals. She has handled 400+ cases of therapist-patient sexual abuse allegations as well as cases involving non-sexual boundary violations. Ms. Jorgenson has published extensively in this area in numerous law reviews and mental health journals. She contributed the Legal Issues information for the Business Ethics chapter.

FRED N. LERNER, D.C., PH.D., F.A.C.O., has been in practice for more than 22 years. He is a chiropractic orthopedist at Cedars-Sinai Medical Center—The Pain Center. He also serves as Chairman of the National Board of Acupuncture Orthopedics. Dr. Lerner wrote the Health Insurance Portability and Accountability Act (HIPAA) section in the Ethical Practice Management chapter.

JODI A. LEWIS, M.S., M.B.A., R.N., L.M.T., has worked in case management since 1992. She worked as a consultant with many hospitals nationwide in implementing case management programs. She co-authored "Nursing Case Management and Quality" in the *Handbook of Nursing Case Management*. Ms. Lewis and Dr. Kathleen Stephens co-wrote the Case Management section in the Ethical Practice Management chapter.

SHAYE MOORE is a teacher, writer and nationally certified bodyworker whose practice is devoted to children and families. She was the recipient of a grant from the Community Health Program Fund of Children's Hospital in Boston, to bring infant massage instruction to disadvantaged young parents. Ms. Moore helped write the sections on dual relationships, working with minors, boundaries and the definitions covered in chapter one.

DIANNE POLSENO, L.M.T., is the former chair of the AMTA National Ethics Subcommittee, is a practicing massage therapist, practical nurse, academic director and teacher at the Bancroft School of Massage. She also leads ethics workshops and has authored numerous articles on ethics. Ms. Polseno contributed information on Sexual Misconduct, Informed Consent and Scope of Practice.

STUART N. SIMON, L.I.C.S.W., B.C.D., has been a psychotherapist for 25 years with experience working with couples, families and adults and organizations. He is a member of the core faculty of Gestalt International Study Center's, Center for the Study of Intimate systems, and a contributing author to several books on psychotherapy. Mr. Simon was a major author of the Boundaries Chapter.

KATHLEEN N. STEPHENS, D.C., L.M.T., has been involved in the alternative health field since 1977. She is the author of *The Stephens Method of Manual Therapy* and teaches her recognized technique nationally. Dr. Stephens also serves as a consultant in Case Management in private practices. She and Ms. Lewis co-wrote the Case Management section in the Ethical Practice Management chapter.

NANCY TAM, B.ED, B.F.A., B.S.W., is a human relations consultant, educational policy analyst, trainer and writer. Her company, Creative Neurons, specializes in mediation, organizational change, adult education and graphic design. She wrote the section on Process Recordings in the Dynamics of Effective Communication chapter.

DIANA THOMPSON, L.M.P., author of *Hands Heal: Communication, Documentation and Insurance Billing for Manual Therapists*, wrote the section on Insurance Issues for the Business Ethics chapter.

RUTH WERNER, L.M.T., has been a massage therapist and instructor since 1984. She is the author of *A Massage Therapist's Guide to Pathology*, as well as many other articles that have appeared in a variety of publications. Ms. Werner contributed to the Touch section in the Sex, Touch and Intimacy chapter.

Acknowledgments

We acknowledge all those individuals whose work and thoughts contributed to creating this book. First our thanks to whose graciously let us use information that they developed: Mark Annett; Virginia Anthony; Lu Bauer; Joan Calgano, J.D.; James Clay; Estelle Disch, PH.D., C.C.S.; Dave Eppley, PH.D., L.AC.; Clyde Ford, D.C.; Steven Hassan, L.M.H.C.; Judy Herman, M.D.; Krishnabai; Whitney Lowe; Shaye Moore; Angelica Redleaf, D.C.; Melissa Soalt; Helene Sorkin, L.AC.; and Janet Yassen, L.I.C.S.W.

We express our appreciation to the following people who shared their stories, gave us ideas, provided information and resources, and critiqued our material: Caroline Abreu; Virginia Anthony; Cindy Banker; Monque Barazone; Elaine Calenda; James Clay; Mary Ann DiRoberts, M.S.W., L.M.T.; Estelle Disch, PH.D., C.C.S.; Dian Fitzpatrick; Robert Flammia; Jackie Galloway; Susan Gottlieb; Rebecca Gwynne; Judy Herman, M.D.; Debbie Jedlicka; Helene Jewell; Janet King, J.D.; Jennifer Kuhn; Karen Manning; Sue Mapel. L.I.C.S.W.; T.C. Merrill; Shaye Moore; Daz Moran; Bill Mueller, L.AC.; Doug Newman, J.D.; Betty Norris; Ken Pope, PH.D.; Angelica Redleaf, D.C.; Julia Riley, R.N.; Mary Ringenberger; Daniel Schmidt; Gary Schoener, PH.D.; Rebecca Stephenson, P.T.; Sandi Straub; Stella Tarnay; Tracy Walton, M.S.W., L.M.T.; Christi Warner; Charles Whitfield, M.D.; Tracy Williams, M.S.; Gary Wolf, J.D.; and Janet Yassen, L.I.C.S.W.

Our deepest thanks go to the peer reviewers: Mark Annett; Elaine Calenda; Dave Eppley, PH.D., L.AC.; Judy Herman, M.D.; Shaye Moore; Bill Mueller, L.AC.; Angelica Redleaf, D.C.; Julia Riley, R.N.; Mary Ringenberger; Rebecca Stephenson, P.T.; Christi Warner; and Tracy Williams, M.S.

We are grateful for the following people who gave their time and expertise editing various drafts and giving input to make this book as accurate and useful as possible: Joelle André; Mary Ann DiRoberts, M.S.W., L.M.T.; Ginevra Fay; Helene Jewell; Fran Knott; James Moe; Shaye Moore; Melissa B. Mower; and Tracy Williams, M.S.

We thank James Moe and Umanga de Silva for their beautiful cover design and interior book layout, and Paul Kraytman for his drawings in the Boundaries Chapter.

Table of Contents

Ethical Principles   1
Key Terms   2
Codes of Ethics   3
Self-Accountability   4
Values Clarification   7
Ethical Dilemmas   9
Resolving Ethical Dilemmas   10
Core Psychological Concepts   14
In Conclusion...   22
Chapter Highlights   23
Discussion Questions and Activities   24

Boundaries   25
What Are Boundaries?   26
Types of Boundaries   28
Boundary Models   30
How Boundaries Develop   35
Boundary Crossings and Violations   39
Why Boundary Crossings Occur   44
Establish, Maintain & Change Boundaries   49
In Conclusion...   50
Chapter Highlights   51
Discussion Questions and Activities   52

Dynamics of Effective Communication   55
Communication Barriers   56
Learning Styles   58
Managing Boundaries   58
Emotions in the Treatment Room   62
Reflective Listening   65
Interactive Speaking   67
Body Language Awareness   69
Tools for Maintaining Boundaries   71
Process Recordings   73
The Assertion Sequence   75
In Conclusion...   81
Chapter Highlights   82
Discussion Questions and Activities   83

Dual Relationships   85
An Historical Perspective   87
Sequential Relationships   88
The Range of Dual Relationships   88
The Risks of Dual Relationships   90
Minimizing Concerns   94
The Special Case of Schools   97

In Conclusion…   98
Chapter Highlights   99
Discussion Questions and Activities   100

Sex, Touch and Intimacy   103

A Psychosocial Overview   104
Touch   106
Intimacy   112
Sex   114
Sexuality   116
Sex and Touch Therapy   119
Sexual Misconduct   127
Desexualizing the Touch Experience   134
In Conclusion…   138
Chapter Highlights   139
Discussion Questions and Activities   141

Ethical Practice Management   143

Professionalism   144
Scope of Practice   145
Standards of Practice   151
Policy Statements   152
Working With Minors   162
Informed Consent   165
Declining Potential New Clients   167
Dismissing A Client   168
The Team Approach   171
Spa and Salon Issues   176
In Conclusion…   176
Chapter Highlights   177
Discussion Questions and Activities   178

Business Ethics   181

Attitudes About Money   182
Fee Structures   184
Tips   187
Barter   188
Gift Certificates   190
Taxes   191
Product Sales   191
Referrals   193
Marketing Materials   194
Legal Issues   196
Insurance Issues   207
In Conclusion...   210
Chapter Highlights   211
Discussion Questions and Activitie   213

Special Considerations In Cases of Trauma   215
Understanding Trauma and Abuse   216
The Core of Trauma and Abuse   218
The Benefits of Touch Therapy   224
Prerequisites for Working with Survivors   226
Body Memories and Flashbacks   231
In Conclusion...   235
Chapter Highlight   236
Discussion Questions and Activities   239

Supervision   241
The Role of Clinical Supervision   242
Essential Elements of Helpful Supervision   249
How to Find a Supervisor   250
Peer Supervision   251
In Conclusion…   252
Chapter Highlights   253
Discussion Questions and Activities   254

Appendix A   Forms   255
Boundary Clarification Exercise Answer Key   256
Client Bill of Rights   257
Sample Oriental Medicine Office Policies   260
Sample Massage Therapy Center Policies   261
Sample School Clinic Informed Consent   263
Sample Massage Therapy Informed Consent   264
Trauma Survivor Handout: Feelings List   265

Appendix B   Specialized Protocols   267
Specific Techniques for Working with Self-Disclosed Survivors of
    Trauma and Abuse   268
BITE Model of Cult Mind Control   276

Appendix C   Codes of Ethics   279
American Chiropractic Association   280
American Massage Therapy Association   283
American Organization for Bodywork Therapies of Asia™   284
American Physical Therapy Association   285
American Polarity Therapy Association   286
Associated Bodywork & Massage Professionals   290
Feldenkrais Guild® of North America   291
International Massage Association Group   292
Kripalu Yoga Teachers Association   293
Nat'l Certification Board for Therapeutic Massage & Bodywork   294
Nat'l Certification Commission for Acupuncture & Oriental Medicine   295
Ontario Massage Therapist Association   296
Trager International   297

Endnotes

Index

1

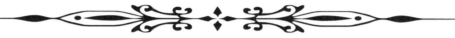

Ethical Principles

- ✦ Key Terms
- ✦ Codes of Ethics
- ✦ Self-Accountability
- ✦ Values Clarification
- ✦ Ethical Dilemmas
- ✦ Resolving Ethical Dilemmas
- ✦ Core Psychological Concepts
- ✦ In Conclusion...
- ✦ Chapter Highlights
- ✦ Discussion Questions and Activities

The topic of ethics can often be confusing, difficult and at times downright baffling. Although debated by philosophers for millennia, agreeing upon what is "good" and "bad" remains difficult. So much depends on the situation. Not all ethical breaches are gross violations of conduct; much unethical behavior is subtle. Furthermore, being ethical is not limited simply to knowing and following ethical codes, laws and regulations. Ethical behavior also involves striving to bring the highest values into one's work and aspiring to do one's best in all interactions: doing the right thing in the right manner for the right reasons and with the right attitude. Tom Peters, acclaimed author of *In Search of Excellence,*[1] sums it up like this: "High ethical standards—business or otherwise—are, above all, about treating people decently. To me (as a person, business person and business owner) that means respect for a person's privacy, dignity, opinions and natural desire to grow; and people's respect for (and by) co-workers."[2]

For somatic practitioners ethics can be especially complex as they encounter ethical issues and dilemmas that do not always have simple, apparent solutions. In many cases practitioners may inadvertently act unethically because they have not considered the relevant issues. Expanding their grasp of ethical principles helps practitioners understand the impact of their behavior on clients and provides the knowledge and tools to act appropriately. The overall purpose of ethics is to guide professional practitioners so that clients' welfare remains the first priority.

This book is written especially for you, the somatic practitioner. Whether you are a massage therapist, acupuncturist, physical therapist, chiropractor, yoga instructor or bodyworker—professional or student—this material can help you to run an ethical practice, prevent many ethical violations from occurring and be equipped to resolve ethical dilemmas when they arise. We begin this chapter with an overview of key terms, basic concepts, practical applications and tools to use in creating an ethical life.

Key Terms

People often confuse the words ethics, values, principles, morals, laws and professionalism, and use the terms interchangeably. While they are closely related, they are not the same. Ethics embodies all of these elements. The following definitions help clarify the differences:

ETHICS is the study of moral principles and appropriate conduct. This can be applied to individuals, groups or professions. In general, ethics in somatic therapies involve behaving honorably, adhering to prevailing laws, upholding the dignity of the profession, respecting each client, staying committed to high quality, working within the appropriate scope of practice, being client-centered and remaining service-oriented.

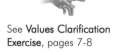

See **Values Clarification Exercise,** pages 7-8

VALUES are tangible and intangible convictions that an individual considers of intrinsic worth. Values are based upon beliefs and attitudes and involve what is desirable rather than what is right and correct. For example, while you know the worth of your services and believe in receiving a fair fee, you may also have a strong value of making your services accessible to everyone regardless of their economic means and therefore incorporate a sliding scale into your fee structure. Individuals do not necessarily agree on what is important as a "value" and may even change their own value structure many times over the course of their life.

PRINCIPLES comprise an individual's code of action and enable a person to behave with integrity. The person of principle modifies her behavior so that each action arises from her deeply held sense of self. For example, a person who acts upon the principle of honest financial dealings may be reflecting his core value of fairness and equality among people. Principles are therefore based at least in part upon one's values. Again they may differ widely from one individual to another.

MORALS relate to the judgment of goodness and badness of human behavior and character. They are often stated in terms of virtues. This shared assessment, undertaken by a group of people, is usually based on cultural or religious standards. Consider the following example of poor character and lack of beneficence: You determine that a client would really benefit by seeing a practitioner in a different field, but you do not refer out because you do not want to lose the income. Also, keep in mind that actions can be judged as moral in one culture and immoral in another. For instance in the Islamic culture a woman is forbidden to be unclothed in a room with a man who is not her husband.

LAWS are codified rules of conduct set forth by a society and are generally based on shared ethical or moral principles. Laws often set the minimum standard necessary to protect the public's welfare and are enforceable by the courts. Specific laws relating to scope of practice may vary by locale. For example, in some locations manually treating the breast is not permitted by law while in other places no such restrictions exist.

PROFESSIONALISM is the quality of the image an individual conveys. Professionalism stems from your attitudes and is manifested through your technical competency, your communication skills, your ability to manage boundaries, your respect for yourself and clients, and your business practices. The term professionalism is related to ethical behavior. High standards of action with clients result in both ethical and professional behavior. Obviously, ethical violations are unprofessional. However, not all unprofessional behavior is unethical. For example, dressing in torn workout clothes when working with a client is unprofessional, but not unethical.

See page 9-10 for more information on **beneficence**.

Codes of Ethics

Codes of Ethics are conduct guidelines. While individuals may have developed their own personal codes of ethics, these codes are most commonly set by professional organizations. Their major functions are to: inform practitioners of appropriate ethical norms and behavior; supply direction for challenging situations; encourage practitioners to provide excellent service; protect clients; and provide a means for enforcing desired professional behavior. Most codes of ethics are broad and vague, partly due to the contextual nature of "right" and "wrong." In most instances research, consultation and self-exploration are required to determine what is appropriate and ethical.

For example, the National Certification Board for Therapeutic Massage and Bodywork (NCBTMB) Code of Ethics states: "Provide treatment only where there is reasonable expectation that it will be advantageous to the client." If a practitioner believes that touch is valuable for everyone she may come to one conclusion ("everyone, regardless of their problems and conditions, should have regular bodywork"). But if a practitioner believes that only certain types of bodywork are good for a particular individual or condition he may come to an entirely different conclusion ("only perform manual lymphatic drainage techniques, not massage, for the condition of lymphedema").

The Acupuncture and Oriental Medicine Code of Ethics states, "I will continue to work to raise the standards of the profession." This leaves room for wide interpretation; one practitioner might think this means affecting public policy or giving public talks while another practitioner simply takes this to mean conducting an ethical practice.

Those are my principles. If you don't like them, I have others.

—Groucho Marx

See Appendix C for sample **Codes of Ethics**.

Only in certain instances do ethics codes clearly dictate the desired behavior. The American Chiropractic Association Code of Ethics clearly states, "It is unethical for a doctor of chiropractic to receive a fee, rebate, rental payment, or any other form of remuneration for the referral of a patient to a clinic, laboratory, or other health service entity."

The American Physical Therapy Association Code of Ethics states that, "A physical therapist shall not engage in any sexual relationship or activity, whether consensual or nonconsensual, with any patient while a physical therapist/patient relationship exists."

Some ethical situations include a combination of the elements of ethics, morals, values and professionalism. For example, one of your values might be to work from home so you can spend more time with your family. But if the zoning laws in your area prohibit home businesses, you would be breaking the law. Engaging in sexual activities with a client crosses almost every element: this behavior is considered unethical and unprofessional. Moreover, it is illegal in many professions. Yet the practitioner who engages sexually with a client obviously has different values and morals, or maybe weak discipline, poor resistance to temptation, or a neurotic compulsion (all of which may conflict with values and morals) that allows the practitioner to justify the behavior.

Self-Accountability

In essence, self-accountability is the cornerstone of ethics. It is about who you are and what you do when no one's watching you. When you have a well-developed sense of self-accountability you are honest with yourself, and you are answerable and fully responsible for what you say and do at all times. You have the ability to look beyond the immediate moment to consider all the consequences and know if you are willing to accept them. You have personal ethics. As individuals it is our capacity for self-accountability that keeps us functioning ethically and responsibly.

Personal ethics is the precursor to professional ethics: you are not likely to be more ethical in your professional life than you are in your personal life. As the saying goes, "No matter where you go, there you are." In other words, you are most likely dishonest in your business affairs if you are dishonest in your personal life. Likewise, if you cannot keep the secret of a friend, your client's confidentiality is at risk.

Ethics is a code of values which guide our choices and actions and determine the purpose and course of our lives.

—Ayn Rand

Always do right. This will gratify some people and astonish the rest.

—Mark Twain

It's OK, Son, Everybody Does It

When Johnny was 6 years old, he was with his father when they were caught speeding. His father handed the officer a twenty dollar bill with his driver's license. "It's OK, son," his father said as they drove off. "Everybody does it."

When he was 8, he was present at a family council presided over by Uncle George on the surest means to shave points off the income tax return. "It's OK, kid," his uncle said. "Everybody does it."

When he was 9, his mother took him to his first theater production. The box office man couldn't find any seats until his mother discovered an extra $5 in her purse. "It's OK, son," she said. "Everybody does it."

When he was 12, he broke his glasses on the way to school. His Aunt Francine persuaded the insurance company that they had been stolen and they collected $75. "It's OK, kid," she said. "Everybody does it."

When he was 15, he made right guard on the high school football team. His coach showed him how to block and at the same time grab the opposing end by the shirt so the official couldn't see it. "It's OK, kid," the coach said. "Everybody does it."

When he was 16, he took his first summer job at the supermarket. His assignment was to put the overripe strawberries on the bottom of the boxes and the good ones on top where they would show. "It's OK, kid," the manager said. "Everybody does it."

When he was 18, Johnny and a neighbor applied for a college scholarship. Johnny was a marginal student. His neighbor was in the upper three percent of his class but he couldn't play right guard. Johnny got the scholarship. "It's OK, son," his parents said. "Everybody does it."

When he was 19, he was approached by an upperclassman who offered the test answers for $50. "It's OK, kid," he said. "Everybody does it."

Johnny was caught and sent home in disgrace. "How could you do this to your mother and me?" his father said. "You never learned anything like this at home." His aunt and uncle were shocked.

If there's one thing the adult world can't stand, it's a kid who cheats...

From: *The Power of Ethical Management*, Blanchard and Peale[3]

> *The measure of a man's character is what he would do if he knew he never would be found out.*
> —Thomas B. Macaulay

A Practical Application for Students

As demonstrated in the story about cheating, this behavior can start at a very young age and continue throughout one's life. School is an environment rife with opportunity for cheating. What you do there lays the groundwork for the rest of your professional career. The student who bends the rules in school is at high risk of bending them in professional life. Your internal moral code, your definition of being truthful, your determination of what's okay in your personal ethics, is first expressed in the school setting.

Cheating is one of the most common ethical problems in schools. Students cheat during exams, forge signatures on practice forms, get other people to do their homework, buy papers, or practice professionally before permissible. The student's thinking process becomes skewed and sounds a little like this: "It's okay to cheat a little, it doesn't really hurt anybody. This is a way for my grades to get better and for me to succeed at school, and it won't have any meaning after I graduate." However, such thinking is faulty. Three facts about cheating at school are clear.

First, cheating is not a victimless crime; in fact, a significant number of people are negatively impacted even by one student cheating. The teacher in whose class the cheating occurred is upset that the trust extended to this student has been betrayed. Fellow students who observed or know about the cheating and kept quiet are troubled about their relationship with that student and feel badly about not telling the teacher. Those students are in a further conflict if they are asked if they were aware of the student's cheating and have to decide whether to tell the truth and implicate themselves for non-action. Students who see the cheating and tell the teacher feel upset or angry at the student and feel guilty for reporting the incident. After the student is exposed other students take sides and often become conflicted and divided. Everyone suffers as a result of this experience. The classroom energy and atmosphere becomes filled with an uneasy tension until the issue is resolved.

If the student is caught, he either denies the cheating and is unrepentant, denies the cheating but feels intense guilt, or admits to the cheating and feels shame, isolation and loss of trust (and sometimes relief). The student may be put on probation or expelled, depending upon his reaction, the amount and quality of the evidence and the school's policy.

Secondly, cheating does **not** help a student succeed at school. The student's grades do not significantly improve and the student does not end up doing better work. How well students do at school is demonstrated through the whole fabric of their behavior: their manner; their sensitivity to others; their understanding of the issues involved; their degree of self-disclosure; and their interrelationships with clients, teachers and other students. The student who cheats is wearing a fabric that does not fit and the impression left is jagged or discordant. Teachers, administrators and other students often have an intuitive sense that something is wrong about this person.

The third fact is that cheating **is** an ethical violation that inevitably spills into professional life, often with disastrous results. Academic dishonesty that is okay becomes professional dishonesty that is okay. For example, in research, the professional fudges the numbers just a little to make the results come out the way she wants. He plagiarizes just a little when writing an article. She hides part of her income and inflates her expenses. He decides it is okay to break laws and regulations he does not like. The student who cheats becomes a poor performing professional whose behavior also undermines the credibility of the profession. The teaching institution that tolerates cheating or turns a blind eye to dishonest behavior joins the student in downgrading the integrity of the profession.

Cheating is a form of lying, dishonesty and deception that erodes the moral fiber of the person who engages in it. The reasons are legion why students cheat: Cheating is often approached in a mindless manner by a student when the academic work becomes too challenging or the student feels he does not need to know this information and does not want to do the work or study. The student may also come from a family or a culture where the groundwork for cheating is set by lying, bribery, tax evasion and other dishonest acts. The student may feel pushed toward cheating when personally or emotionally over-extended, particularly when the consequences of failing are high (e.g., losing financial aid or loss of face within his family). The student who makes the decision to cheat may unconsciously feel desperate about failing and be too ashamed or not know how to ask for help. To create a sense of safety and fairness in the classroom environment, cheating must be stopped. If it is not confronted by the school, not only does an awkward, dishonest atmosphere pervade the classroom environment, but the entire profession suffers.

A Practical Application for Professionals

Forethought and understanding help practitioners avoid a myriad of problems throughout their careers. Awareness of these potential issues and careful consideration assist health care professionals to avoid thoughtless errors in judgment. Below are a sampling of actions and behaviors generally considered unethical by professional codes of ethics.

PRACTICING BEYOND SCOPE OF PRACTICE: Doing spinal adjustments, massage or counseling without appropriate training.

SEXUAL MISCONDUCT: Watching a client undress or hugging a client in a sexual way.

MISREPRESENTATION OF EDUCATIONAL STATUS: Calling yourself a craniosacral therapist after taking a three-hour workshop.

FINANCIAL IMPROPRIETY: Charging a cash-paying client a different fee than an insurance-paying client.

EXPLOITING THE POWER DIFFERENTIAL: Asking a stock broker for financial tips during a treatment.

MISLEADING CLAIMS OF CURATIVE ABILITIES: Telling a client you guarantee her pain will be gone in two sessions.

ACCESSIBILITY: Refusing to adapt your office (or making some reasonable accommodation) for those with physical challenges.

BIGOTRY: Refusing to work on someone due to race, religion, size or sexual orientation.

INAPPROPRIATE ADVERTISING: Using a provocative picture in advertising; presenting misleading qualifications.

DUAL RELATIONSHIPS: Dating a client.

VIOLATION OF LAWS: Practicing out of your home when it is not permitted by law.

CONFIDENTIALITY: Name-dropping famous clients; telling a spouse details about his partner's session.

CONTRAINDICATIONS: Treating a client when you are sick/infectious; ignoring signs of conditions that preclude physical contact.

INFORMED CONSENT: Working on a minor without parental knowledge; treating someone's injury without permission.

> "
> In matters of style swim with the current; in matters of principle stand like a rock.
> "
> —Thomas Jefferson

Values Clarification

A satisfying and balanced life occurs when your values are in synchrony with the way you lead your life and run your business. Invest the time in exploring your values. After all, they are the major conscious and unconscious influences on the decisions you make throughout your life. Many conflicts in one's life, both professional and personal, arise because there is a clash of values either within oneself or among others.

Core Values Assessment

The following exercise helps clarify your core values. Take your time. Ask yourself the following questions and write your responses. We have listed sample responses to stimulate your thinking (if needed). When you finish this exercise, we recommend you discuss it with a fellow student, friend or colleague. Engaging in a dialogue with others is another way to more fully explore your own values.

> "
> I wouldn't have turned out the way I was if I didn't have all those old-fashioned values to rebel against.
> "
> —Madonna
> [Madonna Louise Ciccione]

- **WHAT VALUES ARE MOST IMPORTANT TO ME?**
  Being honest; treating myself and others with respect and kindness; trusting my intuition; appreciating nature; acknowledging people for their support.

- **WHAT ARE THE CHARACTER TRAITS I DEEM ESSENTIAL?**
  The ability to communicate; patience; a sense of humor; the ability to listen without giving advice; honesty; integrity.

- **WHO AND WHAT HAVE BEEN MAJOR INFLUENCES IN MY VALUES DEVELOPMENT?**
  My mother; my father; my third grade teacher; my mentor; Martin Luther King; psychotherapy; my decision to pursue this profession; Outward Bound experiences.

- **WHAT ARE MY ATTITUDES AND BELIEFS ABOUT WELLNESS?**
  If people exercise regularly they live long and healthy lives; good health involves a balanced body, mind and spirit; it takes a lot of work to be healthy; just because you have a disability does not mean you are sick; the best path to wellness is through acupuncture/ massage/chiropractic/yoga.

- **WHAT ARE MY ATTITUDES AND BELIEFS ABOUT MY PROFESSION?**
  It is really the best path to getting and staying healthy; it complements other types of health care; it feels like a good vehicle for me to make a difference in other people's lives; this profession has a proven track record for effectiveness.

- **WHAT ARE THE MOST IMPORTANT PERSONAL CHARACTERISTICS FOR SOMEONE IN MY FIELD?**
  Intuition; empathy; a sincere desire to help others; patience; humor; good personal boundaries.

- **WHAT ARE THE KEY PROFESSIONAL CHARACTERISTICS FOR SOMEONE IN MY FIELD?**
  Hard work; punctuality; skillful touch; professional proficiency; dedication; excellent communication skills; integrity; good professional boundaries.

- **WHAT ARE THE MOST MEANINGFUL ATTRIBUTES OF AN EFFECTIVE PRACTITIONER IN MY FIELD?**
  The ability to connect with people and create a safe environment; the ability to admit mistakes; the ability to recognize conditions in individuals beyond my professional expertise capabilities; investing in continuing education; using high-quality products and equipment.

- **HOW DO MY VALUES AFFECT MY WORK WITH CLIENTS?**
  Everyone should behave responsibly and I therefore charge when people cancel without giving 24 hours notice; one of my values is giving back to the community so I hold a free clinic one day a month; I believe people should participate in their care therefore I discuss my overall treatment plan and give self-care exercises for clients to do on their own.

- **WHICH OF MY PERSONAL VALUES CONFLICT WITH PROFESSIONAL RULES OF CONDUCT?**
  My religion forbids me to touch a person of the opposite sex except my spouse but my profession dictates that I cannot discriminate against any individual; I believe I should be allowed to mention the names of my celebrity clients to my friends and family but the confidentiality code of my profession prohibits it.

- **WHICH OF MY PERSONAL VALUES CONFLICT WITH LAWS OR REGULATIONS?**
  I do not believe the government has any business regulating what I do but my profession says I need a license; I believe that I should be allowed to work out of my home but the zoning laws in my area do not permit home offices.

- **HOW DO MY VALUES ENHANCE MY PROFESSIONALISM?**
  My commitment to open communication with my clients makes me a more effective practitioner; my good boundaries create a safe environment for my clients; my honesty with my clients instills trust in me as a professional and in my profession as a whole.

> *"The greatest homage we can pay to truth is to use it."*
>
> —Ralph Waldo Emerson

Ethical Dilemmas

An ethical dilemma occurs when two or more principles are in conflict, and regardless of your choice, something of value is compromised. At times there might even be several viable options, each with merit and it is unclear as to the most appropriate choice. These situations are troubling and by their nature difficult to resolve.

Two Examples of Ethical Dilemmas

A minor comes to see you for an evaluation. He is in pain from a soft tissue injury and you feel confident that you can relieve his pain after several weeks of treatment. You tell him you need parental permission before you can work on him. He informs you that his parents refuse to let him see you for treatment and he has come to see you without their knowledge. He pleads with you to work on him without getting parental consent.

A client, in discussing her stress, reveals that she is excessive in her corporeal punishment of her child. You feel torn between your client's right to confidentiality and your concern about the welfare of the child which would lead you to report her to the child welfare authorities. (In many areas the law requires that suspected child abuse is reported.)

Conflicting Duties and Rights

The two major principles involved in ethical dilemmas are duties and rights. Almost all ethical dilemmas arise from a clash between the following: two or more competing duties; two or more competing rights; or duties competing with rights.

Duties

A duty is an act or course of action required by position, social custom, law or religion. It is a moral obligation or a compulsion felt to meet such obligation. It is experienced as a deep commitment to act in a certain way.

Two primary duties identified by most health professionals are 1. Do no harm (nonmaleficence) and 2. Do positive good (beneficence). "Not harming" and "acting to benefit" are treated by many practitioners as separate duties with "do no harm" as more compelling if the two conflict in any situation.

A client sees an acupuncturist because she is ill. The client wants the practitioner to give her herbs to help alleviate the problem. The practitioner is hesitant because of the following: the potential negative interactions with medications the client is taking; the possible consequences if the client discontinues the medication; and the possible breach of ethics if the practitioner contradicts the orders from the client's physician.

Rights

Rights can be thought of as very stringent claims. Justice is a basic right: the expectation that all clients will receive equal treatment. An essential client's right is the right to self-determination, meaning clients are free from interference with their personal life and autonomy. A common ethical error occurs if the practitioner tries to override the client's right to self-determination when worried about the client's behavior.

For instance, a chiropractor insists a client change her diet because he "knows" it will help her heal faster from her injury. In this example, the client's right to self-determination clashes with the practitioner's perceived duty to do positive good. Actually, simply mentioning something once fulfills the duty to do good.

The client's right to self-determination always overrides the practitioner's duty unless the anticipated negative consequences are extreme. For instance if your assessment indicates that client has a serious, possibly life-threatening medical condition, and needs to see a doctor, you would more strongly encourage the client to see a specialist even if she is hesitant to do so.

Resolving Ethical Dilemmas

When faced with an ethical dilemma, many of us turn to our formal codes of ethics and relevant laws to guide us. However, the nature of ethical dilemmas is that they are complex and multi-faceted. In addition to ethical codes, laws, organizational policies and the community's expectations, you must also examine your personal values and practical considerations.

According to Mark Annett in the book, *The Scruples Methodology*,[4] whenever you decide to take an action that some might construe as unethical, or avoid tackling an ethical dilemma, then you should be aware that you are taking a risk at three different levels.

"The first level of risk is personal. People are always observing other people's behavior. If you act unethically in one situation then people will assume you might act that way in others. Consequently, people may begin to distrust you and your judgment, even under unrelated circumstances. For instance, if a coworker hears you convincingly lie to a customer then your coworker might think, 'Wow, she is really good at lying. I wonder if I would be able to tell I was being lied to or not.' From that moment on, mistrust begins to build.

"The second level of risk is to your company. People learn by example. If top management is doing things that are unethical then people might get the message that it is okay for them to do the same. For instance, if the company just cheated another company out of $50,000, then my stealing $50 in office supplies does not seem so bad.

"Finally, being unethical also places your industry at risk. For instance, take telemarketers. I will absolutely not give out my credit card information, even to charities. Now, not all telemarketers are unethical. But, the ones that are have so badly damaged their reputation that the whole industry is tainted."

The Six-Step Resolution Model

The following model is helpful in thinking through ethical problems and making decisions. It is adapted from problem-solving processing and steps identified by Corey, Corey and Callahan.[5] Keep in mind that this processing model is just a starting point. In the article *Crossing the Spectrum: Steps for Making Ethical Decisions*,[6] Frank Navran states, "The process alone doesn't guarantee an ethical outcome. Unfortunately, only the decision maker can do that."

1. **IDENTIFY THE PROBLEM**
   A. Gather as much relevant information as possible.
   B. Talk to the parties involved.
   C. Clarify the nature of the problem: legal, values, moral, ethical, or a combination.

2. **IDENTIFY THE POTENTIAL ISSUES INVOLVED**
   A. List and describe the critical issues.
   B. Evaluate the rights, responsibilities and welfare of those affected by the decision.
   C. Consider the basic moral principles of autonomy, beneficence, nonmaleficence and justice.
   D. Ascertain the potential dangers to the practitioner, client and the profession.

3. **REVIEW YOUR PROFESSION'S CODE OF ETHICS AND RELEVANT LAWS**
   A. Determine if this issue violates either the letter or the spirit of applicable laws, regulations or professional codes (on a national, state or local level).
   B. Check if your policies or procedures address this issue.

4. **EVALUATE POTENTIAL COURSES OF ACTION**
   A. Brainstorm lots of ideas. Usually the first few options are based upon your personal values or an emotional response to the issue. Delve deeply for potential courses of action that are not necessarily apparent at first.
   B. Enumerate the benefits, drawbacks and outcomes of various decisions.
   C. Consider the consequences of inaction.
   D. Contemplate how you will feel about yourself when all is done.

5. **OBTAIN CONSULTATION**
   A. Engage in self-reflection. Identify which of your personal and professional values could be impacted by the various actions.
   B. Consider how society and members of your community might view these actions.
   C. Determine the impact it could have on your profession (colleagues or a supervisor can add an outside perspective).
   D. Justify a course of action based on sound reasoning which you can test in a consultation. (It is a serious warning sign if you do not want to talk to another person about actions you are contemplating.)

6. **DETERMINE THE BEST COURSE OF ACTION**
   A. Map out the best way to resolve the problem: Who should be contacted first if multiple parties are involved? Do you need outside support? Do you need to talk to a supervisor?
   B. Consider who, if anyone, should know about the problem (such as a work supervisor, friend, client, doctor, police, professional association, school or colleague).

You'll never have all the information you need to make a decision. If you did, it would be a foregone conclusion, not a decision.

—David Mahoney

Ethics Resolution Scenario: A Practical Application

A chiropractor offers to give you financial remuneration for every client you refer to her. You like the chiropractor's work and occasionally you refer clients to her even with no financial incentive. You are fairly confident you will not yield to temptation and send additional clients for financial motives. You need to decide if you should accept the offer. You are under financial pressure and every dollar helps.

1. **IDENTIFY THE PROBLEM**

    An opportunity exists to make more money. You feel reasonably sure that the financial incentive will not influence your referral decisions. You lean toward saying yes, but want to make sure you have really examined the issue and are acting ethically. This is an ethical dilemma and possibly a legal issue.

2. **IDENTIFY THE POTENTIAL ISSUES INVOLVED**

    You think the critical issue is: Can this action and my desire to earn more money conflict in any way with my duty to do no harm and to benefit the client? Also, would it in any way harm my profession? You list the possible dangers of taking this action.

3. **REVIEW YOUR PROFESSION'S CODE OF ETHICS AND RELEVANT LAWS**

    You review your Code of Ethics and read: "Refuse any gifts or benefits which are intended to influence a referral, decision or treatment that are purely for personal gain and not the good of others."

    You review the chiropractic code and find under the Addendum: Rental Arrangements and Clinic or Laboratory Referrals, "It is unethical for a doctor of chiropractic to receive a fee, rebate, rental payment or any other form of remuneration for the referral of a patient to a clinic, laboratory or other health service entity." "Arrangements in which 'rental fees,' 'rebates,' or free gifts are received in return for patient referrals are, in the ACA's view, unethical and unacceptable in the professional practice of chiropractic." Nothing explicitly states that a chiropractor cannot *offer* a "reward." Individual states have additional rules. For instance in Arizona, Section 32-924, Grounds for Sanction; Hearing; Definition states: "Giving or receiving or aiding or abetting the giving or receiving of rebates, either directly or indirectly."

    After reading the various codes you are not exactly sure that the action you are considering is prohibited. You do not intend to refer purely for personal gain. But you can imagine that the action you are considering wouldn't be seen as acting with honesty and integrity.

    You review the law governing your discipline and find no relevant statutes prohibiting the behavior. By talking to friends and colleagues, you find out that this behavior is viewed as an unacceptable practice in health care.

4. **EVALUATE POTENTIAL COURSES OF ACTION**

    The major courses of action are: accept the offer; propose a change to the offer; and refuse the offer.

    Accept the offer so you would have more financial gain:

    Upon serious reflection, you acknowledge some risk exists that you will be influenced to refer some clients to the chiropractor who only have a borderline potential for benefiting from the referral.

    You also realize that it is possible that the client could suffer emotional harm if he later found out that you were given a financial kickback for the referral. You imagine it would create a general sense of mistrust toward you and the client could not be sure that you did not refer at least partially for your own financial gain. Depending on the nature of the treatment relationship, it could create a small or very large negative impact on the client. It seems quite unlikely that the client will find out, but the fact you do not want him to know the arrangement creates concern in you.

Additionally, you identify a possible risk for the profession if someone finds out then assumes that your discipline is a less than legitimate profession because this arrangement is not sanctioned in many health care professions.

You decide that if you accept the offer that you will disclose to your clients what your arrangement is with the chiropractic clinic.

Propose a change to the offer:

Instead of a direct financial interchange, you could set up a reward system such as: for each referral, the chiropractor gives you a $10 gift certificate for services by any practitioner at the clinic (redeemable by you or someone you designate). A variation on this would be a special reward after certain levels of referral (e.g., a certificate for a full treatment after the third referral). This option feels better to you, particularly since you plan to mainly use those certificates for clients in financial need who could benefit from those services.

This arrangement has similar concerns as the first option. You determine that if you do decide to go with this option that you will disclose the arrangement to your clients.

Refuse the offer:

The major risks involved in taking this offer are: this action could cause harm to clients related to their sense of trust in you and trust in the work you have done with them; the potential for tarnishing your professional image; and violation of your personal or professional code of ethics.

You determine that accepting the offer would cause you significant internal conflict in deciding whether to refer a client to this chiropractor as opposed to another practitioner.

Refusing the offer also could incur alienation from the chiropractor.

5. **OBTAIN CONSULTATION**

Talking to colleagues you get a mixed reaction. Some think it is okay, others do not. Although no consensus exists, you are surprised how strongly several colleagues express their sense that the contemplated action is wrong.

6. **DETERMINE THE BEST COURSE OF ACTION**

You choose to refuse the offer and suggest that you show appreciation for each other's support by extending the professional courtesy of working on each other when needed. You also suggest negotiating a strategic partnership where you offer mutual clients discounted fees.

Ethical Congruency

While there's no right answer to a test for ethical congruence, the following checklist helps clarify your level of ethical conflict. Ask yourself these questions whenever contemplating an action (or inaction) that you find questionable:

1. What does your gut say?
2. Do you get butterflies just thinking about the issue?
3. Do you have doubts?
4. Are you needing to sacrifice any of your personal or professional values?
5. Is it against the law, policies or a professional code of ethics?
6. Is this fair to all concerned parties in the short term as well as the long run?
7. How would it hold up to scrutiny if all the details were made public?

8. How would you feel if the people you hold in high esteem knew your decision?
9. How would you feel if your decision was emblazoned on the headline of your local newspaper?
10. How would you feel about yourself when all is done?

Core Psychological Concepts

To behave responsibly and ethically, every practitioner must intimately understand a number of core psychological concepts. A lack of psychological savvy is no longer a valid excuse for inappropriate behavior. These basic concepts are essential for all practitioners to understand. Practitioners must have a thorough understanding of the meaning of: the therapeutic relationship; power differential; transference; countertransference; projection; repression; and denial. These concepts create the bedrock of ethical decision-making and responsible behavior in all professional and (as a bonus) personal relationships.

The Therapeutic Relationship

The major elements in a therapeutic relationship are: there is a client-centered, fiduciary relationship; the time together is structured; each person has a clear role; the environment is safe; and there is a power differential.

Client-Centered

The therapeutic relationship is a very special kind of relationship and is often referred to as *client-centered*. Client-centered means that every action that the practitioner takes is in the service of the client's needs and not the practitioner's needs. Trouble often begins when the practitioner takes an action just because she feels like it and not because it is therapeutically necessary. Client-centered also means that the client has a voice in the process and must agree to the course of treatment for it to proceed. In the client-centered relationship the client has the right to expect that the practitioner always acts in the client's best interest. When this occurs the client feels safe and attended. The client-centered relationship considers the client as a partner who shares decision-making power.

In *The Power of Touch*, Phyllis K. Davis, PH.D., describes a list of the characteristics of an "effective healer" that includes being motivated by the needs of the client.[7] She emphasizes that creating a space for a supportive and nurturing environment begins with the practitioner's commitment to personal and professional excellence. In this environment, overall health improves and enables everyone the practitioner touches to make a fuller connection with their lives.

Fiduciary Relationship

All health care practitioners have a *fiduciary relationship* with their clients. Fiduciary is a term that's applied to a professional in whom a client places his trust. The client is putting his well-being in the hands of the practitioner and there's an implicit contract that the practitioner places the client's interests above and before the practitioner's. Protecting and maintaining the boundaries of professional relationships is the responsibility of the professional even if the client requests or instructs the professional to behave otherwise.

When a professional deviates from standard practice, which is sometimes necessary and useful to individualize care for a particular client, the fiduciary principle and the client-centered approach remain as the guiding parameters of care. The practitioner/

client relationship and the treatment choices must be continually monitored. Also, because somatic practitioners are in positions of power relative to their clients, the law holds them to a higher standard of behavior than in business relationships with a lower level of a power differential.

Structure

Other elements of the therapeutic relationship are that the time spent together is limited and *structured*. The client comes for a session each week, or some other time interval, for a specific type of treatment. Within a prescribed time frame certain expected activities occur. Each person has a clearly defined role in these interactions. The client comes for help and the practitioner is there to help the client.

Safety

The client has the right to expect that the emotional and physical environment is *safe* and does not include inappropriate personal comments or sexual advances.

Power Differential

It is difficult to understand the therapeutic relationship between client and practitioner without comprehending the dynamics of power in a therapeutic relationship. There is a natural *power differential* in many but not all relationships: between parent and child; between teacher and student; between employer and employee; and of course between health care practitioner and client.

A parent, teacher, employer or health care practitioner has the more powerful position. They are the authority figures whose actions, by virtue of their role, directly affect the well-being of the other. The child, the student, the employee and the client are in the more vulnerable position. In theory, and in ethical practice, the power differential exists for the purpose of bringing benefit to these more vulnerable individuals: the child's well-being should be enhanced by the parent's care; the employee should benefit from the employer's management.

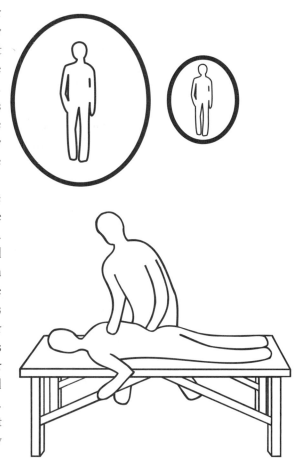

The power differential is inherent in any therapeutic relationship. There is an implicit acknowledgment that the practitioner has more knowledge in this area than the client. In the health care field the power differential is amplified by the physical aspects of practice. The client takes a position—usually lying or sitting—in which he allows the practitioner access to his body. The practitioner positions herself within the client's physical space, often leaning over the client. Furthermore, in many professions the client is partially or fully unclothed. Although draping is used for privacy, the psychological effect of the unclothed client and the clothed practitioner increases the imbalance of power. Finally, as the practitioner's hands make physical contact with the client's body, the client's physical safety is literally in the practitioner's hands.

The Practitioner's Role

The power differential in a relationship such as this requires consideration of two questions. The first seems obvious: How is the person with more power (in this case, the practitioner) handling that power?

The person who holds the power in the relationship may be tempted to misuse that power. The practitioner could take advantage of clients physically, emotionally, financially or professionally. Resentment usually brews when a client is put in an awkward position. Consider the following examples:

- A practitioner is treating a client who happens to be a lawyer and asks, "Since I have you here, could you just answer this quick little question I have about my divorce?"
- A practitioner who is running in a charity race solicits sponsorship during a session.
- During a session the client begins talking about an executive whom the practitioner has wanted to meet and the practitioner asks for a personal introduction.

To maintain an ethical practice, the person in power must regularly say "no" to something she could easily get and must instead choose to pay special attention to the needs of the person with less power. The practitioner must consciously decide to maintain the integrity of the client's boundaries in a situation where the client has significantly relaxed those boundaries.

Clients frequently test boundaries by offering things that may be inappropriate. For instance a client suggests that he tells you about some exciting new stock options while receiving a treatment or a client volunteers to take your computer home to repair it because he sees you are having trouble with it.

The Client's Role

The second question is not so obvious: How is the person with less power responding to the other's use of power?

The answer to this second question may be difficult to determine because of the explicit power dynamics in professional helping relationships. It is the practitioner's responsibility to be aware of how the power differential may be affecting the client's ability to raise concerns.

Consider this: the increased perception of the power differential in a hands-on session puts the client in a highly vulnerable position. The client feels less free to defend against intrusions or to question unexpected behavior by the practitioner. The client may feel uncomfortable about raising concerns, complaining about the treatment process or making requests. The client may find it difficult to say "no" or to question the practitioner's behavior, even if the client feels uncomfortable or mistreated. The client may even refrain from communicating anything that could possibly be construed as negative for fear of reprisal or loss.

The practitioner, not the client, has ultimate responsibility for ensuring that the therapeutic encounter works to the client's benefit.

An active business woman has received massage twice monthly from the same massage therapist for over two years. She recently began having sharp pains in the big toe of her right foot. On one occasion, she mentioned the pain to the practitioner at the beginning of the session in hopes that the therapist would spend some time vigorously working the area. As the massage proceeded, the practitioner moved through the foot area rather quickly.

Disappointed, the client debated about asking the massage therapist to go back to the toe area. She couldn't understand why it was so difficult to ask. After some thought she realized she felt vulnerable lying naked on the table having someone standing over her, touching her body (even though she was covered by a sheet). And asking someone to do something to her (especially on a big toe) might seem silly. She might be imposing, or maybe the practitioner would become upset since it was close to the end of the session. She did not want to appear needy or self-centered.

Finally, the client muttered in a very unsure, child-like tone, "Um, ah, do you think, I mean, would it be OK, could you, um, work on that toe that hurts?"

The practitioner's response? "Sure!"

In this case, even though the client and practitioner had worked together for a couple of years, the client became hesitant to make a request out of a sense of vulnerability, a fear of appearing foolish and concerns over possibly upsetting the practitioner. The psychological effects of the power differential in this case remained unperceived until a need arose requiring the client to make a request. And even after recognizing the effects, the client still asked as a child would for something she is not quite sure she should have.

Because of this psychological dimension, a growing trend in the health care world is to encourage clients to take an active role in the decision-making process of their health care. This is the way most somatic practitioners interact with their clients. Getting clients to take responsibility is not always easy. Unfortunately, it is difficult to reprogram a lifetime of "the doctor knows best." Realize that even though you may be doing your best to foster an atmosphere of equality, the power differential *always* exists on some level in a therapeutic relationship.

Transference

A client seeks treatment hoping, and in most cases believing, that the practitioner knows what's best. Wishing to be helped by an authority figure who possesses greater knowledge, healing ability, and therefore power, the client defers to the practitioner's judgment. Since a power differential exists in any health care or helping relationship, the client is also disposed to responding to the practitioner as he does to other authority figures. In doing so, the client may recreate, in the current helping relationship where he is vulnerable, the same complex elements of similar relationships he has had in the past. This situation is known as *transference*.

Transference is a normal, unconscious psychological phenomenon that inevitably appears during any therapeutic process. Professional helping relationships usually have a strong transference element in which the parent-child relationship is unconsciously re-established. In transference, unresolved needs, feelings and issues from childhood are transferred onto the helper.

Whenever there is a power differential in a relationship, there is a strong potential for transference and countertransference (see next section) to surface in that relationship.

Transference also may occur in other relationships where there is a real or perceived power differential such as with a boss, teacher or clergy.

The power of touch in stimulating transference hasn't been formally studied. But anecdotal evidence suggests that touch, especially when it is intentional and done with care, can quickly create transferential or regressive experiences. When someone in a vulnerable position is touched in a caring way by a person of perceived greater power and authority, the touch often evokes a childlike state and a strong transference. Somatic practitioners daily hear comments from their clients that confirm this reality. Clients frequently disclose very personal information in a first or second session; they often tell the practitioner about their emotional problems, or forcefully demand special treatment. On an unconscious level, clients often expect practitioners to help them in emotional and other areas as well. These are transference reactions and somatic practitioners need to understand and deal with them in a gentle, appropriate manner.

In the mature adult client, these feelings are more likely to be recognized and not control the person's behavior. In individuals who are unaware of or not psychologically able to handle these feelings, transference may become the dominant reality, causing frequent disappointment and rejection in many relationships, often followed by anger and withdrawal. Maintaining clear boundaries is crucial for handling transference occurrences and ensuring that they do not negatively impact the therapeutic relationship.

Signs of Transference

- The client frequently asks you very personal questions.
- The client calls you at home even though your policies state that calls should be placed to your office.
- After only one or two treatments the client is overly complimentary of your work and effuses about what a wonderful person you are.
- The client keeps trying to bargain with you for a reduced rate even when you have clearly stated your policy.
- The client regularly requests that you change your schedule to work at a time that you do not normally see clients to accommodate his schedule.
- Every time you see a particular client she brings you a gift.
- A particular client repeatedly invites you to social engagements and feels rejected when you explain your policy of not socializing with clients.
- At the end of most treatment sessions the client asks you to do just a little bit more and expresses disapproval if you do not comply.
- The client often asks you to help him solve personal problems.
- The client frequently asks you questions in areas that you have previously explained are not in your scope of practice.
- This client often mentions that you remind her of someone.
- The client has difficulty maintaining a physical boundary and attempts to inappropriately hug or touch you at the end of each treatment session.
- The client has great difficulty leaving after the session and tries to engage you in conversation.
- The client gives you details of his personal life, which feel too intimate and makes you uncomfortable.

Countertransference

Countertransference is simply transference occurring in the opposite direction, from the practitioner to the client. The practitioner also carries unresolved needs, feelings and issues into the therapeutic relationship.[8] When these are unconsciously transferred onto the client, it is called countertransference. What happens is that the practitioner begins to feel toward the client the same way the practitioner felt toward someone in his past.

Countertransference is a strong force that can adversely affect the therapeutic relationship if not recognized and properly moderated. The results of unchecked countertransference are less effective therapy, loss of clients, or actual psychological harm to a client. If the practitioner is aware of the phenomenon of countertransference she is more likely to recognize it when it is occurring. This awareness can make the practitioner's responses more appropriate and can facilitate refocusing on the client.

Signs of Countertransference

- There is a strong emotional charge, either positive and negative, toward a client.
- The practitioner's thinking is distorted: she may have an idealized view of or feel very negatively toward a client.
- The practitioner feels irritable or angry with a client for not changing, not improving, or not cooperating with the prescribed treatment plan.
- The practitioner thinks his work is so much better than most practitioners' work or feels his work is totally ineffective and worthless in relation to a specific client.
- A pattern of feeling exhausted, exhilarated, depressed or uneasy when the practitioner sees a particular client.
- Recurring themes such as frequent sexual attraction to clients or the recurrent desire to make friends with clients.
- The expectation of praise and resulting disappointment when clients do not praise the practitioner's work.
- Feeling guilty when a client experiences a painful reaction that lasts for an extended period after the treatment.
- The practitioner frequently experiences anger when a client crosses minor boundaries, questions the practitioner's competence, or otherwise "pushes his buttons" in some way.
- The practitioner undergoes secondary trauma upon hearing painful and graphic stories about a client's past.
- The practitioner frequently helps a client in matters outside the sessions, such as offering rides and introducing the client to social contacts.

If you notice any of these phenomena in your behavior or experience, take this as a signal of something happening on an unconscious level and get help from a supervisor, counselor or psychotherapist.

> When you blame others, you give up your power to change.
>
> —Robert Anthony

See Special Considerations In Cases of Trauma, pages 227-229, for details on **secondary traumatization**.

The Blending of Transference and Countertransference

Taken together, transference and countertransference form a potentially volatile mixture within the inherent difficulties of power differential relationships. Transference and countertransference affect the answers to the questions: How is the person who holds the power using that power; and how is the person with less power responding? When both individuals in a relationship are psychologically mature, there is greater assurance that they use power or handle the other's use of power in a healthful way. Nevertheless, such maturity does not ensure that transference and countertransference does not occur.

The practitioner working with a less psychologically savvy client has an especially serious responsibility, for such a client may be unaware of the transference he brings to the therapeutic relationship. The practitioner must cultivate his own awareness of both transference and countertransference and consciously guard against their effects. Some examples of individuals who are more prone to transference are: a child or adolescent; a client who behaves in a needy manner; a client who has been referred by a mental health professional for bodywork to assist in the processing of psychological issues.

A good goal for practitioners is to minimize the potential for unconscious "acting out" of power issues in the therapeutic relationship. Nevertheless, the person who holds the power in a relationship may have difficulty recognizing both transference and countertransference. Getting supervision on a regular basis gives the practitioner the opportunity to explore these issues, gain clarity and learn methods for dealing effectively and ethically within the situation.

See the Supervision chapter for details.

Defense Mechanisms

People develop ways to cope with situations and feelings they cannot process at the time of the event. These mechanisms are often known as defense mechanisms, which are defined as behaviors that are used to protect the ego from guilt, anxiety, or loss of esteem.[9] These behaviors help the individual to survive the initial experience. However, without resolving the experience the individual may develop unhealthy ways of relating to others. A list from *Therapeutic Communications for Health Professionals*[10] by Carol Tamparo and Wilburta Lindh includes: regression, sublimation, projection, undoing, identification, repression, rationalization, displacement, compensation and denial.

Human beings' growth depends upon the willingness to confront the limits that these defense mechanisms impose. In his book, *The Hidden Dimensions of Bodywork*, psychologist and bodyworker, Ronan M. Kisch, PH.D., states, "As bodywork professionals achieve greater strength through the process of growth and the quality of their presence and touch, they filter back well-being and health, not only to their clients and themselves, but also to society as a whole."[11] Projection, denial and repression are three of the most common defense mechanisms that affect the health of clients as well as somatic practitioners.

Projection

Projection occurs when a person has a thought or feeling that she is not comfortable with and then "projects" it onto others, seeing it as their issue. For example, if a practitioner feels sad, she may experience the client as feeling sad and ask about it. Or, when a practitioner is unaware of feeling angry, she may perceive the client as generally angry, or angry at the practitioner. The primary danger of projection is that the practitioner may not see the client where he is and fails to help the client in an appropriate way. Instead, the practitioner tries to help the client with issues and in ways that the practitioner needs. Keep in mind that projection mostly occurs on an unconscious level.

A practitioner has recently lost a loved one and has been grieving for several weeks. A client comes for a session and isn't as animated as usual. The practitioner makes an assumption that the client is feeling sad and begins to offer words of comfort such as "Don't worry, everything will be okay," or "It's okay to feel sad." The practitioner gives the client a reassuring pat on the shoulder. Then the client responds by saying, "What do you mean? I feel fine." The practitioner then says, "It's normal not to want to admit it when you feel down or sad but this is a safe environment for you." The client is perplexed and leaves wondering what was up with the practitioner.

A practitioner with a great deal of unresolved anger about a recent relationship sees a client for a session. During the session the client makes several requests for a change in the manner in which the treatment is carried out. After each request the practitioner feels uneasy and concludes that the client is dissatisfied and angry with the practitioner. The practitioner also feels a bit hurt and uncomfortable after each request and begins to withdraw. As a result the client becomes more demanding, experiencing the practitioner as not being present. The treatment ends with the client feeling dissatisfied with the quality of the practitioner's work and the practitioner feeling disrespected.

Repression

When people have experiences that are too painful to feel or to bear, they use the psychological mechanism of repression to remove them from the awareness of their conscious mind. For example, the adult who as a child experienced a trauma may have no recollection of the incident ever happening; instead, the memory exists deeply buried in the unconscious. This is frequently the case in sexual abuse cases. Remembering would be too painful, so the memory is repressed.

Repression is a mechanism by which feelings or memories are kept out of consciousness. It is the process of forgetting something or squelching an impulse or feeling: "to reject painful or disagreeable ideas, memories, feelings or impulses from the conscious mind."[12] Note that the mechanism of repression is an unconscious process; repression is not a decision made by the conscious mind but an instinctive reaction to trauma. In some respects the term "amnesia" rather than repression is a more useful description of what happens. Hands-on health care practitioners report that it is common for unconscious memories to surface during body therapy sessions. Practitioners must be aware of this phenomenon and know how to handle this situation when it arises.

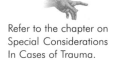

Refer to the chapter on Special Considerations In Cases of Trauma.

Practitioners should also be aware that they could have unresolved repression issues that may affect their professional behavior. Kisch states, "Repression may lead bodywork practitioners to seek personal gratification from professional contacts...or attempt to avoid the clients with whom the issue arises and anxiously hope that they never come back." Repressed awarenesses do not simply go away. "They are translated into somatic tension lodging in the body tissues, covertly robbing the practitioner of peace of mind and precision in work. In turn the tension is somatically transferred to unknowing clients."[13] Unresolved repression in a practitioner affects not only the practitioner but the client as well.

Denial

Denial is an active refusal to recognize or acknowledge the full import or the feeling state of a reality. Denial occurs when a person insists on a distorted interpretation of reality that excludes unpleasant realizations. One can say denial is very similar to repression, but the mechanism of denial requires the collaboration of the conscious mind. The conscious mind goes through many twists and turns to deny the implications of what the person knows to be true. For example, a person who suffers from addictions often admits to the action in question but is in denial about its magnitude or its effects on her life and the lives of her loved ones; an alcoholic may acknowledge the act of drinking, but if he drives drunk and wrecks his car he may deny that this event shows his drinking is excessive.

It is also possible for denial to follow the retrieval of repressed memories. Sexual abuse victims who have recovered memories of traumatic events may, for a time, speak of the events as if they were unimportant, thus denying the impact of the events on their lives.

In Conclusion...

It is always the right time to do the right thing.

—Martin Luther King, Jr.

Despite its complexity, ethical decision-making must be of the highest priority for somatic practitioners. Not only is the credibility of the profession at stake, effective treatment depends on it as well. By cultivating a commitment to the underlying principles of ethical practice, practitioners enhance their ability to identify issues, assume self-accountability, and facilitate the process when confronting a dilemma. Awareness of core concepts also creates a larger perspective. Ethical practitioners understand how ethical choices support the overall healing process and provide deeper professional satisfaction.

Chapter Highlights

- Ethical behavior involves striving to bring the highest values into one's work and aspiring to do one's best in all interactions: doing the right thing in the right manner for the right reasons and with the right attitude.
- The overall purpose of ethics is to guide professional practitioners so that clients' welfare remains the first priority.
- Ethics is the study of moral principles and appropriate conduct.
- Values are tangible and intangible convictions that an individual considers of intrinsic worth.
- Morals relate to the judgment of goodness and badness of human behavior and character.
- Laws are codified rules of conduct set forth by a society and are generally based on shared ethical or moral principles.
- Professionalism is the quality of the image an individual conveys.
- Self-accountability is the cornerstone of ethics.
- Personal ethics is the precursor to professional ethics.
- Cheating is not a victimless crime.
- Forethought and understanding help practitioners avoid a myriad of problems throughout their careers.
- An ethical dilemma is when two or more principles are in conflict.
- A duty is an act or course of action required by position, social custom, law or religion.
- The two primary duties of a health professional are non-maleficence (do no harm) and beneficence (do positive good).
- Clients have the right to expect equal treatment and freedom from interference with their personal autonomy.
- The six steps to resolving ethical dilemmas are: identify the problem; identify the potential issues involved; review the profession's code of ethics and relevant laws; evaluate potential courses of action; obtain consultation; determine the best course of action.
- Core psychological concepts create the bedrock of ethical decision-making and responsible behavior in all professional and (as a bonus) personal relationships.
- The therapeutic relationship is a very special kind of relationship and is often referred to as client-centered, where every action serves the client's needs.
- In a fiduciary relationship there is an implicit contract that the practitioner places the client's interests above and before the practitioner's.
- The therapeutic relationship includes limited and structured time spent together.
- The client has the right to expect that the emotional and physical environment is safe.
- The power differential always exists on some level in a therapeutic relationship.
- Transference occurs when unresolved needs, feelings or issues from childhood are transferred by the client to the practitioner.
- Countertransference occurs when unresolved needs, feelings or issues from childhood are transferred from the practitioner to the client.
- Transference and countertransference are usually unconscious.
- Projection occurs when a person has a thought or feeling that she is not comfortable with and then "projects" it onto others, seeing it as their issue.
- Repression is a psychological defense mechanism to remove experiences from the awareness of the conscious mind when they are too painful to feel or to bear.
- Denial is a defense mechanism to actively refuse to recognize or acknowledge the full import or the feeling state of a reality.

Discussion Questions and Activities

These discussion questions and activities assist you in integrating the chapter's material and provide personal and professional insight. Many of the questions can be done on your own as writing explorations, although ideally you would also discuss them with colleagues. Some of these questions and activities are best done in a classroom setting or in a peer supervision group.

- Make a list of behaviors you deem unethical.
- What are some behaviors, while unethical in your profession, might be fine in others?
- Trace your ethical values from your family history.
- Complete the Core Values Exercise on page 8.
- How do you stay professional when there's a conflict in your values versus laws or codes of ethics?
- How would you handle working with a client when there's a values conflict?
- Where do your personal values conflict with your profession's code of ethics?
- What major problems do you expect to encounter in your practice?
- How do ethics and morals vary in different countries? List specific examples.
- When do your concerns over a third party's welfare take precedence over upholding client confidentiality?
- How does the desire for money influence our ethical decision-making personally and in the society at large?
- Explore a current ethical dilemma using the six-step process.
- Review the professional codes of ethics in the Appendix. Note the differences in complexity, breadth and clarity. Are there any contradictions within a specific profession's code? Can you identify any weaknesses or omissions? How do the various codes relate to one another?
- What conditions might contribute to an inappropriate power differential?
- What types of relationships inherently do not have power differentials?
- What are the conditions that make for a greater or lesser power differential?
- Describe positive and negative experiences you have had in relationships where there is a power differential.
- What are the positive and negative aspects of transference and countertransference?
- Describe an experience when someone has projected their feelings onto you.
- Describe a time when you discovered you had repressed an experience. How did you feel when you realized your prior memory had been different than what had actually happened?
- How will you handle a situation with a client who is in denial regarding his contraindicated condition?
- What other defense mechanisms have you used or have you witnessed others using?
- What unethical behaviors by your colleagues would you feel compelled to report?

2

Boundaries

- What are Boundaries?
- Types of Boundaries
- Boundary Models
- How Boundaries Develop
- Boundary Crossings and Violations
- Why Boundary Crossings Occur
- Establish, Maintain & Change Boundaries
- In Conclusion...
- Chapter Highlights
- Discussion Questions and Activities

S ome types of boundaries are very simple and clear-cut. For instance, all competent surveyors can clearly draw the boundary that separates the property of two neighbors. Unfortunately, that kind of simplicity and clarity does not exist in the relationships between people, especially in practitioner/client relationships. In relationships, a boundary is a limit that separates one person from another. It protects the integrity of each person. A boundary can be as tangible as the skin that surrounds our body or as intangible as an attitude. The primary problem in defining boundaries is that in most instances they are intangible.

Understanding boundaries is crucial to creating an ethical practice and building professional relationships. By increasing your awareness of your clients' boundaries (as well as your own), you can improve the therapeutic relationship and avoid many inadvertent slips into unethical behavior. To begin this process it would be good to clarify the knowledge you already possess. If the following exercise does not seem clear to you, do not worry—it takes time to understand the breadth of this material. And it is an ongoing learning experience.

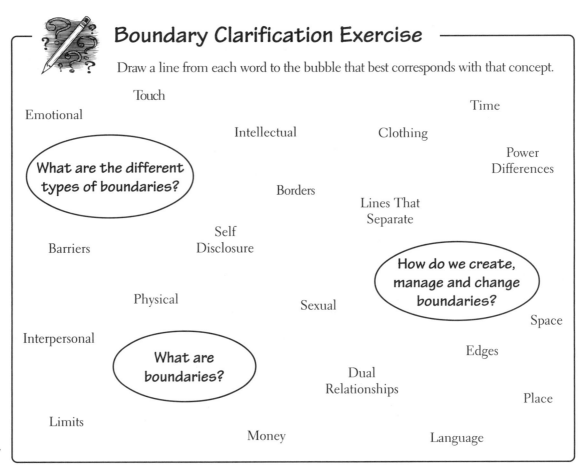

Boundary Clarification Exercise

Draw a line from each word to the bubble that best corresponds with that concept.

Touch

Emotional

Time

Intellectual   Clothing

Power
Differences

What are the different types of boundaries?

Borders

Lines That
Separate

Self
Disclosure

Barriers

How do we create, manage and change boundaries?

Physical   Sexual

Space

Interpersonal

Edges

What are boundaries?

Dual
Relationships

Place

Limits

Money   Language

For **solution**
see Appendix A,
page 256.

What Are Boundaries?

Boundaries separate humans from their environment and from other humans. They are elusive yet personally discernable lines that distinguish you from everything and everyone around you. They define your personal space—the area you occupy which you appropriately feel is under your control.

Most likely, you have had the experience of someone standing too close to you or touching you without your permission. What that person has done, knowingly or not, is invaded your space and crossed your physical boundary. Boundaries are not only physical though. They also protect emotions and thoughts as well. Boundaries provide a sense of safety. They help you to sense how close or far away you want people, both physically and emotionally. Often you are unaware of your boundaries unless they are threatened or crossed.

Each person faces innumerable boundary decisions each day. Whom do you greet with a smile, with a handshake, with a hug, or with a kiss? What information about yourself do you disclose to which people? With whom do you cry when you are sad, or vent when you are angry? To make things even more confusing, the boundaries may fluctuate because they are both idiosyncratic and contextual. Boundaries are idiosyncratic because they reflect each person's likes, dislikes, cultural background, temperament and history. They are contextual because they can change depending on the situation. Behavior that is deemed appropriate at one time may be highly offensive in another setting. For instance you do not touch a client in the same way off the treatment table as you do when he is receiving a treatment because the context is different. Even involving the same person, the context can influence boundaries becoming more fluid or rigid. For example, some people who like to be affectionate in private are very uncomfortable with public displays of affection. Although some interpersonal boundaries are fairly stable, others require ongoing sensitivity to changes in time, place and emotional state.

See Communication Skills chapter for specific **comunication techniques**.

Most people find it stressful to discuss boundary issues. Their upbringing seldom prepares them to do this effectively. In her book, *Parents, Teens and Boundaries*, Dr. Jane Bluestein notes that for most people there has been a severe shortage of healthy role models in this important aspect of family relationships. Furthermore, knowledge of how to set and maintain boundaries "isn't typically a part of a child's education. If anything, most of us have been conditioned *not* to set boundaries as a way to avoid the negative reactions of others."[1] So most clients and many, if not most, practitioners are ill-equipped to freely discuss boundaries.

Negative reactions can occur as part of any personal boundary discussions. People like to think well of themselves. So if you suggest that their behavior is causing you discomfort because they are encroaching on your space, they are apt to feel hurt or angry—or both. Then you must communicate about their feelings *and* your boundary needs. Unless you are a very skilled communicator, you may decide it is not even worth the effort to raise the issue.

Boundary issues between a practitioner and a client are especially sensitive. Helping relationships often require the client to make unusual boundary adjustments. For example, in very few settings other than health care are people expected to undress shortly after meeting practitioners, then permit the practitioners to touch them or insert needles into their bodies. In this vulnerable state they may be expected to tell the practitioners aspects of their life history that they have told no one else, or allow practitioners to manipulate their muscles and bones in ways that are uncomfortable. The health care practitioner is accustomed to these types of boundary adjustments. They are part of his daily work life, year in and year out. For the client, though, these adjustments may be an unusual and stressful experience. In this uncharted territory clients may not even be aware of their own needs, options, or of what constitutes appropriate boundaries and behavior.

Types of Boundaries

The five major types of interpersonal boundaries are: physical; emotional; intellectual; sexual; and energetic.

The Physical Boundary

In day-to-day human interactions people regularly monitor their physical boundary—usually without being aware of it. For example, when standing in line at the bank or milling around with strangers on a public transportation platform, with little effort they all find the appropriate "comfortable" distance to keep—their physical boundary. In the American culture the majority of people prefer a space in front and back that extends about an arm's length from the body (approximately two to three feet). The space deemed comfortable at the sides of the body seems narrower for most people, about a foot or so.

In nearly all human interactions the physical space contained within this invisible line may expand or shrink depending on the individual's level of comfort and safety. People generally allow someone they like and know well to move closer to them than someone they do not know. However, if they are upset about something or angry with another person, the limit of the boundary changes dramatically. For instance, if you feel fear toward someone, you may create more distance from that particular person. If you feel safe with someone and you feel sad, your boundary may change to allow that person to be very close. When there is a perceived threat to the boundary, monitoring becomes more heightened. For instance, being on an elevator with only one other person who has an unkempt appearance and a menacing look may cause uneasiness. Most often, people purposely attempt to create some small measure of personal space in an effort to minimize the discomfort of having their physical boundary crossed. These changes in the physical boundary may occur instantaneously.

Physical boundaries also vary in a professional setting. When a somatic practitioner is in an actual session, it is appropriate to be in physical contact, yet during the pre- and post-session, that same physical contact is inappropriate. As another example, clothing which often serves as a protective boundary may be removed to some extent in the treatment setting. The physical boundaries also shift depending on the part of the body being treated and the intensity of the treatment. For instance working in the mouth may elicit thoughts such as, "Get out of my mouth!" whereas working on the hand or shoulders is usually less threatening. The setting modifies the boundary.

While a physical boundary may be more tangible than other types, it must always be carefully considered.

> " Good fences make good neighbors....
> "
> —Robert Frost

The Emotional Boundary

In many ways people are defined by their emotions and how they feel in the moment. The people we love, the things that make us afraid, the sadness and losses in our lives, and the situations that bring us joy, are major components of our personal identity. To reveal our feelings means that we have decided to trust another with an important part of ourselves, and thereby create a kind of intimacy with that person. The emotional boundary may change with each situation; and it influences whether a person expresses his feelings and how he chooses to do that with others.

Consequently, it is important to be conscious of your own and your clients' emotional boundaries. If not, and boundaries are crossed, it can be as painful (or even more painful) as a violation of our physical boundaries. For example, everyone knows the anger, anguish and shame that occurs when someone reveals a personal confidence to others. The actual content of what is revealed is often less significant than the sense of violation that occurs from the betrayal of trust.

The Intellectual Boundary

Like emotions, a person's thoughts, beliefs and opinions form a significant part of her identity. They help to create a world view and define an individual as different and separate from others. If our belief system is accepted, encouraged and validated, or even respectfully challenged, we feel respected and validated. If our ideas and beliefs are ridiculed, criticized, ignored, dismissed or punished, our sense of self may be shaken, and we may become hesitant to speak openly about our ideas. For instance, it might be challenging to remain open with a fellow practitioner if, after you shared some of your deeply-held beliefs about wellness, he responded with, "You don't really believe that, do you?!"

Realizing that we are the victim of propaganda, dogma or indoctrination may also leave us feeling violated because intellectual boundaries have been disregarded.

The Sexual Boundary

The sexual boundary can be defined in several ways and be thought of as a subset of the physical or the physical and emotional boundaries. Sexual boundaries are created by determining with whom, when, where and how we wish to express our sexuality. Any of these boundaries can be treated respectfully or violated.

The sexual boundary is also determined by the context of the relationship. Health care professionals should not have sexual relationships with their clients. Period. Issues of crossing sexual boundaries in the health care professions are of such significance and concern that they have led to numerous laws, regulations and professional ethics statements regarding inappropriate sexual behavior with clients and in the workplace. Violation of the sexual boundary can be a violation of the law. Know the requirements of your state or regulatory board. Ignorance of the law is **not** a defense.

Violating the sexual boundary with a client can violate all the other boundaries as well. Respecting it is not only the ethical choice, it is the healing choice as well.

The Energetic Boundary

Most everyone who works with human bodies comes to understand over time that practitioners are affected by the emotional and mental states of clients. Awareness of these effects is the first step toward understanding that there is a constant flow of energy around every human being, and that the energy patterns of one person can influence those of another.

The human body is composed of materials that conduct electrical currents. The processes within the body require chemical reactions, and the body actually generates an electromagnetic field. We are energetic beings who need to maintain our energetic boundaries just as we maintain our physical, emotional, intellectual and sexual boundaries. The practitioner who develops this skill works with clients with more safety and greater respect. He protects his own energy from the influence of the client's energy, and he does not allow his own energy to inappropriately cross the client's energetic boundary.

In his book, *Beyond Technique*, Ronan M. Kisch, PH.D., describes the phenomena of psychophysical stress causing psychophysical toxins. Since clients come specifically to

Respect for emotional boundaries is essential to any healthy relationship.

See the chapter on Sex, Touch and Intimacy.

the practitioner to relieve stress, the practitioner is "constantly bombarded with clients' psychophysical toxins."[2] This can be detrimental to the practitioner's health and well-being, especially if the practitioner is particularly sensitive to "extra-sensory experiences."

Some people who enter somatic professions do have "somatic, intuitive personalities." Those abilities may not be readily known to the practitioner, but develop along with the sense of touch. Unprepared for this type of energetic intimacy, the practitioner may struggle with issues of reality versus fantasy and when to share what she perceives. By understanding the concept of the energetic boundary, practitioners can learn to maintain it for their own well-being and that of their clients.

Boundary Models

In this section we draw from the work of family therapist Salvador Minuchin, M.D.[3] and Gestalt Theory[4] to help make the often amorphous concept of boundaries more concrete. We look at how boundaries function under different circumstances in human interactions and how that awareness is useful in the somatic practitioner's work. With fuller awareness you can consciously make adjustments in your own boundaries and behavior, thus preventing only a conditioned response.

Context determines which boundaries are the most appropriate. For instance, if you feel compassion for a client, it may be appropriate for your boundary to be thinner and more "permeable" to allow you to feel more empathy. If you feel threatened in a therapeutic situation, it may be more useful for your boundary to thicken and become more "rigid" to protect you. These models also give a conceptual picture of what happens when a boundary is crossed or when you feel you are doing just the right thing for a client.

Personal Boundaries

Minuchin describes the nature of boundaries as a continuum of permeable to rigid. The degree of permeability also represents vulnerability. The following series of diagrams illustrate selected points along that continuum.

Permeable

A permeable boundary allows information and feelings to flow easily in and out without barriers. Diagram A illustrates a permeable boundary by a series of dots surrounding the figure. In this state a practitioner working with a seriously ill client may feel empathy and the boundary might become more permeable while she gently and compassionately works with the client. If the practitioner becomes identified with her own feelings of loss or sadness and is overwhelmed by the client's pain, a permeable boundary may interfere with the practitioner's effectiveness. In a different situation a practitioner might encounter a client who is very strong and dominant. In this case, the practitioner with a permeable boundary may lose a sense of identity, subordinating her opinions and beliefs to the client.

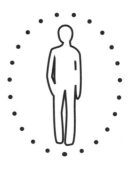

Diagram A
Thin/Permeable

Semi-permeable

In the middle range of the continuum is the semi-permeable (also referred to as flexible) boundary represented by a series of dashes around the figure (Diagram B). This boundary indicates a flexible relationship with the outside world. Allowing closeness if appropriate and keeping someone at a distance when necessary characterizes this boundary.

A flexible boundary is useful when scheduling appointments with a client whose work limitations, illness, or children's needs are involved. On the other hand, inappropriate flexibility can interfere with the therapeutic relationship. For instance, excessive flexibility in scheduling which interferes with your personal time may lead to resentment and models a lack of self-care. Also, even though a limit is usually set for the length of a session, flexibility in the boundary would be called for if the client had an extreme physical reaction to part of the treatment and more time was needed.

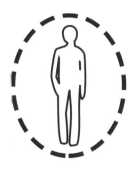

Diagram B
Semi-Permeable/
Flexible

An example of this is when a practitioner's boundary overly accommodates a client who suffered a traumatic history (and needs steady, consistent limits about boundaries and behavior).

Rigid

At the far end of the continuum is what could be described as a rigid or thick boundary[5] which is very firm and distinct (Diagram C). A rigid boundary severely limits the flow of information and feelings moving in or out. This is illustrated by a solid line that encircles the figure. In this case the person is well protected from external harm or stimuli but may feel isolated. This boundary is often valuable when someone is berating or attacking you.

A firm boundary is necessary when a client attempts to engage a practitioner in constant conversation or attempts to elicit too much personal information. If a practitioner is treating a terminally ill client, a thicker boundary may be

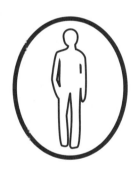

Diagram C
Thick/Rigid

needed to maintain objectivity. However, if the practitioner's boundary becomes too rigid and he becomes distant, the therapeutic relationship is negatively affected.

Doing your best work is difficult if your history and belief systems contain certain prejudices about people (e.g., race, size, sexual orientation, eating habits, smoking, drinking and philosophy) because prejudice makes for a rigid boundary.

Interactive Boundaries

The Gestalt theory views boundaries from an interactive perspective. They are described as existing in relationships between individuals. The three interactive situations useful in understanding the client/practitioner relationship are: meeting at the boundary; crossing the boundary; and being distant from the boundary.

Meeting at the Boundary

In Diagram D one person is meeting another at the boundary. This is illustrated by two figures whose boundaries touch each other. In regards to client and practitioner, the point of contact (where they touch) occurs when the practitioner communicates in a way that the client can easily receive and understand. For example, using the appropriate amount of pressure during a treatment meets the client at his boundary. Sometimes the interaction pushes at the boundary, moving it slightly but never crossing it.

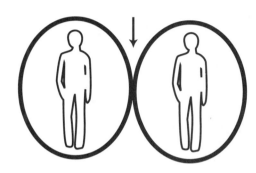

Diagram D
Meeting at the Boundary

Boundary Crossing or Violation

When the boundary is crossed or violated, as in Diagram E, the boundaries overlap. The arrow illustrates that the boundary of one person (A) is crossing the boundary of the other (B). The boundary is considered crossed or violated when the person (B) experiences discomfort or perceives being attacked. Asking inappropriate or invasive questions or hurting the client by applying too much physical pressure are examples of this situation.

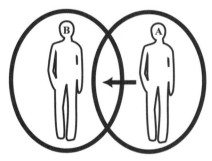

Diagram E
Boundary Crossing

Distance From the Boundary

In Diagram F the figures are separated by a considerable space indicating no meaningful contact. The individuals have difficulty communicating and there is hesitation and coolness in the interaction. Communication attempts are incomplete and unsuccessful. The practitioner's comments and questions may seem out of context or irrelevant to the client which contributes to a sense of isolation and separation between them.

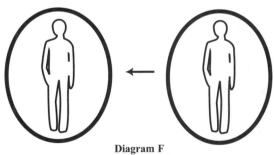

Diagram F
Distant From the Boundary
No Real Contact

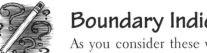

Boundary Indicator Exercise

As you consider these various models you may be assessing where your characteristic boundary lies along this continuum and how your boundaries function in interactions with others. This exercise, adapted from the work of Charles Whitfield, M.D.,[6] helps you understand how your boundaries function. Circle the answer which most accurately represents how you react in these situations. Answer as honestly as you can; do not choose the answer you think is "correct" as there is no right answer.

1. **It is difficult for me to say "no" to people I am close to.**
   Usually   *Often*   Occasionally   Seldom   Never
2. **I feel my happiness depends on other people.**
   Usually   *Often*   Occasionally   Seldom   Never
3. **I tend to take on or feel what others are feeling.**
   Usually   *Often*   Occasionally   Seldom   Never
4. **I would rather attend to others than to myself.**
   Usually   Often   *Occasionally*   Seldom   Never
5. **It is hard for me to make decisions.**
   Usually   *Often*   Occasionally   Seldom   Never
6. **I trust others easily.**
   Usually   Often   *Occasionally*   Seldom   Never
7. **I feel anxious, scared or afraid.**
   Usually   Often   *Occasionally*   Seldom   Never
8. **I put more into relationships than I get out of them.**
   Usually   *Often*   Occasionally   Seldom   Never
9. **I spend my time and energy helping others so much that I neglect my own needs & wants.**
   Usually   *Often*   Occasionally   Seldom   Never
10. **I tend to take on the moods of people close to me.**
    Usually   Often   *Occasionally*   Seldom   Never

Add up your responses in each of these categories to determine where your tendencies lie. The statements where you circled **USUALLY** or **OFTEN** are the areas of your boundaries which are on the permeable side. Where your response was **SELDOM** or **NEVER** indicates aspects of your personality that tend toward the rigid side. Statements where you circled **OCCASIONALLY** indicate a semi-permeable boundary. If you answered most or all questions with **NEVER** you may not be aware of your boundaries. Underline or circle the key words or phrases to which you answered **NEVER**, **USUALLY** and **OFTEN**. These are indicators of potential boundary issues.

The various models described are useful in learning about boundaries. But models by their very nature are guides, and cannot be taken literally. In reality our boundaries are in constant flux. They can quickly change from rigid to permeable depending on the situation and context (as in the following example). Moreover, our boundaries may combine qualities. For example, a person can simultaneously have a permeable boundary and a partially rigid boundary.

Once again, it is essential to remember that one type of boundary is no better than another. Each person needs all of these types of boundaries according to the situation and context. Boundaries need to be contextually appropriate. People experience difficulty with boundaries when they become stuck in a single mode or when the boundary doesn't match the context.

A Day in the Life of a Practitioner

By taking examples of common occurrences and compiling them into one practitioner's day, it is easy to observe how boundaries can fluctuate. This imaginary massage therapist and her partner have an infant son and in-home childcare. The practitioner works out of her home office.

1. Permeable

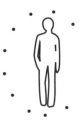

The practitioner sits with her baby and nurses him. Her boundaries are wide open and she merges with the baby.

2. Less Permeable

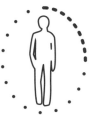

She and her partner are very close. Her partner awakes with a back pain and she lovingly offers to work on her partner's back. They feel very close and in love—almost merged but not quite.

3. Part Flexible—Part Rigid

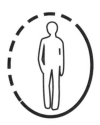

The practitioner greets a new client in her home office and as the treatment session begins the client asks very intrusive and personal questions about her life and her family. She would like to remain open to the client but feels herself pulling away and closing down at times during the session.

4. Permeable, Flexible and Rigid

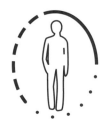

The next client is a Vietnam veteran. As she begins to work on his head and neck, he lapses into a flashback. This has never happened to the practitioner and while she feels great empathy for the client, she is also apprehensive and afraid she may not handle the situation well.

5. Semi-Permeable and Permeable

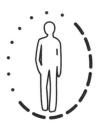

In her afternoon break a close friend drops by to visit. Her friend's father suddenly died in an accident and the friend begins to cry uncontrollably as she talks. This reminds the practitioner of her own father's death two years ago and she quietly begins to cry as well.

6. More Permeable

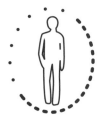

Her third session is with a 12-year-old girl who has headaches. This girl was referred by a physician. While taking the history from the girl and her father, it emerges that the mother has been physically abusive to the child. As the practitioner works with the girl, she is focused yet feels tender and sad.

7. Less Flexible

The next client arrives late for the third time and the practitioner becomes annoyed. Lateness is not something she tolerates well.

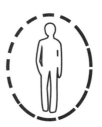

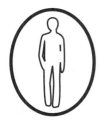

8. Rigid

This same client makes a sexual comment during the treatment. They talk about it and clear the air, but the practitioner continues to feel wary of this client.

9. More Rigid

The practitioner receives a call from someone wanting sexual services. She attempts to educate the caller about her professional services, and the caller becomes irate and obscene. The practitioner gets filled with anger during this interaction and her boundary becomes rigid and thicker.

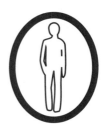

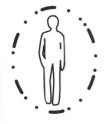

10. Flexible and Permeable

As she closes her office, her partner returns home and they embrace. They sit together processing what happened during her difficult day ending with the disturbing telephone call. The practitioner becomes calm, they laugh together and begin to enjoy the evening with their child.

As is evident in this example, boundaries can dramatically shift many times throughout a day, depending on the situation.

Remember that these models are designed to assist you in better understanding your own responses and behaviors in relation to boundaries. Boundaries are not as clear-cut and simple as the theories suggest. It is more realistic to think of boundaries as multifaceted and multidimensional.

How Boundaries Develop

Boundaries are innate, developed and learned. By innate we mean that there seems to be a genetic quality to the types of boundaries humans develop. Many characteristics of personality and boundaries are discernable in children at very young ages. For example, traits of reticence or of openness are often observable very early in life, and appear to have little to do with learned behavior or environmental influence. Research on studies of twins separated early in life and tested as adults, suggests that the quality of their boundaries are quite similar.[7]

However, many boundaries (socially appropriate as well as self-defeating ones) are learned early in life. Boundary development is influenced by experiences with the environment, family, teachers, neighbors, culture and the world as a whole.

Environmental Influences on Boundary Development

The environmental influences include both the culture at large and the culture within the family. However, the family's influence on boundaries is always influenced by cultural ethnicity, societal mores, social class, laws and educational experiences. In this section we look at the effect of family and culture on boundary development.

The Family

Boundaries emerge and become shaped through relationships with a close circle of caretakers such as parents or other significant individuals who help raise the child. This occurs gradually and primarily unconsciously. All families are guided by both spoken and unspoken rules—sometimes in conflict. Among the factors in family life that shape early boundary development are: privacy; physical contact; emotional expression; intellectual freedom; sexual attitudes; and sensitivity.

A family's attitudes about each of these areas are themselves influenced by culture and family history. Clearly there are different ethnic norms about each. For example, in some cultures emotions are expressed loudly and passionately, while in others such explosiveness would be inappropriate and frightening. Similarly, there are different ethnic/cultural expectations about issues such as privacy and physical contact. Therefore, it is important to consider each of the following areas within the context of ethnic or cultural expectations.

PRIVACY: In some family environments a right to privacy is clear and guides behavior about dressing and undressing, bathroom privacy and the right to personal space. In other family settings the code of accepted behavior may be entirely different; doors may always remain opened, or even if closed a family member may enter a room at any time without requesting permission. If the family style is one that provides for privacy, a person's boundaries may move easily from permeable to rigid within the whole range of boundary interaction. However, if there is limited privacy, a person may develop rigid or distancing boundaries as a way of creating privacy. Or he might have mostly permeable boundaries, having lost a sense of privacy.

PHYSICAL CONTACT: Demonstrating physical affection in some families is a significant part of family relationships. Physical contact, if present, occurs in varying degrees and may be expressed through hugging, physical playfulness, kissing and holding hands. In some families open and warm contact is expected and children are included without inquiring whether touch is wanted; in others children are asked if they want physical touch. Some families experience little physical contact among family members; hugging may be very rare and children rarely witness physical affection expressed between their parents. These behaviors influence how the child responds to her body's physical boundary and what characterizes her degree of comfort with physical contact as she grows into an adult.

EMOTIONAL CONNECTION AND EXPRESSION: Emotional connection is the process by which a person is known emotionally within the family. Emotional expression refers to how emotions are dealt with in the family. Is it common for emotions to be expressed, or is this rare? Are certain emotions acceptable and others not? Do emotions explode or modulate according to the situation? Is emotional expression acknowledged and attended to, or avoided? Is there emotional warmth or coolness in the family? Some families maintain a wide range of emotional connection and expression, while in others it is rather narrow. These factors influence how humans set emotional boundaries as they grow and mature.

INTELLECTUAL EXPRESSION: Some families support intellectual development while others suppress this natural expression of human curiosity and exploration. In one family a child's independent thoughts and ideas are encouraged and heeded with attention and care. In another family no forum or space is provided for this self-expression to occur. In the extreme circumstance a young person may be berated and their ideas ridiculed.

SEXUAL ATTITUDES: Parents transmit their feelings about sexuality in both overt and subtle ways. Children have many questions about the sexual parts of their bodies: they may engage in sex play, touch themselves, and later may begin to masturbate. How parents respond to these situations gives the child early cues to parental sexual attitudes. Sexual attitudes are cemented into the child's belief system through the parents' attitudes and beliefs about premarital sex, sex education, how comfortable they are talking about sexuality, religious influences and whether they feel sexuality is something to feel guilty about or to enjoy.

SENSITIVITY: Hypersensitivity in childhood may be a sign that the child's energetic boundaries are weak or underdeveloped. A hypersensitive child can be a challenge for any family. Some sensitive children quickly learn to hide, deny or repress their sensitivity because the family shames, ridicules or ignores it. On the other hand, the child whose sensitivity is acknowledged and nurtured can learn how to connect with that sensitivity without being overwhelmed by it. These skills form the basis for successful management of energetic boundaries in adulthood. Being highly sensitive is an advantage when understood and directed. Somatic practitioners who have this increased sensitivity often sense when energy is stuck in a particular tissue, direct their energy flow as they work and are receptive to what the body is communicating.

If the elders have no values, their children and grandchildren will turn out badly.

—Chinese proverb

The Culture at Large

While we could identify any number of cultural institutions and influences, the most significant impact on boundaries comes from schools, the media, religion and religious groups, and voluntary social organizations.

SCHOOLS: As children enter the primary grades, their daily lives typically become more structured. Children are required to gain greater control over their bodies. For example, the expectations that groups of children move through hallways in an orderly fashion, or maintain an organized classroom, require increased physical boundary maintenance by the child, and an increasing awareness of other's boundaries.

As the child begins to explore and learn in a structured environment, performance expectations increase. At this early age, and in a new environment, a child's thoughts and intellectual boundaries are particularly vulnerable.

Consequently, depending on the philosophy and competence of the teacher, the school and often the school system, the development of a child's intellectual boundary is supported or inhibited. For example, a second-grader had raised her hand to answer a question, and was told that she wouldn't be called on because "she always had the right answer." In a similar situation, a third grade child was told that he wouldn't be acknowledged because, "You're only raising your hand to get attention!" In these two situations the adults relaying their childhood stories recalled that it was months in the first case and years in the second before each child felt comfortable contributing ideas in class.

MEDIA: Everyone is susceptible to both overt and subliminal messages that print and broadcast media convey. Sexuality is often used as a tool to deliver an advertiser's message and is a predominant theme in the television and motion picture industry. Teenagers in particular are regularly influenced by sexual images, complicating their own boundary development pertaining to when and how they want to be sexual. Ultimately, this can make it difficult for them to develop or respect anyone's sexual boundaries.

At the same time media images have supported a highly polarized view of men and women. Women are often imbued with the ability to understand and manage a range of emotions, with diminished intellectual competence. Men are typically portrayed with intellectual and physical prowess, but with a narrow range of emotions.

Of particular concern for health care practitioners is the number of television and motion picture scenarios in which inappropriate dual relationships are presented in a positive light. These include lawyers, doctors and psychotherapists having sexual or other types of intimate, dual relationships with their clients. Presenting these unethical relationships with humor makes them more damaging. When responsibly and purposefully developed, the media can also teach the importance of healthy boundaries.

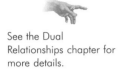

See the Dual Relationships chapter for more details.

RELIGION AND RELIGIOUS GROUPS: Most religious organizations have some sort of adjunct school or social group that focuses on child development. Whether overt or covert, there are often specific messages regarding human sexuality, the role of free thinking and emotional expression. Key to children's emotional or intellectual boundary development is how they are taught to deal with strong feelings (sadness, anxiety, fear, anger, joy, serenity and love), or thoughts that may not be congruent with the organization's teachings.

This is also true when considering how children are taught to think about their bodies. Is the body simply a vessel for the spiritual self, or is a child taught to value the body in its own right? How are questions about the body handled? Religious organizations play a pivotal role in many people's boundary development.

VOLUNTARY SOCIAL GROUPS: Social groups such as scouts, camps, after-school programs and sports often become an integral aspect of children's lives and social education, and consequently their boundary development. The leaders serve as strong role models and are often unaware of the influence of seemingly insignificant comments and actions. For instance, if an adult leader makes statements about sexuality, it can impact the children who look up to the leader. This of course will then have an effect on the child's sense of a sexual boundary. One individual recalled his experiences in the scouts as the first clear communication from an adult about homophobia:

> "At the age of 12 I had already begun to feel that I was different—you know, odd. Then I heard my scout leader making jokes about 'boys that like boys,' and it was the first real proof from an adult that I knew and liked that I was strange. It was horrible. From then on, I knew that I would have to keep this secret to myself."

Youth sports are extremely popular. Boys and girls of school age through college are offered year-round opportunities to play sports such as soccer, basketball, baseball, softball and football. How coaches deal with these young athletes impacts their physical and emotional boundary development. When coaches encourage children to ignore injuries, or to push beyond their bodies' appropriate limits, they are teaching children to ignore their physical boundaries. One man who had played football in his youth remembered injuring his knee. The coach told him to get up and keep playing since there was "no time for injuries on this team." From that day forward, he tried to numb his body—thickening his physical boundary—so that injuries wouldn't interfere with his athletic success. Similarly, if the message is conveyed that certain feelings are "weak" (e.g., crying, apprehension or fear), coaches encourage children to devalue their emotional boundaries. Through awareness, sensitivity and modeling, coaches and other organizational leaders can empower children to develop appropriate boundaries.

Boundary Crossings and Violations

A *boundary crossing* is a transgression that may or may not be experienced as harmful. Often the difference in degree that makes an action shift from being considered a boundary crossing to a violation is minute. It is also relative: what is a mere boundary crossing to one client may be a major violation to another. A *boundary violation* is a harmful transgression of a boundary. Differentiating a boundary crossing from a violation needs to be done on a case by case basis taking into account the context and facts of the situation. "The difference between a harmful and a non-harmful boundary crossing may lie in whether it is discussed or discussable; clinical exploration of a violation often defuses its potential for harm."[8]

No boundaries are inherently right or wrong, yet when confronted with someone whose boundaries are different from ours, we may become uncomfortable and consequently judgmental. At these times, identifying our own discomfort helps us avoid creating value judgments about other people's boundaries. For instance some cultures use personal questions in an attempt to create safety. This behavior is normal in that culture.

Most health care practitioners would agree that the boundaries between the client and practitioner must be respected. There is also agreement about the nature of gross boundary invasions such as sexual exploitation of any kind. However, while sexual abuse is egregious, there are far subtler kinds of intrusions which are harmful both to the client and to the treatment relationship. Unlike sexual abuse, these intrusions may occur without such clarity, leaving the client or the practitioner unable to recognize or articulate them.

These kinds of subtle intrusions are not usually the result of intentionally invasive behavior. More often they occur because the practitioners do not completely understand personal boundaries. Practitioners may also lack awareness of how boundaries are affected by the power dynamics in the professional helping relationship.

The foundation of any therapeutic relationship is an implicit contract between the client and the practitioner which defines appropriate behavior. To act inappropriately is to break the contract. To avoid violating a client's boundaries a practitioner must only do what is included in the professional contract. Several distinct areas hold the potential for boundary violations on the part of the practitioner including: the kind of physical touch permitted by the client; probing for personal or private information about the client's past; the use of intimate words; and value judgments about the client's body or lifestyle. Each of these behaviors is a way of crossing a client's boundary physically or verbally. To do so without permission is at best an intrusion or at worst a violation.

These same actions, if done with co-equals (friends, peers and colleagues), do not usually have quite the same impact. Co-equals by definition have equal power and do not have an implicit contract about certain kinds of boundaries.

Everyone commits minor violations and allows others to do the same. Consider the following examples: someone may put his arm around you when you do not expect it or want it; you might interrupt someone who is having an important telephone conversation; and a loved one may call you sweetheart when you are angry and do not want any closeness. Though these "violations" may be annoying and intrusive, and even feel hurtful, they typically do not do serious damage. This is because as co-equals, no implicit power dynamic keeps us from defending ourselves. You can tell the loved one not to call you sweetheart; the person on the telephone can ask you to not interrupt; and you can find a kind way to remove the person's arm from your shoulder.

> *Never ruin an aopology with an excuse.*
>
> —Kimberly Johnson

See pages 15-17 for more information on the **power differential**.

> *He who has never made a mistake is one who never does anything.*
>
> —Theodore Roosevelt

Scenarios

The following scenarios serve to clarify what constitutes crossing a boundary.

Inappropriate Touch

> For several months Steve has been giving weekly chiropractic treatments to his client Gail for chronic pain. The treatments have been going extremely well. Since Gail had unsuccessfully tried several other approaches, both client and practitioner have been excited about the progress being made. As they are saying goodbye after a particularly good session Steve spontaneously gives his client a hug. Touch to this point has been limited to the treatment. Not wanting the hug, Gail tenses but says nothing.

Although Steve's hug was a sincere and warm gesture toward Gail, it was also a boundary crossing. Steve may have decided that a hug was fine in the moment, and that a hug would not have felt invasive to him. Boundaries are idiosyncratic so he cannot be sure what the experience is like for his client. Gail did not want a hug. Possibly the hug made her uncomfortable, confused and even afraid. Although Gail has invited touch in the form of therapeutic manipulations, she hasn't invited any other kind of touch. Since Gail did not want a hug, Steve crossed Gail's boundary without her permission.

For whatever reasons, Gail did not express her discomfort. She may not have wanted to offend Steve, feeling concerned that future treatments could be jeopardized. She may even have felt that a hug was somehow expected of her.

The point here is not that practitioners should never hug their clients; rather, that it may be difficult for clients to refuse if a practitioner initiates a hug. A non-violating crossing could go like this: After the session Gail asks for a hug. If Steve is comfortable with the idea, he responds by giving one. In this case he is crossing Gail's physical boundary only in response to a clear invitation. In other words Steve would be certain that it was wanted. Whenever a practitioner hugs a client, many decisions about the hug needs to be made in an instant: how close; how long; is there full body contact; and will there be movement or stroking while hugging. There are not easy solutions for this. The practitioner needs to determine how to make sure the hug stays in the friendly, professional hug category.

Careless or Uninvited Words

> Joan is working for the first time with her new client Sarah who has come for physical therapy to build strength. During the course of the treatment, Joan notices that Sarah has a dark mole on her back. Without asking for permission to give her opinion, Joan says to Sarah, "Are you aware that you have a huge, hairy mole on your back!" and proceeds to inform her of the potential dangers of moles and suggests several methods of treatment for the problem.

It is easy to imagine that Joan thought she was being helpful to Sarah by pointing out the mole of which Sarah might not even have been aware. However, it is neither feedback nor professional judgment that Sarah has invited. It is quite possible that Sarah would feel injured and insulted, as anyone might if told something uncomplimentary about her body without her asking. Because Joan did not have explicit permission to offer feedback about Sarah's body, Joan committed a boundary crossing.

This example demonstrates how words that convey any type of judgment are an intrusion. A fine line exists between increasing a client's awareness of a potential physical problem and overstepping your role. Joan could have said, "Is it okay with you if I point out things I notice such as bruises, bites, rashes or moles—particularly those in areas that might be difficult for you to see?" If Sarah were to agree, Joan could be much more diplomatic in describing the mole. Then instead of immediately proceeding to tell Sarah about the implications and steps to take regarding the mole, Joan should wait for Sarah's response. Sarah might say, "Oh, yes, I've had that since I was a child. I had my doctor check it out and she says it's fine." If Sarah doesn't respond, then a simple statement such as, "You might want to have a dermatologist check this out" would suffice. Joan could also ask Sarah if she is interested in learning more about moles or if she would like recommendations (such as a referral to a dermatologist).

In some circumstances a boundary crossing is necessary. A practitioner has a responsibility to inform the client if certain things are noticed. For example, when a practitioner notices facial bruises or a pattern of multiple bruises the issue of domestic violence must be considered. The practitioner must use her judgment in determining if the bruises seem like a normal occurrence or something meriting concern. The client may think the concern is silly, but it is better to be safe. A practitioner might say, "I noticed you have several bruises. Health care practitioners are obligated to inquire if you're in a situation where someone is hurting you. If this is the case, I want you to know that there are many resources to help you and I can provide you with referrals."

Without invitation, even compliments or words of affection may put a person in an awkward position. To be called by intimate names (e.g., sweetheart, honey), or to be told you are attractive or appealing by someone you know and trust, generally makes you feel good. However, without trust, safety and the appropriate context, words like these feel invasive. And in the treatment relationship where power is so unbalanced, they almost always serve to confuse the professional boundary.

We know stories about every type of health care practitioner who unintentionally offended a client by making uninvited comments (positive or negative) about the client's body. Significantly, when this type of boundary crossing occurred in one of the first few sessions, none of these clients went back to the practitioner (we assume because they were too upset or angry).

Dual Relationships Leading to Sexual Misconduct

After several months of treatment, Tracy's client Chris expresses a personal interest in Tracy by making subtle, sexual comments. Tracy finds the client attractive and begins to fantasize about a social relationship. Chris invites Tracy to go out for coffee and they meet after the next session. They decide to see each other socially and become friends. After several dinners the friendship develops into a casual sexual relationship. The professional relationship continues for a few more months, sometimes becoming sexual during the treatment sessions. The treatment relationship slowly ends in several months but the two enjoy each other for six more months until the relationship ends suddenly when Chris realizes that Tracy is also dating someone else. Chris feels betrayed and angry, seeks psychotherapy and ends up suing Tracy for professional sexual misconduct.

See the Dual Relationships chapter for more details.

See the Sex, Touch and Intimacy chapter, pages 127-134 for details on **sexual misconduct**.

This is a clear case of sexual misconduct. It also demonstrates the rapid move along the continuum from a client/practitioner relationship to friendship to a sexual relationship. There were several strong indicators of boundary violations along the way that could have signaled Tracy to seek help or to stop the process: when Chris began to make subtle, sexual comments; when Tracy noticed an attraction to Chris and began to fantasize a social relationship; when the invitation to coffee and then dinner was made. By the time they decided to become friends the slide to sexual misconduct was almost complete.

When Chris began to make sexual comments, Tracy could have stopped it and opened a conversation by saying, "I notice that you're making some personal comments to me with sexual innuendos. This makes me a little uncomfortable and I am wondering if there's something else behind it?" If Chris then says, "I think that I would like to be friends with you," Tracy could have responded by saying, "I feel flattered but in my professional life I avoid mixing my personal and professional relationships. This feels more professional, protects my clients and makes life simpler."

When Tracy noticed an attraction to Chris and began to fantasize about a social relationship, that was a red flag to immediately seek professional or peer supervision. Most practitioners have occasionally felt attracted to a client but when it progresses into fantasizing this indicates that a boundary has been crossed in the practitioner's mind. If Tracy had sought help at this time, the following would have become clear: strong boundaries needed to be put in place or the client/practitioner relationship terminated.

Two other choice points came when Chris invited Tracy to coffee and when Tracy accepted. Both of these occurrences indicated that the relationship was about to change in a manner that was not strictly professional. Going out to coffee with a client that the practitioner has been having fantasies about and who has made sexual comments is a clear recipe for trouble and eventual disaster. At this moment Tracy could have said, "Thank you for the invitation but my policy is to refrain from developing social relationships with my clients." Or Tracy could have said, "I find myself interested in developing a personal relationship with you also but if this were to occur I could no longer work with you in a therapeutic role. If you want to develop a social relationship with me, we need to end our professional relationship first. We need to consider this decision very carefully and perhaps get some outside help."

Some disciplines have strict guidelines about the length of time between a therapeutic relationship ending and a social relationship beginning. Getting supervision before acting on this impulse is highly recommended.

Inappropriate Self-Disclosure

Before working on her new client Jim, Susan hands him a history form to fill out. Jim becomes somewhat annoyed and suggests that they skip the history and proceed with the massage therapy session. Susan explains that to do her work well a history must be taken. Jim remains truculent but agrees.

It seems obvious that taking a history helps a practitioner in working with clients. However, in this example, taking the client's history makes him feel upset and invaded in some way. Although the reasons are not yet obvious, it is apparent that Jim is not comfortable with the history. Perhaps he generally feels uncomfortable disclosing information about himself. Maybe he feels unsafe revealing particular pieces of his personal history. He might even have difficulties reading. Whatever the cause, it is reasonable to interpret his resistance as an attempt to establish a boundary. The practitioner's insistence may serve as a threat to the boundary he is trying to establish.

Jim's agreement may be the result of feeling intimidated. Perhaps he believes that the therapist knows best, or fears that without acquiescing he will not get his treatment. A boundary crossing has occurred because Jim wasn't offered a real choice about giving a history. Susan could have chosen other options: do the history and intake verbally; pare down the intake form—checking off the questions that are vital to providing an appropriate, safe treatment; and ask Jim if he wants to discuss his reluctance to filling out the history.

Remember that because boundaries are unique to each person, what constitutes crossing a line is different for different people. What feels like decent respectful behavior to one client (taking a medical history) may feel like a violation to another client like Jim. Therefore, even the most careful and respectful practitioner must be willing to learn about and assess each client individually.

Energetic Complications

Arianne was a somatic therapist who was unaware of her energetic sensitivity to others and did not believe that another person's energy could influence her energy level and her health. However, once she was out of school and well into her practice, she began to feel fatigued and experienced several ailments. Her ankle became painful for no apparent reason. She got sick frequently. She began to have headaches and temporomandibular joint problems. Finally, she noticed that her ailments generally corresponded directly to new clients' symptoms when she began working with them.

Upon reflection she realized that some type of energy transfer might indeed be happening and that she might be taking on her clients' issues. Still skeptical, she nevertheless decided to practice the techniques her school taught her for re-establishing the boundary of her energy field. Her physical ailments stopped.

Arianne now makes meditation, specific centering techniques and better health practices a part of her daily routine. She gives credit to her mental awareness and her daily discipline for overcoming her skepticism about energetic boundaries and for keeping her more healthy.

This scenario demonstrates the danger of excessively permeable boundaries. Practitioners are the ones who most often suffer energetic complications from overly permeable boundaries. Clients are rarely aware of this reaction in the practitioner unless the practitioner mentions it. If the client does find out, she usually feels uncomfortable for any number of reasons including guilt for "causing" the problem and uncertainty about the practitioner's ability. However, energy transference can go both ways.[9] The client can take on the energy and ailments from the practitioner. The situation can be easily avoided if the practitioner makes a habit of focusing the mind through simple meditation techniques and visualization.

Why Boundary Crossings Occur

Most practitioners genuinely intend to maintain clear boundaries and act ethically. Subtle boundary crossings generally occur for several reasons: a lack of understanding of boundaries in general; the practitioner is not aware of her own boundaries; the practitioner may not comprehend or pay attention to a particular client's boundaries; the practitioner may make incorrect assumptions about a client's ability to communicate when a boundary has been crossed; and the practitioner may choose to ignore certain therapeutic boundaries. This section explores how each of these may have been involved in the boundary transgressions described in the previous scenarios.

Without a good understanding of the nature of boundaries, and their own boundaries in particular, practitioners might assume that clients feel the same way they do. Consequently practitioners may do things such as move too close physically or emotionally, or offer unwanted advice. It is unlikely that the practitioner who offered unwanted feedback about the mole in the second scenario did so callously (although flippantly). More likely she was trying to offer good advice or inspire confidence by demonstrating her expertise. However, without understanding that unwanted advice may seem invasive, she obliviously created an intrusion.

Similarly, in the first scenario, it is likely that Steve's initiation of a hug was based in his belief that what felt appropriate for him would also apply to Gail. Steve lacks a conceptual understanding of boundaries: a hug might have a different meaning to a client than to a practitioner. He did not realize that while his own boundaries allow for an easy expression of affection, Gail's may not. This confusion was also true for Susan in the fourth scenario. Had she been in touch with her own boundaries, she might easily have realized that the client, Jim, was trying to establish a boundary.

Sometimes practitioners choose not to explore their boundary issues before going into practice. Luckily, Arianne's bodywork delivered no known detrimental effects to her clients during the time before she established her energy boundary. Arianne overestimated her abilities and beliefs. She found out that she needed to take another look at her boundary issues altogether and was willing to do so.

In the third scenario, Tracy's desire for a social relationship with Chris turned into a gross violation of therapeutic boundaries. Sometimes practitioners ignore the precepts of ethical client/practitioner interactions, attempt to bend the rules, or simply believe the rules do not apply to them. This manifests most often when in dual relationships (having more than one type of relationship with the same person). While dual relationships are not necessarily harmful, they are often difficult, and effective management requires attention and careful consideration.

As demonstrated in all the scenarios, practitioners need to get more information about a particular client's boundaries and learn more about their own. Getting this information is important work that can also be difficult. Patience and good communication between client and practitioner are required to discuss issues which may feel very personal and private to the client. Those issues might also appear threatening for the practitioner.

Difficulties In Identifying Boundary Crossings

A practitioner may mistakenly assume clients know how to identify when their boundaries are being crossed. In reality some clients may not initially be aware of this type of discomfort. Their personal history with emotional distress, physical pain, or abuse may have taught them to deny these feelings. Therefore, in another version of the first scenario, it is possible

> *Everything we do seeds the future. No action is an empty one.*
>
> —Joan Chittister

that a different client might not want a hug, and not be aware of it. In this case the client would feel uncomfortable afterwards but not know why.

The practitioner may also mistakenly assume that when clients are aware that their boundaries have been intruded upon, they are then willing to talk about it. In some cases, past experiences have taught people to avoid conflict by remaining quiet, even if they are uncomfortable. Others may simply feel it is not worth the effort. For example, neither Gail (the huggee in the first scenario) nor Sarah (who had the mole in the second scenario) told the practitioner how she felt.

In addition to personal histories, the power dynamics of the treatment relationship often make it difficult for clients to talk about their discomfort to a practitioner. The point here is that practitioners should not rely on clients speaking up to ensure that boundary crossings and violations do not occur.

Steps to Avoid Boundary Crossings and Violations

Practitioners make mistakes. Given the power that is accorded to health care professionals, they often feel enormous pressure to know everything that a client needs. This pressure may lead practitioners to avoid acknowledging mistakes to themselves or to others. Yet if the practitioner wants to learn about boundaries and identify when crossings or violations occur, it is useful to remember that even the most skilled and careful practitioners make these errors. In fact, by noticing mistakes when they occur and speaking about them with clients, practitioners are demonstrating awareness and respect for their clients' boundaries.

> Nothing is more important to the future of an idea than the first step you take to try it out.
>
> —O. A. Battista

With this in mind you can take several steps to avoid boundary crossings or violations, and to identify and correct them when they occur. These actions include:

- Increase empathetic awareness of clients' experiences.
- Take action to better manage your own and your clients' energy fields.
- Enhance skills for identifying clients' behaviors that indicate crossed boundaries.
- Ask questions that identify when clients' boundaries may have been violated.
- Teach clients how to identify and establish their own boundaries.
- Encourage clients to articulate their experience.

INCREASE EMPATHETIC AWARENESS OF CLIENTS' EXPERIENCES. Increasing empathy means that the practitioner regularly works on expanding awareness of what the client may be experiencing. In the first scenario Steve gave Gail a hug because he wanted to, not because he was attending to her needs. If Steve increases his empathetic awareness, he will be more considerate of how Gail might experience touch that is separate from the treatment. He will also pay attention to what Gail is and is **not** asking for.

TAKE ACTION TO BETTER MANAGE YOUR OWN AND YOUR CLIENTS' ENERGY FIELDS. In contrast to Arianne who had taken on her clients' ailments, practitioners can take action to better manage their own and their clients' energy fields by developing the skill of directing energy consciously. For example, Arianne might take a few moments before each session to clear her thoughts and energy. She may create and use a ritual to focus her mind before she places her hands on a client's body. Once the session is complete, she may utilize various focusing techniques that revitalize her energy field. Because she is aware of the existence of her own and her clients' energy fields, she is a more effective practitioner who ensures the safety of her clients.

ENHANCE SKILLS FOR IDENTIFYING CLIENTS' BEHAVIORS THAT INDICATE CROSSED BOUNDARIES. Because clients cannot always articulate the fear and discomfort that accompany unwanted boundary crossings, practitioners must become better at identifying behavior that indicates an intrusion. If the client cannot easily set a boundary, or tell the practitioner when they feel crossed, their indirect verbal or nonverbal behavior may provide clues. For example, if Jim (the client who resisted giving his history), had felt comfortable enough to set a boundary, his response to the request for a history might have been to calmly say, "I'd really prefer to skip the history. I don't feel comfortable right now saying a whole lot about myself. Perhaps we could do it another time." However, without such emotional clarity and verbal skill, clients may set the boundary indirectly. If the practitioner had understood that Jim's stubborn behavior was his best attempt at setting a boundary, she could have helped him set the boundary more easily and directly. This scenario illustrates these concepts:

> **Jim:** "I really don't see why I have to give you all this information. I just came here to get a massage."
>
> **Susan:** "I realize that. However, getting the information helps me give you the best possible treatment."
>
> **Jim:** "Well, I don't understand that. And I don't really care. I just want a massage."
>
> **Susan:** "You know, to do my job well and to make sure I don't miss anything, I really do need a history. But I do understand that giving a history is something you don't want to do. Perhaps you can tell me....is there a particular reason you don't want to do a history?"
>
> **Jim:** "Yes."
>
> **Susan:** "Do you feel comfortable enough to tell me why?"
>
> **Jim:** "Not really."
>
> **Susan:** "Well how about this? There is some basic information I need to know before we proceed. How about if we just go over those questions at this time? Then if you like the treatment, and decide you want future sessions, we can schedule a little extra time before your next session to complete the history. Also if you like I can give you an intake form for you to fill out at home and bring it back at your next session."

At this point Jim may accede. Either way, Susan's message to him is that while a history is important, she is willing to respect his boundary. Further, she has communicated that she is open to learning more about his reluctance when Jim feels comfortable. This also communicates respect for his boundary.

ASK QUESTIONS THAT IDENTIFY WHEN CLIENTS' BOUNDARIES MAY HAVE BEEN VIOLATED.
Practitioners must learn to ask questions when they feel they have violated a client's boundary.

> **PRACTITIONER:** "I just realized that for the past several minutes I've been asking you some very personal questions that aren't actually an integral part of the medical history. Have any of them made you uncomfortable?"

Of course this type of intervention only works if the client identifies her discomfort. If the practitioner suspects that the client might avoid conflict by not acknowledging the problem, the practitioner may simply have to make a statement:

> **PRACTITIONER:** "I just realized that for the past several minutes I've been asking you some very personal questions. Let me apologize if any of them made you uncomfortable."

TEACH CLIENTS HOW TO IDENTIFY AND ESTABLISH THEIR OWN BOUNDARIES. Practitioners can prevent boundary crossings and violations by teaching clients to identify and establish their boundaries. This encourages clients to be aware of what feels right and wrong for them in all aspects of the professional relationship. This training begins from the first moment of contact with the client: the practitioner establishes an environment of choice which teaches clients to identify their boundaries.

> **PRACTITIONER:** "Regarding disrobing, people feel comfortable getting a massage in a variety of ways. Some people remove all their clothes before getting under the sheet. Others choose to leave their underwear on or wear a smock. Still others feel most comfortable leaving their clothes on. Do what's right for you. I'm going to leave the room for a few minutes, and while I'm out please choose what feels best for you."

Asking specific questions often helps clients identify their boundaries.

> **PRACTITIONER:** "I'm going to show you a diagram of a back. Are there parts of your back you would prefer I focus on or avoid?"   -or-
>
> **PRACTITIONER:** "Occasionally pain is experienced in the process of relaxing the muscles. I want to work with you to limit discomfort. How do you typically respond to pain? If it becomes too painful, do you grimace quietly or would you tell me so I would know to reduce pressure or stop?"

ENCOURAGE CLIENTS TO ARTICULATE THEIR EXPERIENCE. Establishing an atmosphere of choice encourages clients to pay attention to their boundaries and articulate their experience. Depending on the client's answers, the practitioner might inquire further. This allows for more refined understanding of the client's boundaries and encourages the client to notice any feelings of violation. Continuing from the same example:

> **PRACTITIONER:** "Would you grimace quietly or would you tell me so I would know to stop or change my technique somehow?"
>
> **CLIENT:** "Come to think of it, I probably wouldn't say anything. I've had treatments from other people and I guess I sort of hang on during the real painful parts. I've always assumed that good work would most likely elicit some pain. Is that true?"
>
> **PRACTITIONER:** "Not always. If you're in so much pain that you're tensing against it, it may be counterproductive."
>
> **CLIENT:** "Well, the truth is I guess I do sometimes put up with more pain than I really want to. It just never occurred to me to ask anyone to go easier."
>
> **PRACTITIONER:** "Now that we've established it's okay, will you tell me when I'm working too hard?"
>
> **CLIENT:** "I'm not sure."
>
> **PRACTITIONER:** "How about if I check in with you regularly and I ask you if you're comfortable with the intensity? Would that make it easier?"
>
> **CLIENT:** "Maybe. Let's try."

These types of questions teach the practitioner about clients' boundaries. Note that they also teach clients to pay attention to, and learn about, their own boundaries. It is clear from the above scenario that when this type of interaction goes well, both the practitioner and the client benefit.

Discovering Your Boundary Issues

Oftentimes as health care practitioners you may be unaware of when you are overstepping boundaries with clients. You may feel uneasy about your relationship with a particular client, yet the reason eludes you. This checklist (adapted from the work of Estelle Disch[10]) helps you illuminate boundary issues with one or more of your clients. To do this exercise imagine a problematic relationship that you are having or have had with one of your clients. Place a checkmark next to the statements that apply to you in this situation.

1. ____ This client feels more like a friend than a client.
2. ____ I often tell my personal problems to this client.
3. ____ I want to be friends with this client when treatment ends.
4. ____ I think the goodbye hugs last too long with this client.
5. ____ Sessions often run overtime with this client.
6. ____ I accept gifts or favors from this client without examining why the gift was given.
7. ____ I have a barter arrangement with this client that is sometimes a source of tension for me.
8. ____ I sometimes choose my clothing with this particular client in mind.
9. ____ I have attended small professional or social events at which I knew this client would be present without discussing it ahead of time.
10. ____ This client often invites me to social events and I don't feel comfortable saying either yes or no.
11. ____ Sometimes when I'm touching this client during our regular sessions, I feel like the contact is sexual for either or both of us.
12. ____ This client is very seductive and I often don't know how to handle it.
13. ____ This client owes me a lot of money and I don't know what to do about it.
14. ____ I have invited this client to public or social events.
15. ____ I am often late for sessions with this particular client.
16. ____ I find myself cajoling, teasing and joking a lot with this client.
17. ____ I am in a heavy emotional crisis myself and I identify so much with this client's pain that I can hardly attend to the client.
18. ____ I allow this client to comfort me.
19. ____ I feel like this client and I are very much alike.
20. ____ This client scares me.
21. ____ This client's pain is so deep I can hardly tolerate it.
22. ____ I enjoy feeling more powerful than this client.
23. ____ Sometimes I feel like I'm over my head with this client.
24. ____ I feel that I am the only person who can really help this client.
25. ____ I often feel hooked or lost with this client and advice from colleagues and former teachers hasn't helped.
26. ____ I often feel invaded or pushed by this client and have difficulty standing my ground.
27. ____ I feel overly protective of this client.
28. ____ I have been doing things for this client that I don't usually do with other clients.
29. ____ I sometimes have a drink or use recreational drugs with this client.
30. ____ I'm doing so much on this client's behalf I feel exhausted.
31. ____ I am reluctant to discuss certain client/practitioner interactions in my peer supervision group.
32. ____ I accommodate this client's schedule and then feel angry/manipulated.
33. ____ This client has invested money in an enterprise of mine or vice versa.
34. ____ I have hired this client to work for me.
35. ____ I find it difficult to keep from talking about this client with my close friends and colleagues.
36. ____ I find myself engaged in a lot of self-disclosure with this client—telling stories and carrying on peer-like conversation.
37. ____ I feel emotionally drained after working with this client.
38. ____ My body, especially my arms, feels heavy after working with this client.

If you check off any of these items, boundary issues may be interfering with your ability to work effectively and ethically and we highly recommend you seek professional supervision to assist you in developing stronger boundaries.

We suggest that you periodically do this exercise to give you insight into areas where you might want to further your knowledge or get support.

Establish, Maintain & Change Boundaries

Change Agents

Eight of the major areas to consider in establishing, maintaining and changing boundaries are: location of service, interpersonal space, appearance, self-disclosure, language, touch, time and money. Including these issues in a policy statement and addressing them at the beginning of the treatment relationship, lessens the possibility of inappropriate, embarrassing, harmful or legally damaging situations.

Location of Service

Treating a client in a professional office sets a different contextual boundary than treating the client in her home or in an office located in your home. Always create a professional environment regardless of your office location. If you are in your home or making a visit to the client's home, more attention must be given to establishing and maintaining appropriate boundaries. For example, it is helpful for home offices to have a separate entrance and separate bathroom facilities. If this is not possible, eliminate as many personal items as possible from the "office area."

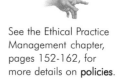

See the Ethical Practice Management chapter, pages 152-162, for more details on **policies**.

Interpersonal Space

Note the distance you allot when talking with your clients before and after sessions. Be mindful of the height differential. Do you stand while clients are seated or lying on a table? Do you sit on a higher stool or table? Being at the same height helps level the power differential. If crossing a boundary is required, act with awareness and respect as you move through this zone. Create an appropriate space boundary by maintaining a physical distance that makes both you and the client comfortable—always defer to whomever requires the greater space.

Appearance

The way you dress establishes a certain tone and carries a message to those you meet. Your primary goal is that your clothing and appearance foster feelings of trust and safety in your clients. Professionalism involves dressing appropriately for your daily work and maintaining good hygiene. Boundaries are clearly defined by uniforms, but many practitioners have varying degrees of formality in their dress code. Care is needed to avoid overly informal, revealing, or sexually provocative clothing. Modify your appearance for the therapeutic relationship (e.g., tie back long hair, trim fingernails).

Refer to Appendix A, pages 260-262 for sample **policy statements**.

Self-Disclosure

Self-disclosure occurs when a practitioner reveals professional or personal information about himself. Decisions about this must be made carefully. Completely avoiding any disclosure may create an unnecessary distance from a client. Too much self-disclosure often institutes an inappropriate closeness.

Appropriate professional disclosure includes describing training and experience to instill confidence in a client. An example of appropriate personal disclosure is sharing a personal experience that communicates empathy and understanding regarding the client's present situation. Self-disclosure creates a danger to the boundaries of the relationship when the practitioner reveals information which is not pertinent to the health care relationship and which may result in the client feeling uncomfortable or inappropriately close to the practitioner. Self-disclosure is a powerful factor in regulating the emotional distance between practitioner and client. In all cases self-disclosure must be guided by a belief that the information revealed is helpful to the client.

Language

Language is one of the most potent means for creating and maintaining healthy boundaries. The words you choose, your voice intonation, timbre and overall skill as a communicator are vital aspects in creating effective boundaries. Clients are more likely to know what they can expect from you and understand your expectations of them if you are respectful, articulate, clear and have a sincere and honest tone of voice. In this way a clearly defined boundary is created. Conversely, if you are imprecise, unclear, hesitant or insensitive, expectations of both parties are more likely to be cloudy and the boundaries unclear.

Touch

The type of touch either establishes a sense of safety and reassurance or it makes the client feel uneasy, apprehensive and uncomfortable. The practitioner needs to be very sensitive to the physical boundaries of touch both on and off the treatment table. A major touch boundary is the actual depth of touch. Working or probing too deeply or too lightly may be perceived as inappropriate. Another example of touch boundaries concerns greeting and saying goodbye to a client. In general the more conservative approach of shaking hands is advised. Make certain it is appropriate (and beneficial) before hugging a client or putting a hand on the client's shoulder or back.

Time

How you deal with time delineates your boundaries. In personal relationships the time spent in social interaction is usually very flexible; clear limits are not often stressed. A distinguishing feature of professional relationships is the limit placed on the time spent with clients. Clients often test the seriousness of your boundaries by asking for more time at the end of a session, coming late and expecting a full session, or canceling without adequate notice. Your responses to these situations either builds or weakens the client's trust.

Money

Money also helps to establish professional boundaries. The exchange of money reinforces the business nature of relationships. Friends do not pay to help each other. Be clear about your financial interactions. Boundaries are altered if a client owes you money over a long period of time or if a client never pays for sessions.

In Conclusion...

The foundation of an ethical practice is built upon establishing, maintaining and respecting personal and professional boundaries. A large measure of your professional success will be determined by the clarity with which you communicate expectations, the integrity in how you manage the business aspects of your practice, and the delicacy and grace with which you acknowledge the pain and vulnerabilities of your clients. Honoring your own boundaries and the boundaries of your clients promotes understanding and healing.

Chapter Highlights

- By increasing your awareness of your clients' boundaries (as well as your own), you can improve the therapeutic relationship and avoid many inadvertent slips into unethical behavior.
- Boundaries define our physical, sexual, intellectual, energetic and emotional space.
- In nearly all human interactions the physical space contained within this invisible line may expand or shrink depending on the individual's level of comfort and safety.
- In many ways people are defined by their emotions and how they feel in the moment.
- A person's thoughts, beliefs, emotions and opinions form a significant part of her identity.
- The sexual boundary can be defined in several ways and be thought of as a subset of the physical or the physical and emotional boundaries.
- Issues of crossing sexual boundaries in the health care professions are of such significance and concern that they have led to numerous laws, regulations and professional ethics statements regarding inappropriate sexual behavior with clients and in the workplace.
- There is a constant flow of energy around every human being, and the energy patterns of one person can influence those of another.
- Context determines which boundaries are the most appropriate.
- Boundaries fluctuate between permeable, semi-permeable and rigid.
- A permeable boundary allows information and feelings to flow easily in and out.
- A semi-permeable boundary indicates a flexible relationship with the outside world.
- A rigid boundary severely limits the flow of information and feelings moving in or out.
- In regards to client and practitioner, the point of contact occurs when the practitioner communicates in a way that the client can easily receive and understand.
- Boundaries need to be contextually appropriate.
- Boundaries are innate, developed and learned.
- Boundaries are influenced by family and culture.
- Boundaries emerge and are shaped through relationships with caretakers.
- There are different ethnic and cultural expectations about issues such as privacy and physical contact.
- Other areas distinctly developed early in life within the familial setting are privacy, physical contact, emotional connection and expression, intellectual expression, sexual attitudes and sensitivity.
- Schools, the media, religion and religious groups, and voluntary social organizations also greatly affect boundaries.
- A fine line exists between boundary crossings and violations.
- The difference between a harmful and a non-harmful boundary crossing may lie in whether it is discussed or discussable; clinical exploration of a violation often defuses its potential for harm.
- Several distinct areas hold the potential for boundary violations on the part of the practitioner including: The kind of physical touch permitted by the client; Probing for personal or private information about the client's past; The use of intimate words; Value judgments about the client's body or lifestyle.
- Boundary maintenance is always the responsibility of the practitioner.
- It is crucial to have the skills to identify boundary crossings and the knowledge and confidence to remedy the situation.

- Subtle boundary crossings generally occur for several reasons: Lack of understanding of boundaries; The practitioner is not aware of her own boundaries; The practitioner may not comprehend or pay attention to a particular client's boundaries; The practitioner may make incorrect assumptions about a client's ability to communicate when a boundary has been crossed; The practitioner may choose to ignore certain therapeutic boundaries.
- The power dynamics of the treatment relationship often make it difficult for clients to talk about their discomfort to a practitioner.
- By noticing mistakes when they occur and speaking about them with clients, practitioners demonstrate awareness and respect for their clients' boundaries.
- Actions practitioners can take to avoid boundary crossings or violations include: Increase empathetic awareness of clients' experiences; Take action to better manage your own and your clients' energy fields; Enhance skills for identifying clients' behaviors that indicate crossed boundaries; Ask questions that identify when clients' boundaries may have been violated; Teach clients how to identify and establish their own boundaries; Encourage clients to articulate their experience.
- There are eight major areas to consider in establishing, maintaining and changing boundaries: Location of service, interpersonal space, appearance, self-disclosure, language, touch, time and money.
- Treating a client in a professional office sets a different contextual boundary than treating the client in her home or in an office located in your home.
- Create an appropriate space boundary by maintaining a physical distance that makes both you and the client comfortable.
- The way you dress establishes a certain tone and carries a message to those you meet.
- Self-disclosure must be guided by a belief that the information revealed is helpful to the client.
- The words you choose, your voice intonation, timbre and overall skill as a communicator are vital aspects in creating effective boundaries.
- The practitioner needs to be very sensitive to the physical boundaries of touch both on and off the treatment table.
- A distinguishing feature of professional relationships is the limit placed on the time spent with clients.
- The exchange of money reinforces the business nature of relationships.
- The foundation of an ethical practice is built upon establishing, maintaining and respecting personal and professional boundaries.

Discussion Questions and Activities

- Describe the experiences in your culture, environment or family that have influenced the development of your boundaries.
- What are your clients' cultural considerations?
- Identify behaviors that might indicate that a client's boundaries have been crossed.
- Describe the cultural diversity of your practice.
- Make a list of questions that would help a client identify when boundaries have been crossed or violated.
- What professional or personal situations make you uncomfortable because your boundaries have been crossed?
- List actions to take when a client's boundaries have been crossed.
- Write or discuss in small groups: What areas of boundary management might be difficult for you and how can you address them?
- Spend several days noticing your thoughts and how they affect your mood. Keep a journal on your reflections. Ask yourself: How does separating your mood from your thoughts influence your boundaries?
- What are some boundaries that are idiosyncratic to your cultural background (e.g., touch, disclosure)?
- What are the areas in which you might be in danger of disregarding boundary signals?
- Imagine that you and a number of your colleagues are meeting to create a series of exercises (or curriculum) on how to prevent, detect and correct boundary crossings and violations. Create exercises for each of the following:
  1. Describe how practitioners can increase their empathetic awareness of the client's experience of an inappropriate boundary crossing.
  2. List ways to enhance practitioners' skills at identifying client behaviors that indicate crossed boundaries.
  3. Develop questions that help clients identify when their boundaries have been crossed or violated.
  4. Create an activity that teaches clients how to identify their own boundaries.
  5. Identify practitioners' behaviors that may encourage clients to articulate their discomfort when they feel invaded.

3

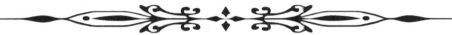

Dynamics of Effective Communication

- Communication Barriers
- Learning Styles
- Managing Boundaries
- Emotions in the Treatment Room
- Reflective Listening
- Interactive Speaking
- Body Language Awareness
- Tools for Maintaining Boundaries
- Process Recordings
- The Assertion Sequence
- In Conclusion...
- Chapter Highlights
- Discussion Questions and Activities

Clear communication is the foundation of successful professional relationships. A minimum of misunderstanding and a maximum of creative interaction occurs when we accurately transfer information about what we think and feel. Yet effective communication is often a challenging process. Having what seems to be a simple verbal exchange between two or more individuals is dramatically more complicated than we might assume at first. Each person engaging in the exchange brings to it a unique personal history, with individual perceptions, beliefs, emotional patterns, sensitivities, personality, likes and dislikes, educational training and so forth. Add to this multitude of factors all the subtleties involved that fall outside the spoken word such as body language, feelings and the environment. The words we speak may seem simple enough and we might feel quite clear about what we are saying, but the dynamics of speaking are subject to misunderstanding and misinterpretation. Learning to communicate effectively in every aspect of our lives is a major task and one that is an ongoing process.

Mastering communication skills takes study, time, patience, good teachers and a safe educational setting. This chapter provides you with proven concepts and tools to assist you in developing your communication potential. We explore communication barriers, enhancing effectiveness by communicating in a variety of styles, increasing awareness through the use of self-evaluation tools, incorporating reflective listening and interactive speaking, understanding body language, maintaining practitioner boundaries, and honoring client boundaries.

Some practitioners have received extensive training in many of these ways of communicating. If that's the case for you, we hope this information provides a useful review plus some practical application tips. Others have received little or no training in these skills. They may wish for a more in-depth treatment of each skill than is possible in this chapter. Book-length treatment of some of these skills can be found in Robert Bolton's *People Skills: How to Assert Yourself, Listen to Others and Resolve Conflicts.*[1]

Communication Barriers

One way to understand effective communication is to be aware of the barriers that prevent it. Words are imprecise vehicles of communication. The 500 most frequently used words in the English language have 12,078 separate and distinct meanings in *The Oxford English Dictionary*. On average that's 24 meanings per word! People have to guess at what is meant by a word—usually from the context in which it is used. Often they are right; sometimes they are not.

The biggest problem with language is that the meaning of words is in people, not in dictionaries. Each of us projects our own meanings onto the words we say and hear. For instance, a practitioner and client agreed that the practitioner would be called only "in an emergency." This may seem to be a clear communication, but it became evident that each had very different ideas of what constituted an emergency. The client called at all hours of the day with questions that the practitioner did not consider emergencies. As the eminent philosopher Alfred North Whitehead put it, "The success of language in conveying information is vastly overrated...."

Another problem in interpersonal communication occurs when we try to express what we are thinking. Because we do it every day, it seems easy and we feel quite competent at it. However, if we read an exact transcript of what we have said, we might find that our thoughts came out in a jumble, or that the language conveyed judgment instead of empathy. The meaning may not have been nearly as clear as we thought it was. In writing it often takes several drafts to achieve clarity; however, when we converse with people, they receive the unedited first draft, which often leaves much to be desired. The listener does not always get the message we intend. It can be like talking on the telephone when the wire has been cut and our meanings and intentions do not get through; or when static occurs and the listener gets only half of the words, plugging in imagined words and interpreting what he hears to his own satisfaction.

The choice of words is not the only challenge to effective communication. According to Stuart Simon,[2] "Whether or not information crosses over from the speaker to the listener depends less on what you say than how you say it. Every message is composed of two parts: the visible part of what you say and the invisible part of how you say it. A mere handful of visible defensive behaviors cause most of our everyday communication problems." These behaviors might include a blaming tone, a condescending manner, putting others down, name-dropping, and bragging, to name a few.

> A first-time client told a massage therapist he was feeling tense in his shoulders and back. Beginning to work on the client's back, the therapist exclaimed, "Wow! You really ARE tight, aren't you!" The client stiffened, felt put down and humiliated, but said nothing. He didn't return to this therapist for further treatment.

The therapist's comment did not communicate anything useful. A useful statement might have been, "Would you like me to tell you when I feel tension in certain areas?" or, "I feel what you're describing, it's a little bit tense here," or, "I feel some tension here; let me know if it's too much pressure as we work on it." In these communications the therapist affirms the client's sensitivity and body awareness, and works with the client to help release the tension that is found.

A person's verbal message is also accompanied by non-verbal signals that may distort or even contradict the intended message. Even when a person's words are emphatic, if the accompanying body language appears too laid back or the facial expression seems incongruent with what the person is saying, the message may not be taken seriously. If you have ever seen someone expressing irritation or anger with a big smile on the person's face, you probably got a feeling of dissonance because these two aspects of the communication were in conflict.

Communication breaks down at the listener's end, too. Researchers found that people listen four to five times faster than people speak. The listener has spare time to become bored and may mentally drift off to other thoughts. Without even realizing it, the listener may miss important elements of the message. Furthermore, we all listen through filters that screen out some messages and distort others. Our concerns, needs, moods, roles, prejudices and other factors color what we hear. The possibility for error increases when the speaker, the listener, or both experience strong feelings about the message.

Communication barriers can be overcome if you possess certain skills and information such as: listening; addressing a variety of learning styles; setting boundaries (prominent among them saying "no" when wishing to); asking for what you want when you have a need; saying "yes" without reservation; giving and receiving positive and critical feedback in a constructive manner; appropriately expressing and receiving irritation and anger; noticing destructive, dysfunctional patterns in ourselves and others; and developing a sense of empathy so that our communication timing is in sync with those around us.

"
If the person you are talking to doesn't appear to be listening, be patient. It may simply be that he has a small piece of fluff in his ear.
"
—Winnie the Pooh
(A.A. Milne)

Learning Styles

A multisensory approach is the best way to communicate information effectively. Most people prefer to take in information by one of three methods: auditory, kinesthetic or visual.[3] Awareness of a person's preferred learning style helps to determine the best way to communicate with that person. If you speak your information using the auditory channel, some individuals understand perfectly while others immediately forget what you said. If it is possible to show the information (by demonstration or written materials), you assist the visually oriented segment of the population. Another group takes in information best by having a kinesthetic experience. This may be accomplished if you tell a story which makes an emotional connection for the person or stirs the person in some visceral way. The kinesthetically-oriented person often learns best by physically doing an exercise or role-playing a situation so it is learned from the inside out.

Current learning theory asserts that people learn through an even broader spectrum. Howard Gardner[4] identified eight major intelligences (and is currently exploring a ninth): Verbal/Linguistic; Logical/Mathematical; Visual/Spatial; Bodily/Kinesthetic; Music/Rhythmic; Intrapersonal; Interpersonal; and Naturalist. No wonder that communication is laden with difficulties! Knowledge of learning styles and types of intelligences helps us further appreciate that good communication is a complicated process. This knowledge also helps us to become more effective and efficient in our communication.

If you know an individual's preferred mode of learning, you do not have to use every method to communicate. Without extensive training in communication theory and learning, however, it is often difficult to be certain how others take in information. Therefore it is safest to communicate using as many methods as possible. For instance, if you are explaining a certain problem or condition to a client, it is best to tell him verbally, write it down, give him a handout, have him ask you questions, have him do the activity if it is something physical, and then ask him to explain it so you can check for understanding. Be even more thorough by requesting that the client tell you or show you what you did in the previous meeting to verify his retention. It is common to use several of these methods of communication and to still have the person show you or tell you something completely different at your next meeting. In this case you may have missed the primary method of communication or the individual may simply need more repetition to learn and retain information.

Managing Boundaries

Boundaries are negotiated and maintained through communication—through words, body language and behaviors. Our well-being in life and our competence as practitioners stems in large measure from our ability to communicate our boundary needs with others and our competence in listening and responding to others who are communicating their concerns to us.

Since people feel strongly about many boundary issues, communication about these matters is prone to misunderstanding. Setting a boundary about wearing shoes on your carpet or not calling after 9 P.M. is easy for most practitioners to do. However, emotionally charged issues such as money, body odor, repeated lateness, or intrusive questions are more challenging.

" No one would talk much in society if they knew how often they misunderstood others. "

—Johann von Goethe

In short it can be difficult to communicate effectively about boundaries in any relationship and it can be especially challenging in therapeutic relationships. Recognizing the communication pitfalls surrounding boundaries reminds practitioners how vigilant and skillful they need to be when communicating about areas of vulnerability. Fortunately, there are ways of approaching these matters with sensitivity and clarity.

The Power Dynamic

As discussed earlier in Chapter One, the power dynamic in the practitioner-client relationships escalates communication problems. The practitioner's knowledge and status put her in a superior position in relationship to the client. This often impacts the way people deal with boundary issues. For example, the power differential may so affect boundaries that a client may not speak about boundary concerns because of a fear that these concerns seem foolish, trivial, or cowardly; the client may become overly compliant out of fear that raising issues will be perceived as disrespectful, resulting in poorer service; a client may resent the practitioner's power and become angry, challenge the practitioner's competence, and undermine the treatment; and a client may agree to something for fear of losing the positive connection with the practitioner.

In some therapeutic relationships the practitioner actually feels less powerful than the client and therefore has difficulty communicating well.

> A physical therapist had a client who was a well-known surgeon. The therapist was in awe of this client's training and expertise, and her work with him was tentative. She found herself reluctant to point out his lifestyle stresses that were contributing to his low back pain or to strongly recommend exercises to do at home. She felt relieved when the surgeon stopped booking appointments with her.

See pages 15-17 for more information on the **power differential**.

The power differential can also adversely affect practitioners if they are uncomfortable that the differential exists at all. These practitioners often find themselves being lax about boundaries in an attempt to put themselves and their clients on an "even footing." If you find yourself too often deferring payments for sessions, extending session times even when your schedule is tight, booking outside your regularly established hours, and making home visits when you do not want to, consider whether you are really comfortable with the power dynamic of your role as practitioner.

Communicating Respect for Client Boundaries

When a health care practitioner flagrantly violates a client's boundary, miscommunication is rarely the source of the problem. Flagrant means that it is a clear legal or ethical violation. Making sexual overtures to a person in one's care is an example of a flagrant boundary abuse. This is a breach of ethics rather than poor communication.

Professional Codes of Ethics provide practitioners with a basic framework for establishing boundaries in health care settings. Despite the seemingly comprehensive nature of ethical policies, however, there are always "gray areas" of conduct where practitioners must navigate for themselves. Communication skills are crucial for protecting the client and the practitioner by clarifying and negotiating these boundary concerns to enhance the comfort and effectiveness of the treatment. Here are some actions you can take to help clients be more open about their boundary concerns.

Treat the Client as a Person, not an Object

This would seem too elementary to even mention but in varying degrees many practitioners and organizations treat clients in depersonalizing ways. The focus is often on what makes the organization's or the practitioner's work easier rather than on what makes the client more at ease in the process. Clients are sometimes subjected to bureaucratic intake procedures and needlessly long waits for service. Receptionists and others may respond to clients in a perfunctory manner. When the client finally gets to the practitioner, she may be treated as an object once again.

> A client was treated at a holistic clinic that is known for its technical excellence. The contact pattern with a number of practitioners was always the same. The client was shown to a room to wait. Upon entering the room the practitioner walked past the client as if the client wasn't present in the room. Without acknowledging the client, the practitioner read notes about the case from the files. Finally, after several minutes of treating the client as nonexistent, the practitioner would begin the assessment. It was a very efficient process—and a very impersonal one. It certainly didn't pave the way for the client to raise sensitive boundary concerns or even to be a vital participant in the communication about his own treatment.

It is not easy for a caregiver to be engaging, truly interested and responsive day after day, year after year. No one does it perfectly. However, sincere and clear communication is an important key to boundary maintenance and to effective treatment. If a client feels he can talk to a practitioner, he is much more likely to feel comfortable addressing boundary issues.

One of the best ways to treat clients as human beings is to reveal your own human-ness: admit your mistakes. All practitioners have moments when, through no fault of their own, their best attempts to honor the client's boundaries fail. Drapes slip, hands fumble, hair brushes over a client's face, and accidents happen. The best response is to treat the client with respect by immediately and clearly communicating about the incident.

> When working on a male client's thigh, a female polarity therapist leaned across the table and accidentally brushed the client's testicles. The therapist straightened up and placed both her hands on the client's arm near his shoulder; "I'm sorry," she said. Her reassuring touch and her simple apology allowed the session to continue without incident.

> A male chiropractor started to work on a prone female client, who was wearing a gown opened in the back. He placed one of his hands on her lower legs and the other hand on her upper back. All of a sudden, with a cry of shock, the client said, "Doctor, what's going on?" The chiropractor looked down and saw that his tie had fallen between the client's thighs. In an even and professional voice, he said, "I'm sorry; my tie slipped and is touching you. Let me keep my hands where they are while you turn your head to see for yourself." The client saw that the chiropractor was telling the truth; because of his clear and honest communication, she relaxed and the treatment continued.

Set Policies and Practices that Protect the Client

Let the client know at the outset that you want to make the experience as safe and comfortable as possible. Describe policies designed to safeguard the client's well-being, such as confidentiality, lateness, no shows, payment policies, and so forth. Invite questions or comments. Close by saying that while you will not knowingly do anything to make the client feel ill at ease, each of us has different comfort levels about certain procedures. You might say something like, "Let me know if you ever feel uncomfortable about what we are doing."

See Appendix A, pages 260-262 for sample **policy statements**.

Foster Appropriate Self-Disclosure

Self-disclosure refers to how much personal information is exchanged between the practitioner and the client. A client usually discloses personal information to the practitioner as it relates to the presenting problem. This gives the practitioner the relevant information for proper assessment and treatment. There is also a level of self-disclosure from the client to the practitioner which may be excessive and inappropriate. A client can move quickly into transference with the practitioner and proceed to share all kinds of personal and sensitive information. The client may also be lonely, have no one to talk to, or may have very loose boundaries when it comes to communicating personal information.

The client often views the practitioner as all-knowing and expects advice and input that is not in keeping with the practitioner's training and areas of expertise. Many traditional and complementary hands-on health care practitioners are commonly asked questions as if they were psychotherapists. Deal appropriately with this type of self-disclosure to avoid trouble as the relationship develops.

For instance the practitioner might say, "I can be a good listener but what you appear to be asking me about isn't in my field of expertise. It would be unethical for me to give you any type of advice. I would be happy to refer you to a good therapist regarding this matter."

On the opposite side of the equation, what the practitioner reveals about herself may significantly affect the quality and ongoing viability of the relationship. Sometimes a personal self-disclosure by the practitioner to the client can be a powerful therapeutic intervention, or simply an act of kindness.

If you go back to the maxim of the client-centered relationship and ask yourself why you are revealing the information, the answer tells you if this is for the benefit of the client or the practitioner. For example, if the client begins to cry as he tells the practitioner that his teenage daughter is using drugs and failing in school, causing enormous pain and stress, the practitioner might respond by saying, "My son had a similar problem and it was one of the most painful and difficult things I have ever had to go through." This brief personal disclosure might help the client know that the practitioner really understands. If, on the other hand, the practitioner launches into a 15-minute story about how her son was abusing drugs, stealing and lying, the client might feel overloaded and invaded by the practitioner's problems. This second self-disclosure was primarily for the benefit of the practitioner. In this circumstance the client would be unlikely to return.

Many clients report that appropriate self-disclosure by the practitioner have been among the most important moments in the therapeutic interaction. When done well and expressed at the right moment, they help to establish trust and safety in the ongoing therapeutic relationship.

While you can learn much by listening carefully to what people say, a great deal more is revealed by what they do not say. Listen as carefully to silence as to sound.

—Dee Hock

Emotions in the Treatment Room

Hands-on techniques can elicit emotional responses in some clients. Practitioners must know how to communicate with clients when emotional expression occurs in the treatment room. A client may cry, have an anxiety reaction, or become angry in a session. What the practitioner says and how he says it in response to these emotional expressions affect the therapeutic alliance with the client. Many practitioners discuss this with clients prior to sessions, particularly if their type of work is prone to elicit emotions or if the client's history suggests emotional volatility.

Practitioners who are not prepared for emotional responses might not react in a manner that provides the necessary safety for clients. Also practitioners might get drawn into inappropriate responses. Sometimes the boundary between the roles of somatic practitioner and psychotherapist become blurred. Kylea Taylor states in her book, *The Ethics of Caring,*[5] "Certain intense and profound experiences in clients can produce subtle and powerful [responses] in therapists. These experiences tend to make boundaries more diffuse, confuse roles, intensify transference and trigger surprisingly compelling countertransference."

Refer to Special Considerations In Cases of Trauma, pages 215-239.

Sometimes just touching a particular area triggers an emotional response associated with a past occurrence. If this occurs, the client might want to discuss it with the practitioner. Allowing expression is usually fine but encouraging it, asking questions, or interpreting it often exceeds the practitioner's scope of practice. A different course of action is required if a client experiences a flashback.

During an emotional release it is important to keep clients focused on the present moment. You can suggest that the client breathe into the area, relax, and perhaps open his eyes. If a client appears in great distress, ask if the client wants to continue the session or stop. If the client wants you to work on the area, you must proceed carefully. Keep in mind the significant difference between assisting a client in letting go of a thought, memory or feeling that has surfaced, and promoting an emotional reaction or release.

Checking in with clients is appropriate but refrain from asking questions that probe into the cause of their emotional expressions. Examples of potentially inappropriate questions include: "Do you know why you felt sad when I touched your leg?" "Were you thinking of someone in particular when you began to feel anxious?" "Do I remind you of someone in your family or your past?" Avoid playing the role of an armchair psychiatrist. Emotional release is a gray area where professional boundaries are easily crossed. Intent is of primary importance.

The bottom line is that unless a practitioner has strong communication skills, knowledge and training in working with the emotional reactions of clients, she should defuse the situation and change the focus of the session with a statement such as, "This seems to be an area in your body where a strong experience is being held. Should I move to a different area?" The practitioner may take the opportunity to explain that emotional experiences are often held in the body and mention that counseling or therapy can be beneficial in processing the emotional issues that come up in touch therapy.

Clients normally have a variety of physical and vocal responses (usually unconscious) to treatments. The following sections offer communication guidelines to protect the therapeutic encounter when specific emotions place the relationship at risk. If the practitioner finds the magnitude of a client's emotional expression overwhelming, she has the responsibility to bring at least temporary closure to that interaction. Calling a time-out, leaving the room, or stopping the session are all appropriate responses. In such circumstances achieving some distance ensures safety and enables the practitioner to maintain professional and ethical behavior.

Sadness

The first step for interacting with a client who begins to cry during a session is to acknowledge the emotion. Ask if the client he wants to take a short break, end the session or have you continue working. Most sessions can proceed if a client is gently crying. If the client wants a short break, ask if he prefers you to stay in the room, or if he would like some time alone. If the client wishes to be alone, you leave the room for five minutes or so and then check on the client. A client may want the practitioner to stay in the room and sit by quietly. If so, it is usually a good idea to refrain from conversation and make physical contact only if the client requests physical contact in some way.

Fear and Anxiety

Anxiety is elicited by touch therapy when more energy is moving in the body than the person can tolerate. Anxiety and fear reactions may include: holding the breath, clenching fists, gripping the jaw, involuntary shaking, feeling numb, skin discoloring (going white in the face), sweating, nausea, distracting behaviors, erratic movements, and avoiding eye contact. Anxiety can arise from a thought, a feeling or a sensation. If you notice that a client has become anxious or afraid, the pace of the treatment should be slowed down or stopped and the anxiety discussed. The practitioner might say: "I may be way off here but I notice that you seem a little anxious. Is this correct?" If the client answers yes, the treatment should be temporarily discontinued until the issue is discussed and resolved if possible. Keep the focus on what needs to be done to foster a sense of safety and diminish the anxiety reaction so that the session can proceed.

A safe technique to lessen anxiety by involving the person's thinking process is to discuss the physical sensations. Inquire if the client is willing to try something that might help him feel better. Pose a series of questions that focuses the client's energy and diminishes the physical experience of anxiety. Such a dialogue might go like this:

> PRACTITIONER:
> Where do you feel the anxiety in your body?
> CLIENT:
> I feel it in my chest and my abdomen.
> PRACTITIONER:
> Is the sensation getting more intense or less intense?
> CLIENT:
> It's getting a little stronger.
> PRACTITIONER:
> Is the sensation moving anywhere?
> CLIENT:
> Yes, I feel it down my arms as well.
> PRACTITIONER:
> Do you feel the sensation in your legs?
> CLIENT:
> No.
> PRACTITIONER:
> Do you feel it in your neck?

The most important thing in communication is to hear what isn't being said.

—Peter Drucker

Dynamics
of Effective
Communication

CLIENT:

No.

PRACTITIONER:

Is the sensation getting larger or smaller now?

CLIENT:

I only feel it in my chest now.

PRACTITIONER:

Can you describe exactly what it feels like?

CLIENT:

It's like a cold wind running up and down in my chest.

PRACTITIONER:

Are you more comfortable sitting up than when you were lying down?

CLIENT:

I feel much more comfortable; it seems to be disappearing.

Another option is to stop the treatment session. If the client is undressed, allow him to dress. Being fully clothed and sitting face-to-face often lessens the power differential or at least diminishes the client's feeling of vulnerability.

Annoyance and Anger

Communicating with a client who exhibits a strong emotion such as annoyance or anger is challenging for most practitioners. At the moment this occurs it is essential for the practitioner to listen and to acknowledge what the client is saying and experiencing. The first step is to determine whether the expression is an emotional response related to a past experience or an expression of a currently felt experience that is directed at the practitioner.

When the annoyance or anger is directed at the practitioner, it is crucial that the client be acknowledged (unless the client is totally out of control and yelling). Whether the practitioner agrees with the client is not relevant; the practitioner needs to be quiet, listen, and take in what the client is saying. If the client is angry with the practitioner the reason could be that the client has mistaken information, misunderstood what was said, or is undergoing a transference reaction.

If the practitioner determines that the client's annoyance or anger is not an immediate response to the practitioner, then these emotions may be the result of a conscious or unconscious memory or flashback from the client's past. When this occurs, the practitioner should proceed carefully and seek supervision if needed.

If the practitioner becomes upset, feels immobilized or defensive it is best not to react at all but tell the client that he wants to think about what the client has said and respond later. When the session ends, this is the time to immediately consult a supervisor or trusted peer. If the practitioner made a mistake, did something inappropriate or inadvertently crossed a boundary, an acknowledgment and an apology would be the appropriate response in the next meeting. If the client's concerns were appropriate, the practitioner should take steps to correct the problem and tell the client.

If the client was mistaken about the facts or misunderstood something, this information should be shared with the client at the next meeting along with an acknowledgment of how the practitioner's actions could have been misinterpreted. If the client was undergoing a transference reaction, allotting a cooling off period may allow the incident to be discussed more easily when it is approached at the next meeting. This is, of course, the most difficult and delicate situation to handle. Kindness and clear communication are essential.

What you do speaks so loudly that I cannot hear what you say.

—Ralph Waldo Emerson

See Ethical Principles, pages 17-20, for details on **transference and countertransference**.

Reflective Listening

Reflective listening is a key skill in effective communication[6] and is the foundation for helping you understand and honor your clients' boundaries. Reflective listening, also called "active listening," is an integral part of several communication methods referred to later in this chapter. It is also an important skill in and of itself.

Words convey only part of a communication message. It is not enough for a listener to comprehend what a speaker is saying—the listener needs to understand what the message *means* to the speaker. That entails understanding what is said from within the speaker's *frame of reference*.

Each of us sees the world a bit differently. Our personal perspectives color everything we hear or see. The bottom line is that many times we hear the *words* a person says but miss the implications. We do not understand "where the other person is coming from." Because of this pitfall in interpersonal communication, practitioners often miss when a client raises a boundary issue or miss the significance of the client's concern.

> A male acupuncturist who took a "whole person" approach to health care was conducting an annual physical with a female client. After discussing diet, exercise and other matters, he asked, "Do you have a satisfactory sexual life?" She replied, "I don't know if that's relevant."

From the acupuncturist's frame of reference, it was indeed relevant to his assessment and treatment, and he proceeded to explain why and then asked the question again. He was responding to what the client *said* but missed what she *meant*. She was trying to find a polite way of saying that the topic of sex was off-limits.

The effective practitioner transcends his frame of reference sufficiently to understand the client's perspective. Listen not only to the client's words but *through* them to the meaning behind the words.

A reflection is a brief statement of the essence of the other person's message, stated in the listener's own words. Listen to the person's whole message and then summarize it in a word, a phrase, or a sentence. Seldom should your reflection be more than one sentence. You do not have to repeat every idea—just the key meaning. Find the core of the message and reflect that succinctly and in your own words.[7]

To familiarize yourself with reflective listening, use starter phrases such as:

> *You* think…
> *You* feel…
> *You're* saying…
> *Your* point of view is…

The words YOU, YOU'RE and YOUR in the above phrases are italicized as a reminder that you are attempting to express the other person's point of view by restating the other person's message in your own words. Since every word has many meanings, using your own words to summarize what the client said helps you check if you have correctly identified the client's intention. Even more significantly, it makes it more likely that you will search for the meaning behind the client's words.

In response to the client who said, "I don't know if that's relevant," the practitioner might have reflected, "You aren't sure it's relevant." However, if he forced himself to substitute another word or phrase for the key word *relevant*, he might have focused more

Dynamics
of Effective
Communication

on the client's outlook. When he reflected that statement without using the word *relevant*, he came up with a restatement that was closer to the client's real meaning: "It seems like this is something you don't want to talk about."

Listeners often focus too much on content and miss the feeling aspects between the lines. Yet, feelings can be as important as the content of a message.[8] This is especially true of boundary issues. A listener must be especially aware of feeling words and body language that provide clues about the speaker's emotions.

The following are examples of common statements and body language that occur in a treatment setting and the possible feelings or messages behind these communications:

- **Client says, "I can't really describe it."** The client: feels it is none of your business; lacks awareness; doesn't know terminology.
- **Client sighs**: The client is: bored; indifferent; or relaxed.
- **Client looks down or away.** The client: is shy; doesn't know how to respond; is embarrassed; gave a less than honest response; discounts what you said; is lost in thought.
- **The client's body tightens.** The client: suddenly feels pain; is cold; is experiencing an unpleasant memory or emotion; is feeling defensive; is restraining a belch; feels the work is too deep.
- **Client says, "Do you think you could do that a little differently?"** The client: doesn't like what you are doing; wants you to work lighter or deeper; feels uncomfortable; senses that you are distant and is attempting to bring you to the present moment; feels that what you are doing does not match the expectations.
- **The client's chest collapses downward.** The client is experiencing: fear; withdrawal; sudden depression; meditative breathing.
- **The client grimaces.** The client: is expressing disapproval or condescension; is trying to prevent a sneeze; nose itches; has an unconscious tic.
- **The client laughs at inappropriate moments.** The client is: experiencing discomfort or embarrassment; covering for being sad; thinking of something funny.
- **The client says, "It gives me a funny feeling."** The client: is uncomfortable and doesn't know why; cannot determine whether this is a "good" or "bad" sensation; isn't sure about your intention; doesn't really like the treatment but feels you know best and doesn't want to hurt your feelings; is expressing that he wants you to stop.
- **The client tilts head to the side.** The client: is confused or in disbelief; cannot hear well; is doing a neck stretch.
- **The client does not maintain eye contact.** The client: is upset with you; has difficulty communicating; cannot think while making eye contact; is showing respect (in many cultures it is inappropriate to look directly into another's eyes).
- **The client squirms.** The client: has a full bladder; feels sexually aroused; is in an uncomfortable position; experiences discomfort with the work.

Reflecting feelings is more a matter of the heart than the head. If your reflection is made in cold, matter-of-fact tones, the person likely will not feel understood. When reflecting feelings, capture the mood of the speaker and reflect this with your tonal quality and facial expression as well as through your words.[9] When your whole being is in harmony with the other person's emotions, a reflection of feeling communicates empathy. When reflecting feelings, it is often desirable to tie them to what seems to trigger the feelings. Filling in the blanks of this statement often does the trick:

You feel _____ about _____.
       (feeling word)   (content)

For example, "You feel *reluctant* about *continuing to discuss this.*"

Of course there are other ways of linking feelings and content in one brief reflection: "This is *upsetting* for you to *talk about.*"

When you are reflecting, choose understatement. Do not say, "You are scared to talk about this," if *timid* is more accurate.

When listening, back up your reflecting with a posture of involvement. Give your physical attention to the person by facing him, leaning slightly into the conversation, maintaining eye contact, and nodding your head from time to time.

Reflective listening encourages the other person to say what is on her mind. It helps the client finish a train of thought, rather than jump from topic to topic. It creates an empathetic climate where the client feels freer about discussing difficult concerns such as boundary topics. Furthermore, it builds a sense of safety that may enable the client to adjust his boundary so especially sensitive issues can be expressed. Skillful reflective listening and a sound ethical stance are your best allies in helping protect client boundaries.

Interactive Speaking

Clients feel more comfortable bringing up boundary issues when there is considerable two-way communication in the treatment sessions. All too often, though, there is a preponderance of one-way communication between the practitioner and the client. It is easy to see how this can happen. Clients have a problem they cannot solve so they seek someone to help them. They are likely to expect practitioners to run the show. Practitioners, quite naturally, want to be helpful, and from their perspective that often means coming up with solutions and imparting those solutions to their clients. So, from both sides of helping relationships, there may be assumptions that lead to fairly one-sided communication with clients feeling disempowered.

There are many reasons why dialogue is preferable to monologue. Two-way communication creates a milieu where clients are more likely to share their boundary concerns.

Interactive Speaking is a simple three-step method that promotes two-way communication. The steps are:

        Speak ➡ Invite ➡ Reflect.
        (Recycle as needed)

SPEAK: Say what you have to say. Keep it short. Thirty to 60 seconds is best. You can add to your statement in later cycles of Speak ➡ Invite ➡ Reflect. Keep the speak portion brief during each cycle of this method.

INVITE: After you have made your point, invite the other person's response. Often a pause is all it takes to solicit the other person's opinion. It is useful to ask a checking question.

Here are some examples of checking questions:

"What's your reaction?"
"Sound OK?"
"Any problems with this?"
"What do you think so far?"
"How does this sound to you?"

REFLECT: From time to time as the other person responds, succinctly restate the essence of what she is saying. When the other person comes to the end of what she has to say and you have reflected, the ball is back in your court.

Informed Consent Discussions

The informed consent discussion uses Interactive Speaking to encourage clients' input on boundary issues. Clients are more likely to discuss their boundary concerns when they are engaged early and often in low-threat conversations about matters of potential concern to them. Informed Consent Discussions are a good way of doing this. In these conversations the practitioner explains (1) *what* she will be doing in the next procedure or part of the session, (2) *why* it is recommended, and (3) *how* it impacts the client. For instance, one topic might be how much discomfort is likely to be experienced during the technique or procedure. This information is divided into small segments and each segment initiates a Speak/Invite/Reflect cycle.

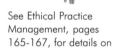

See Ethical Practice Management, pages 165-167, for details on **informed consent**.

See Appendix A, pages 263-264, for sample **informed consent forms**.

A client is receiving a series of Rolfing® treatments. One of his concerns is jaw pain.

PRACTITIONER SPEAKS:
I think it would be helpful to do some work inside your mouth. This is the most effective way to manipulate the fascial membrane of the jaw muscles.

PRACTITIONER INVITES:
Would this be okay with you?

CLIENT RESPONDS:
I'm not sure. Will it hurt? How hygienic is it?

PRACTITIONER REFLECTS:
You feel apprehensive about this course of treatment.

PRACTITIONER SPEAKS:
I wear sterile gloves while working in the mouth. Some people do experience discomfort. The goal isn't for you to feel pain, but to soften the fascial restrictions. If it becomes uncomfortable, raise your hand and I will stop.

PRACTITIONER INVITES:
[Practitioner pauses]

CLIENT RESPONDS:
If that's the case and you think it will help me—let's try it.

Informed consent interactions are important, not only for major matters like a decision to do heart bypass surgery but also the innumerable less consequential issues that come up in health care relationships. For example, when a woman's breast requires some treatment, or when a technique performed high on the inner thigh close to the genital area is deemed necessary, an informed consent discussion is invaluable. At virtually every step of a session, these discussions let a client know what is going to happen and how she is likely to be affected. Because the practitioner is proactive in apprising the client about matters that could be of concern, the client has a background for agreeing to go forward with or expressing concerns about the intended technique or procedure. This process provides a natural context in which to discuss boundary issues as needed. In addition to facilitating discussions about boundaries, the increased participation in the treatment process makes it more likely that the client will do her part to make it a success.

Body Language Awareness

Though we should know better, we oftentimes act as if communication is primarily a verbal process. We become so focused on the words a person is saying that we do not pick up on significant nonverbal messages coming our way. This is an unfortunate oversight since a person's body language may reinforce what the person is saying, send a contradictory message, or signal something important that has not been verbalized. For instance a shiatsu practitioner might ask a client if the amount of pressure is too much. The client may answer "No, the pressure is fine, I need it." But the client may grimace, tense up or actually jump while being treated at that particular depth of pressure which crosses a threshold of discomfort.

> *Your expression is the most important thing you can wear.*
>
> —Sid Ascher

A male client scheduled a massage and informed the practitioner that he was participating for the first time in a long distance bicycle race and was working out to get ready. He wanted the practitioner to assist in the process with bi-weekly massage. The practitioner knew that special attention would need to be paid to the hips, buttocks and legs, and that stretches were critical. The practitioner explained to the client that these areas would need to be worked on and that special stretching techniques would be used. The client was appropriately draped while work was done on these areas.

With one particular stretching technique, the practitioner was on the table utilizing body weight to stretch the client's legs apart. The client tensed and the practitioner noticed that his facial expression indicated anxiety but he said nothing. The practitioner asked if everything was okay and the client nodded yes but said nothing. The client remained ill-at-ease through the rest of the session. As the client was ready to leave the practitioner asked about booking the next session. The client uncomfortably glanced at the practitioner, mumbled a bit, and left. A few days later, the practitioner placed a follow-up call to the client. The client admitted that during the session he was concerned about the way the practitioner was hovering over him and separating his legs, but he couldn't say anything. He stated that although he felt the practitioner was doing appropriate work, he didn't like being so openly exposed. He didn't want to have another session if this is what he was going to have done. He then said that he didn't want to question the practitioner's expertise and would feel bad if he insulted the practitioner.

Clients are often reluctant to express themselves in words for many reasons including their personal styles, their limited contact with the professional, the inherent power dynamics of the therapeutic relationship, their cultural backgrounds, limited knowledge of what is appropriate, and the potentially stressful nature of asserting personal boundaries. Therefore, practitioners need to be aware of body language since clients may be hesitant to express themselves verbally—especially on sensitive matters like boundary issues.

Additionally, verbal and nonverbal communication tend to convey different types of content. Though there is considerable overlap, words impart facts while nonverbal language is more likely to express feelings. Because boundary issues basically reflect how we *feel* about one another's behavior, responding to nonverbal messages is a key to understanding and honoring a client's boundary concerns. For example, if a client feels uncomfortable being fully disrobed but feels obligated, she may demonstrate discomfort by clinging to a gown or pulling the draping linen up to cover more of her body.

Follow this four-step variation on Interactive Speaking when responding to a person's body language:

Observe ➡ Understand ➡ Reflect ➡ Invite.

OBSERVE: Whether you are speaking or listening, observe the other person's nonverbal communications. Notice physical reactions to what you say or do. Be aware of ways the person's body language is different than it typically is. Is he more subdued than usual? More energetic? More hesitant when speaking? More quiet than usual?

UNDERSTAND: Discern what the body language signifies. To grasp what nonverbal signals mean, consider them in context—preferably multiple contexts. Here are some to consider: the history of the therapeutic relationship; the substance or impact of what is currently being discussed; what is characteristic behavior for this person; similarities and differences of the person's past reactions to other practitioners.

A client went for her first session with a physical therapist. After the treatment, the client felt better and sincerely thanked the therapist. Making an assumption based on the client's gratitude, the therapist moved toward the client to give her a hug. Immediately the client pulled back and held out her hand. "Oh, you're one of those," the therapist said. The client never returned. This therapist not only misinterpreted her client's verbal communication but also made a judgment about what the client's body language meant. Expressing that judgment was offensive to the client.

Realize that when you are reading a person's body language, *you are always making a hypothesis*. The best you can do is infer what the other person's behavior means. If a person crosses his legs or arms, it may indicate defensiveness; or, he may merely be temporarily shifting to a more comfortable position. When a person's body language seems at odds with what's being said, the mixed message may indicate ambivalent feelings, that the person is out of touch with his feelings, or the person is reluctant to speak about certain concerns.[10] Whatever you infer from the behavior within the known context, treat your interpretation as a hypothesis. Remember, reading body language is an inexact art—not a precise science.

REFLECT: When you sense that a client's nonverbal communication suggests a boundary concern, it is often appropriate to reflect what you have observed. To review, a reflection is a succinct restatement of what a person says. When reflecting body language you say what you see. Sometimes it is useful to mention the context in which the body language occurred.

For instance, a neuromuscular practitioner had been working with a client weekly. The client was in a recent car accident, the third one in five years. During the session, the practitioner gave the client an opening to talk about the accident's effect on her body and movement. Immediately the client's body tensed. The practitioner reflected, "When I asked if you wanted to talk about the accident [context], your muscles suddenly tensed

Attention to body language can unlock the meaning of the client's unspoken message facilitating understanding and clarity in the therapeutic relationship.

[observation]." After giving that opening for the client to talk, the practitioner paused to listen. In this case the client chose to remain silent.

One has to be sensitive about reflecting body language that suggests a boundary issue, and it is sometimes advisable to be less direct. This can be accomplished with a third-party statement instead of a reflection. A third-party statement attributes to a third party the kind of thoughts and feelings the client may be experiencing. In the above example, the practitioner could have said, "Some people find it helpful to discuss such incidents and describe in detail the injury and its effects, while other people prefer to keep the focus of the session strictly on relaxing their body."

INVITE (a response): Often only a pause is required. After you reflect the person's body language or make a third-party statement, be silent and wait for the client to speak. If the other person doesn't speak right away, extend the pause. It often takes time to mull over thoughts and emotions. Usually the client responds. If the client remains silent, you have at least two options. Use a verbal invitation such as, "Help me understand what's going on." Or say what you are seeing and what you think the *current* body language (e.g., the silence) means. For instance, you could say, "It seems like you'd rather not talk about this. It might be more relaxing if I just focus on the treatment." Beware of the further discomfort an overly extended pause may cause. The client may feel pressured to respond and become resentful.

Tools for Maintaining Boundaries

Clients are not the only people with boundary concerns. Practitioners also must safeguard their own space for both personal and professional reasons. It is easy to see how a practitioner's quality of life deteriorates when he is lax about maintaining boundaries. Many clients are needy people who become so absorbed with their own needs that they become oblivious to yours. Consequently, clients may overrun your boundaries in numerous ways: missing appointments; showing up without an appointment; calling you at home; attempting to develop a friendship; being delinquent on payments; making overtures for physical intimacy; and using verbally or physically aggressive behavior.

Maintaining your own boundaries protects your professional competence too. The boundary concerns already mentioned impact your effectiveness as a practitioner. Practitioners suffer burnout when they do not shield themselves from excessive client demands.

The Proactive Principle

Boundary-wise practitioners are proactive in addressing boundary issues. They make many of their limits clear in the initial phases of the client/practitioner relationship. There are two advantages to this. Proactive discussions prevent many boundary crossings and violations from occurring since the boundaries and consequences are made clear up-front. Also, before-the-fact discussions are usually far less stressful to the client. If you wait until a client crosses your boundary before speaking about the issue, the client is likely to feel guilty, hurt, angry, or even betrayed because he broke a "rule" that was never overtly stated. After-the-fact discussions often trigger negative feelings that not only make the boundary discussion more difficult, but also make your work harder by straining the therapeutic relationship.

Practitioners need to be aware of projection!

See Ethical Principles, pages 20-21, for details on **projection**.

The right to be heard does not automatically include the right to be taken seriously.

—Hubert Humphrey

A client misses an appointment. The practitioner expects the client to pay and sends a bill. The client arrives for the next appointment with the bill in hand.

CLIENT SPEAKS:

I don't understand why you billed me for this session.

PRACTITIONER SPEAKS:

I sent you a bill because you didn't show up or call to cancel.

PRACTITIONER INVITES:

I assumed that you realized you're responsible to pay for the appointment time. Did you have a different understanding?

CLIENT RESPONDS:

I never thought about it and you never told me about that policy.

PRACTITIONER REFLECTS:

You feel you shouldn't have to pay because I didn't make my policy explicitly clear.

PRACTITIONER SPEAKS:

Because of my poor communication, I'll waive the charge this time.

This is an example of why it is vital to have written policies that are reviewed with clients.

Before a problem arises, it is helpful to figure out *where* your boundaries lie as well as your *rationale* for placing your boundaries where you do. In his book, *Back to One: A Practical Guide for Psychotherapists*,[11] Sheldon Kopp discusses several boundary issues and why he draws the line where he does. For example, Kopp doesn't take emergency calls from clients: "The only time the switchboard operator is to buzz through for me is if there is an urgent call from my wife or from one of my kids. That's my boundary." Here's the rationale. Kopp works with "well-functioning people…for whom the focus of therapy is more a matter of growth than of problem solving." In this context at least, Kopp says, "There are no other emergencies in my profession. I only run the therapy; my clients run their lives. Should clients attempt to make their emergencies mine, I accept no responsibility for intervening in their crises. At such times of distress in their lives, just as I do they must turn to family, to friends, or to community crisis intervention services (such as the police, the fire department, the local hospital emergency room, etc.)."

You might not draw the line where Kopp does and you may disagree with his rationale. Two people of the same profession often have significantly different boundaries. We cite this example because of the mental clarity Kopp had not only about his boundaries, but also about the personal and professional reasons those boundaries made sense to him.

A massage therapist had a history of injury to her hands from working too deeply. After her recovery she practiced her communication skills to set a clear boundary when clients asked for deeper work. "The kind of work I do doesn't become deeper through pressure," she would say. "I've found that slow and gentle work allows most of my clients to relax in a deeper way. We can try this method and if you don't like it, I'll be happy to give you a referral."

The likelihood that you will defend your boundary is strengthened when you have thoughtfully worked out the rationale for where you draw the line. If you believe sound reasons exist for where you put the border, it is easier to explain and maintain the limits you have set. With boundaries as with so many other matters, it is unwise to overdo a good thing. While it is desirable to have a clear sense of one's boundaries prior to interacting with a client, there are times when situational variables need to be considered. For example, if your client is involved in a car accident on the way to an appointment at your office, it would be an extreme action to charge the client for missing the appointment even though you have a 24-hour cancellation policy.

One aspect of being proactive is taking time for self-reflection and analysis. It is desirable to be proactive, yet most people need experience and practice. All practitioners have had experiences with clients where the outcomes were less than desirable. Learn from these experiences to hone your skills and change your future behavior.

Process Recordings

Process recordings are an effective tool for guiding a practitioner's self-development and for analyzing and maintaining boundaries. Practitioners can identify strengths and areas for improvement by reflecting upon different practice issues such as conducting an interview, performing hands-on techniques, and clinical decision-making. A process recording is generally the recollection of a certain time period within a therapeutic session or therapeutic relationship. The recall of this time period can be done by various means including one's memory, audiotape recordings or videotaping. Written consent is required from the client if you make audiotape or video recordings of the session.

Process recordings allow you to reflect on your work and to make conscious choices about how you communicate.

Awkward or Challenging Moments

Process recordings are an excellent reflective tool when issues emerge in therapeutic practice such as: setting boundaries; managing conflicts; dealing with difficult clients; and resolving ethical dilemmas. They can clearly play a pivotal role in the development of mature, insightful and reflective practitioners. In a process recording you seek to understand the thoughts and feelings that shape your decisions. Reactions and dysfunctional patterns of behavior may be transformed into responses and choices which provide you with a basis for personal growth and a sense of empowerment.

A basic process recording involves revisiting a time period during the session. The decision to revisit the chosen time period, from a few seconds to several minutes, is based on a number of factors. It is often useful to revisit a time period when the therapist remembers feeling awkward or challenged. Moments of awkwardness are often key indicators for growth areas. For example, practitioners often feel awkward when they do not know how to respond appropriately to a situation or a question that arises during a therapeutic session, such as inadvertently undraping a body region or feeling challenged when a client disagrees with their recommendations in a medical report submitted for an insurance claim.

Also, process recordings can be used regularly to self-evaluate a variety of skills related to levels of clinical reasoning. A practitioner could purposefully select a focus area to assess, such as clinical decision-making in a series of sessions to better understand the effectiveness of treatment planning for clients. The efficient use of time when interviewing and assessing clients to determine a treatment plan is a common area for development. In this case process recordings are useful for noting if certain assumptions led the practitioner down the "wrong path" because an important detail was overlooked or specific tests were not performed during the initial assessment of the client.

Scripts

Process recordings resemble a dramatic script. When revisiting the chosen time period or focus area in a session, the practitioner records the content (what was actually said or done between the practitioner and the client with observations of voice delivery, body language, physical action and spatial boundaries) and the process (the practitioner's inner monologue of thoughts, feelings and impressions during the conversation or interaction between the practitioner and the client). Be aware of the congruency of a practitioner's words with feelings, thoughts and actions.

After reviewing the process recording (alone, with a colleague or in a peer supervision group), certain communication patterns, emotions, behavioral tendencies, assumptions, values and beliefs may emerge which provide the basis for a deeper understanding of a practitioner's process. This information is invaluable for practitioners interested in self-awareness and empowers them to make new and informed choices. Process recordings are a useful way for practitioners to "tune into themselves and clients" and to develop effective client-practitioner relationships. They enrich the practice experience.

Process Recording Scenario

The following is an example of an excerpt from a written process recording. In this scenario, the practitioner has seen the client once a week for nearly three months with stress reduction as the primary goal. The client appears to be interested in a relationship with the practitioner outside of the clinical setting. So far, the practitioner has avoided the client's overtures by changing the topic of conversation or pretending not to understand the client's request. In this session, the practitioner is confronted by the client again.

> CONTENT:
> Client: "Could I have your home telephone number in case I want to reach you over the weekend?" (rummaging in her purse for a pen and a checkbook)
> PROCESS:
> I know she's interested in me personally. I can't sidestep her forever. How am I going to handle this? (pretending to review client's chart)
> CONTENT:
> Practitioner: "Ummm, I'd really prefer that you call me at my office number. You've got my business card, right?" (still pretending to read the chart)
> PROCESS:
> I'm being polite. I hope she doesn't keep pushing for my home number. (I'm averting direct eye contact with her but I hear my voice fading out)
> CONTENT:
> Client: "Why can't I have your home number?"
> (she makes direct eye contact with me, smiles and hands me a check)
> PROCESS:
> Here she goes again. It's time to make a stand. She acts like I'm supposed to be on call 24-7!!! Arghhh!!
> CONTENT:
> Client: "Come on, don't be so uptight. It isn't like I would call you at 3 in the morning... (she laughs) unless, I really was in pain and needed an emergency appointment."
> (she's standing over me as I sit at my desk; her notepad is on my desk and her pen

> is poised to write.)
> "So what's your number?" (stares me straight in the eyes)
> **PROCESS:**
> I don't like confrontation. Why can't she just take a hint and stop trying to find out what my home phone number is??!!
> **CONTENT:**
> Practitioner: "I'm running late. Can we talk about this next week?"
> (ushers her out the door)

Upon reviewing this process recording, the practitioner became aware that a more direct approach was required with this client. The practitioner realized that his people-pleasing approach had created a situation where he felt obliged to say "yes" to his client's requests. In short, he did not like the feeling of disappointing people. The practitioner decided to seek professional counseling around these issues and develop assertiveness skills.

The Assertion Sequence

It would be great if all you had to do to protect your boundaries was to clarify them in your own mind and make the boundaries known to other people. Unfortunately, it is not that simple. Sometimes you think you have an agreement, but flaws in the communication process obscure the meaning. At other times your meaning is crystal clear to the client but because his needs are strong, the client crosses your boundary. With some clients, this may happen repeatedly. The Assertion Sequence minimizes misunderstandings and boundary crossings.

"Assertive" language communicates clearly with minimal emotional content. Assertive language contrasts with "passive" language which communicates undertones of inadequacy, and low self-esteem and with "aggressive" language which communicates undertones of anger. An assertive person maintains dignity, self-worth, self-respect and self-satisfaction without dominating or belittling other people.[12]

Communicating assertively lessens the chance that your interactions go awry. Following are examples of passive, aggressive and assertive statements.

A practitioner declining a tip:
> (**PASSIVE**)
> Oh, why did you have to do that?
> (**AGGRESSIVE**)
> What do you think I am, a waitress?
> (**ASSERTIVE**)
> I appreciate your thoughtfulness, but I've chosen not to accept tips.

A practitioner requesting payment from client who forgets to pay:
> (**PASSIVE**)
> I really hope you pay me next time.
> (**AGGRESSIVE**)
> If you don't bring your checkbook next time, I won't treat you any more.
> (**ASSERTIVE**)
> Please put a check in the mail to me tomorrow. My policy is to expect payment at the time of the session, so please be prepared for our next appointment.

> " A "no" uttered from deepest conviction is better and greater than a "yes" merely uttered to please, or what is worse, to avoid trouble. "
>
> —Gandhi

The Assertion Sequence is a series of increasingly forceful conversations that helps a practitioner effectively protect her boundaries. There are four stages in the sequence:

- Agreement Discussion
- Follow Up
- Confrontation Meeting
- Termination

The more effective you are in the early stages, the less likely you will use the later ones. Dealing with boundary crossings is much easier if you clearly state your expectations up front about policies such as: when and how you expect to receive payment; how you deal with tardiness; what you charge for uncancelled appointments; socializing with clients out of the office; and wearing a perfume in your office. In fact, with many clients the first step is all you need. However, when a client is not honoring your boundaries, it is generally appropriate to move stage by stage through the sequence. With very serious boundary violations it may be appropriate to skip one or more stages. Use Interactive Speaking in every stage of the sequence.

Assertion Sequence Stage I: Agreement Discussions

The Agreement Discussion has five components:

- What
- Why
- Consequences
- Obstacles
- Recap

One or more of the last four components may be omitted if it is not one of your critical boundary issues or if the boundary is not likely to be tested. If you discuss several boundary issues with a person, take the issues through the components one at a time. Throughout these discussions make a special effort to be clear and concise.

WHAT: Let the client know what you expect (e.g., "I am paid at the conclusion of each appointment"). State the issue positively—say what specific behavior you want in a nonjudgmental way,[13] not what you do not want. Sometimes, for clarity's sake, it helps to distinguish those behaviors you want from those you do not. In those cases describe the desired behavior first: this (behavior), not that (behavior).

Avoid abstractions and judgments because they are a major cause of miscommunication. Rather than saying, "It's important for you to be on time," be specific and say, "Our session begins at two o'clock sharp."

Speak with assertive rather than aggressive or submissive body language. Use a tone of voice that conveys that you mean what you say and expect it to happen. Condense your statement into a single compact sentence. Once you have said that sentence, pause or verbally invite the other person to speak. Then listen carefully, reflecting any concerns the client may have (e.g., "Does that sound reasonable to you and is that something you feel comfortable with?").

WHY: Give your reasons for wanting the behavior you requested. Social psychologists remind us that people are much more likely to heed requests that are accompanied by a rationale than requests with no reasons given. State the rationale briefly. For example, "I have four children and only have five hours to work each day. My clients are busy people and it upsets me if I keep them waiting." Avoid rambling on, it may sound like a lecture and become annoying.

There are times when it may be inappropriate to state the rationale. If, for example, you sense that the client grasps the rationale without your mentioning it, skip this component. Later in the discussion, if you sense that the rationale needs to be mentioned, you can do it at that time.

CONSEQUENCES: If a boundary issue is meaningful to you, establish *consequences that follow logically* from the transgression. For example, many practitioners have a policy that clients pay for appointments they miss.

Here are three steps to protect some of your boundaries with logical consequences:

1. Tell the person *in advance* what the particular consequences are for the specific behaviors. In phrasing the message you may wish to use the formula, "If you don't cancel your appointments at least five hours in advance [description of the behavior you wish to prevent], I will charge you for the treatment if I can't fill the appointment [statement of the consequences]." Avoid emotionally loaded words. Keep your statement short. Provide an opportunity for the client to respond. For example "Is that agreeable?"

2. State logical consequences in a very matter-of-fact manner. Later, if the client does the undesirable behavior, the consequences are set in motion in the same emotionally neutral manner. If you become emotional about the infraction, and say something like, "I told you what would happen if you missed an appointment," the other person is likely to feel he is being punished rather than experiencing a logical consequence. Punishment can trigger a variety of dynamics you want to avoid, including damaged rapport, disempowering submissiveness, increased resistance, or a spiraling power struggle. So it is wise to objectively discuss consequences.

3. Finally, apply consequences consistently. The effectiveness of this method hinges on the client's belief that if she does such and such a behavior, this consequence automatically follows.

OBSTACLES: If you think the client may have difficulty meeting your boundary, ask him to identify possible obstacles to doing so; "Do you see anything that might prevent you from giving me enough notice if you need to cancel an appointment?"

Do not solve the problem yourself. Let the client figure out how to surmount the obstacle. Then wait patiently until he figures out how to resolve the situation. He will be more committed to implementing the solution if he figures it out himself.

RECAP: To make sure accurate communication has occurred, ask the client to summarize the discussion about this boundary issue. You could say something like, "Let's be sure you and I are on the same page. Please describe your understanding of the agreement."

When you finish discussing one boundary issue, move on to the next. Remember, you do not need to employ every component on every issue. Depending on the situation, you may only have to do the first component on each issue and ask the client to recap at the end of the discussion.

Assertion Sequence Stage II: Follow Up

If you have gained clear boundary agreements in Stage One of the Assertion Sequence, the other three stages may not be necessary. If, however, you have experienced problems with some issues, or if you are concerned that a particular client may not live up to one or more agreements established in Stage One, verify the issue in question. There are several ways of doing this. Use the approach that seems most fitting.

REINFORCE DESIRABLE BEHAVIOR: When the person does as agreed, thank her for it. This affirms the person and serves as a reminder that the issue is important to you. For instance, you might say, "I really appreciated your calling me with ample notice when you had to cancel your appointment," or, "Thank you for not wearing cologne at your appointments."

PROVIDE ONGOING REMINDERS: Ideas to consider for reinforcing your policies include: print carefully worded reminders of cancellation policies on appointment cards; include payment options on bills; and hang small, tasteful signs in the office that describe basic expectations. Although it is a more delicate matter to give verbal reminders of agreements that have not been broken, it is sometimes advisable to do so to avoid later misunderstanding and conflict. For example, you could say, "It's always best to arrive a little early for your appointment, so you have time to transition from your day and relax. And we have an excellent selection of reading materials to peruse while you wait."

Practitioners walk a fine line in protecting their boundaries. On the one hand, they have legitimate needs to guard. On the other hand, if they overemphasize their concerns, they may seem more absorbed in their own issues than they are in helping clients. This balance is influenced by the varying degrees clients understand and respect boundaries.

BROKEN AGREEMENT DISCUSSION: If a client does not keep an agreement, remind him and re-affirm the agreement. After you bring up the issue, be sure to listen. Step into the client's frame of reference. Based on what you learn, adjust the original agreement or re-establish the initial agreement.

For example, a client forgets your policy about fragrance and wears heavy cologne. You could say, "I notice you're wearing cologne today. I ask everyone not to wear fragrances because some of my clients are chemically sensitive. Is this a problem for you?" Discuss with the client what the difficulty is and negotiate a new agreement (e.g., working on that client first thing in the morning before she puts on cologne or booking the client in the last appointment slot of the day).

Most boundary issues are successfully managed by stages one and two of the Assertion Sequence—Agreement Discussions and Follow Up. In situations that persist despite your best efforts in the initial stages, it is time to confront the issue directly.

Assertion Sequence Stage III: Confrontation

This is perhaps the most demanding type of boundary discussion you will encounter. Though confrontation meetings are difficult, they are effective when well done. Confrontation is used when a client persistently violates a boundary. Occasionally a separate meeting may be necessary when there is a serious violation even though it may be the first time the client has done it.

In a confrontation meeting you get right to the issue and send your message in a single three-part sentence. Listen reflectively to the other person's point of view, and diffuse some of the defensiveness and excess emotionality that often occurs. In the space of this chapter we can only give a condensed explanation. Before conducting a confrontation meeting, you may wish to consult Robert Bolton's *People Skills*.[14]

The three points you want to convey in a confrontation message are behavior, feelings and effect:

BEHAVIOR	When you agree to (describe the agreed-upon behavior) and don't,
+	
FEELINGS	I feel (state your feelings)
+	
EFFECT	because (state the tangible effect on you)

For example:

BEHAVIOR
When you agree to be on time and arrive 30 minutes late

FEELINGS
I feel upset and frustrated

Effect
because there isn't ample time to give you what you deserve in a session and do my best work.

The wording of the message is so crucial that it is often helpful to write it out, edit it carefully, and memorize it. When you say this carefully prepared message, do it with assertive, not aggressive, body language.

You may not like what you hear because the client is likely to respond defensively, but attempt to understand anyway—from the client's point of view. Reflect both the feelings and the thoughts as often as necessary. For instance in the example above the late client might say, "When my meetings run late, it's really difficult to arrive here exactly on time, especially when there are important people at the meeting." You might respond, "What I hear is that it's difficult for you to leave meetings if they run late. It also seems like it's upsetting to you and you don't know how to tell the people in the meeting that you have prior commitments. Is that accurate?"

Listening may uncover reasons for changing the agreement. However, if you have satisfactorily performed stages one and two (Agreement Discussion and Follow Up) those reasons will have already surfaced. When it is your turn to speak again, make a transition, and then repeat the same assertion message. Most people are reluctant to repeat the same message, but that works far better than paraphrasing or winging it. After all, the client did not get your message the first time. So it is appropriate to send the same message again. Transition from the client's statements using words, such as "You think (summarize her point of view in a phrase), but I still have this problem. When you agree to . . . and don't do it, I feel . . . because . . . ." Then reflectively listen again.

Often the client comes up with excuse after excuse. Sometimes she dredges up your shortcomings to show that you are not perfect either. Do not dispute what is said—it only diverts you from your boundary discussion. Keep sending your message in a single sentence prefaced by a transition sentence and keep on reflectively listening to the client's defensive responses. Recycle as often as needed until you find reasons for adjusting the agreement, or the client recommits to the original agreement. When you have a recommitment to the agreement (or, in rare instances, an adjusted agreement), be sure the client does a recap at the end. Set a time in a week or two to discuss how the agreement is working.

It may seem counterintuitive to spend so much time in a confrontation meeting listening to the other person's defensive responses, and as a result, many people are reluctant to do it as described. Yet those elements of the method that are most counterintuitive are the very ones that make it effective. After skillful implementation, evaluate its effectiveness.

Assertion Sequence Stage IV: Termination

See Ethical Practice Management, pages 168-170, for details on **ending a client/therapist relationship**.

Nearly all boundary crossings and violations may be handled effectively using the first three stages of the assertion sequence: Agreement Discussions; Follow Up; and Confrontation Meeting. If there are repeated violations after a well-conducted confrontation meeting, it is time to consider terminating the therapeutic relationship. The circumstances are so varied that it is impossible to suggest a generic approach when it seems fitting to end the relationship. When a client repeatedly crosses or violates your boundaries, you should work with your supervisor or a trusted colleague to figure out whether and how to terminate your work with the client.

After-the-Fact Agreement Discussions

Unfortunately, not all boundary issues can be discussed in advance. Preventive discussion of some issues may sound presumptuous. People will wonder about a practitioner who, a few minutes after meeting a new client, declares, "I expect that clients don't make sexual advances toward me." Furthermore, though there are many kinds of boundary crossings and violations that occur in a professional's lifetime, only a few are likely to occur in a particular relationship. It would be offensive for a practitioner to be so self-protective as to reel off 50 no-no's in the first meeting with a client. The best way to communicate the boundaries and guidelines for your practice is to have clients read a policy statement just prior to their first session and then go over it with them.

See Ethical Practice Management, pages 152-162, for details on **policies**.

If you discover a boundary that you realize was never stated or discussed has been crossed, get an after-the-fact agreement. You conduct an After-the-Fact Agreement Discussion much as you would the agreement discussions covered earlier. A key difference, though, is to start out by saying something like this: "I know we never discussed this before so you had no reason to believe this could be of concern to me…" Then, using Interactive Speaking, tell the What, the Why, and perhaps explore potential Obstacles, and close by asking for a Recap. (Consequences are rarely an appropriate component in after-the-fact discussions.) For example, "I make it a policy never to socialize or go out with any of my clients. I find that it interferes with my objectivity in providing effective treatment for clients. Very recently, my profession has come up with an ethical guideline which states that it is unethical to have personal, intimate relationships with clients. This is probably something you're unaware of and I know you were being kind when you invited me to accompany you to the museum."

See Appendix A pages 260-262, for sample **policy statements**.

When you say up front that you have never discussed this matter before, you decrease the likelihood that the client feels blamed by you. When people think they are being blamed, they tend to react with feelings of guilt, embarrassment or anger—any of which impedes the therapeutic relationship and makes the boundary discussion more difficult. Even with the disclaimer that the person had no way of knowing this was a concern of yours, an after-the-fact agreement discussion could trigger considerable defensiveness. So be careful to sense and reflect the client's feelings.

Respect, empathy and affirmation need to be the foundation of all communication, but particularly throughout the stages of assertion. As a professional, it is your duty to manage ethical behavior through your communication whether written, verbal or non-verbal. When communicating with a client, look at the situation from his frame of reference. Genuinely considering the client's point of view not only shows empathy and respect, but also models good communication. Ultimately, clients are more receptive to what you say when communication is clear and affirms your boundaries.[15]

In Conclusion...

Human communication can be a complex process, subject to misunderstanding and confusion. The challenges are intensified in the therapeutic relationship. Knowing that positive human contact is a healing force, ethical somatic practitioners work to develop their communication skills. You enhance your relationships with clients by understanding the dynamics of communication and using proven tools to clarify and maintain professional boundaries. After all, the success of the therapeutic relationship depends on the healthy connection between you and your client.

We hear only half of what is said to us, understand only half of that, believe only half of that, and remember only half of that.

—Mignon McLaughlin

Chapter Highlights

- Clear communication is the foundation for successful professional relationships.
- Effective communication is a challenging process.
- The listener does not always get the message we intend.
- Enhance effectiveness by communicating information in a variety of styles.
- Every message is composed of two parts: the visible part of what you say and the invisible part of how you say it.
- The skills and abilities that make our communication effective include: listening; addressing a variety of learning styles; setting boundaries; asking for what we want when we have a need; saying "yes" without reservation; giving and receiving positive and critical feedback in a constructive manner; appropriately expressing and receiving irritation and anger; noticing destructive, dysfunctional communication patterns in ourselves and others; and having a developed sense of empathy so that the timing of our communication is in sync with those around us.
- Most people prefer to initially take in information by one of three methods: auditory, kinesthetic or visual.
- Knowledge of learning styles and types of intelligence helps us to be more effective and efficient in our communication.
- Boundaries are negotiated and maintained through communication—words, body language and behaviors.
- Communication skills are crucial for protecting the client and the practitioner by clarifying and negotiating boundary concerns to enhance the comfort and effectiveness of the treatment.
- Treat the client like a person, not an object.
- Set policies and practices that protect the client.
- Foster appropriate self-disclosure.
- Self-disclosure refers to how much personal information is exchanged between the practitioner and the client.
- Excessive self-disclosure from the client to the practitioner sets up a strong transference reaction.
- Appropriate self-disclosure from the practitioner to the client may enhance the therapeutic relationship while excessive self-disclosure may be detrimental.
- What the practitioner says and how he says it in response to the client's emotional expressions affect the therapeutic alliance with the client.
- Allowing emotional expression is usually acceptable but encouraging it, asking questions, or interpreting it often exceeds the practitioner's Scope of Practice.
- Unless a practitioner has particular communication skills, knowledge and training in working with the emotional reactions of clients, she should defuse the situation and change the focus of the session.
- Reflective listening is also called active listening.
- Reflective listening creates an empathetic climate where the client feels freer about discussing difficult concerns such as boundary topics.
- A reflection is a brief statement of the essence of the other person's message, stated in the listener's own words.
- The feeling behind the message may be as important as the content of the message.
- Interactive speaking is a three-step method to promote two-way communication. The steps are: speak; invite; and reflect.

- Informed consent discussions explain: what the practitioner does during the procedure; why it is recommended; and how it impacts the client.
- A person's body language may reinforce what the person is saying, send a contradictory message, or signal something important that has not been verbalized.
- Though there is considerable overlap, words impart facts while nonverbal language is more likely to express feelings.
- When responding to a client's body language follow the four-step process of: observe, understand, reflect, invite.
- Maintaining your own boundaries protects your professional competence.
- Proactive discussions prevent many boundary violations from occurring since the boundaries and consequences are made clear up-front.
- Process recordings are an excellent reflective tool when issues emerge in therapeutic practice such as: setting boundaries; managing conflicts; dealing with difficult clients; and resolving ethical dilemmas. They can clearly play a pivotal role in the development of mature, insightful and reflective practitioners.
- Assertive language communicates clearly with minimal emotional content.
- The Assertion Sequence is a series of increasingly forceful conversations that can help a practitioner protect her boundaries effectively.
- The assertion sequence has four stages: the agreement discussion; follow up; confrontation meeting; termination.
- The more effective you are in the early stages of the assertion sequence, the less likely you'll use the later ones.
- If you discover a boundary that you realize was never stated or discussed has been crossed, get an after-the-fact agreement.
- Mastering communication skills greatly enhances your ability to negotiate boundary concerns with both clients and co-workers.
- Your overall competence as a practitioner includes not only your hands-on skills and scientific information but also your ability to communicate effectively.

Discussion Questions and Activities

- What are your communication strengths and weaknesses?
- Visit http://surfaquarium.com/MIinvent.htm to take Walter McKenzie's "Multiple Intelligences Survey" and learn more about your learning style.
- Identify boundary concerns that you may be uncomfortable discussing.
- How might the power differential affect client-practitioner communications?
- Are you comfortable with the power dynamic of your role as practitioner? Perhaps too comfortable?
- Describe how effective communication skills diminishes the power differential.
- What are some of the ways that health care practitioners treat clients in a depersonalizing manner? Think back to your own experiences as a patient.
- Create a list of questions that help keep clients present when they are experiencing emotional release.
- Identify the types of clients' emotional expressions that would make you feel uncomfortable. Role-play these situations.
- Consider various ways you could handle a situation with a client when your emotions seemed unmanageable at the time.

- What types of self-disclosure might be useful from the practitioner to the client?
- When is practitioner self-disclosure destructive to the therapeutic relationship?
- Identify the types of client self-disclosure that make you uncomfortable.
- How might you handle excessive client self-disclosure?
- Practice reflective listening.
- How might you kindly and gently tell a client that he has a strong body odor?
- How would you recommend that a client seek counseling or therapy?
- List some examples of noncongruent body language.
- Take a history from a client using the reflective listening model.
- Script an Informed Consent discussion using the Interactive Speaking Model.
- Role-play the following topics using all four stages of the Assertion Sequence:
    A client who is frequently late.
    A client who did not show up for the last appointment and did not cancel.
    A client who keeps forgetting to pay you.
    A client who frequently insists that you work during non-scheduled hours.
- Identify client interactions when you felt awkward or challenged. Do a Process Recording for each instance.
- List the communication skills you have effectively used in your life.
- What areas of communication do you want to improve? How do you see yourself making those changes?
- Give examples of when and how poor communication has affected your life.
- Depict how clear communication is essential for a successful practice.
- Keep a communication journal for at least a week. Note your observations including communication barriers, learning styles, boundary issues, reflective listening, interactive speaking, informed consent, body language, and assertion techniques.
- How might you represent effective communication symbolically or rhythmically?
- Interview five or more people in your life and ask them to share their perspective on your communication skills.
- When someone uses a communication barrier with you, how do you redirect the conversation to make it more productive?
- What are some ways you can improve your listening ability?
- Practice "Interactive Speaking: Speak, Invite, Reflect." Note which parts are more difficult or easier than the others for you.
- Design a policy statement for your clients that reflects the boundaries important to you.
- Explain the difference between aggressive and assertive in your own words.
- Describe a situation or person you can use for a model of effective communication.

4

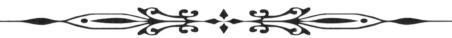

Dual Relationships

- An Historical Perspective
- Sequential Relationships
- The Range of Dual Relationships
- The Risks of Dual Relationships
- Minimizing Concerns
- The Special Case of Schools
- In Conclusion...
- Chapter Highlights
- Discussion Questions and Activities

The term *dual relationships* describes the overlapping of professional and social roles and interactions between two people. Human beings naturally develop multiple relationships in various arenas—among family, friends, neighbors, employees, employers, professional peers, clients, students and teachers. It is clear that people often fit into more than just one of those categories and that certain individuals play a mixture of roles. The classic depiction of a dual relationship is when two persons who interact professionally develop other roles of social interaction. For example, you and a working colleague discover a mutual interest in tennis and begin to play together, or you and your teacher develop a longstanding friendship. Dual relationships also develop in the other direction, from the social to the professional realm: you and your sister decide to go into business together; or a social acquaintance or a friend seeks your professional services. In small towns or rural communities dual relationships are even more common because of the limited numbers of people and choices for professional services.[1]

Dual relationships commonly consist of many layers and encompass a number of professional and social components. Some dual relationships evolve easily and naturally, and initially seem relatively simple. Upon closer examination, their dynamics can be surprisingly complex with ramifications ranging from vital and stimulating to tragically harmful. Potential benefits enrich dual relationships when both parties are emotionally developed and able to handle the multiple roles without confusion. The major benefit is a fuller experience of each other, including shared talents and gifts.

Dual relationships can also enhance the therapeutic relationship. The better you know a person, the easier it is to navigate his idiosyncrasies. For instance, you might take the same communication skills class with a client and thereby gain increased compassion and understanding for each other. Also, you might discover the client's communication weaknesses and take different action in the treatment setting. If you were on the same volleyball team as a client, you might notice how the client uses her body and adjust your treatments to help her to avoid injuries. In this case as well, the dual relationship can assist the therapeutic relationship.

Unfortunately, judging one's ability to successfully juggle multiple roles is often very difficult and problematic. Failure to navigate the risks involved in a dual relationship can result in financial, educational, social or personal loss. Conscious consideration and discernment are important prior to engaging in a relationship of this nature, and clinical supervision is strongly recommended.

In the health care setting it is the practitioner's responsibility to be educated and informed about the nature of dual relationships, and it is the practitioner who is accountable for informing the client about the parameters and possible impact of entering another dimension of the relationship. The power differential that exists in a helping relationship demands that the practitioner behave ethically by clearly defining and maintaining relationship boundaries. This concept appears fairly straightforward on the printed page. However, the work of a helping professional often occurs within complex sets of relationships where boundaries and matters of authority take on shades of gray. We examine the nature of this complexity in this chapter. We begin by looking at how an awareness and understanding of dual relationships started.

> *Whenever you do a thing, act as if all the world were watching.*
>
> —Thomas Jefferson

See the Supervision chapter for details, starting on page 241.

See Ethical Principles, pages 15-17, for details on the **power differential**.

An Historical Perspective

Awareness of the risks involved in dual relationships in health care has evolved slowly over the past 30 years, beginning in the field of psychology. At the beginning of the 20th century, the situation was often handled in a fairly loose manner. Doctors had social relationships with their patients and there was not much clarity or agreement about whether dual relationships were a good or a bad idea. Awareness of the risks of dual relationships was limited to the idea that doctors should not treat their own family members because their judgment might be clouded.

In the 1940s and '50s, much debate sprung among different schools of psychology about the limits and propriety of dual relationships. Consensus gradually moved toward strict rules. Psychotherapists did not treat members of the same family or even patient's friends. It was generally felt that the temptations within dual relationships were too big and falling prey to them was too much of a risk—therefore all dual relationships were to be avoided. In the early 1960s, with the advent of what is referred to as the *Human Potential Movement*, attitudes and cultural norms began to loosen, and some of the advantages of dual relationships emerged. For instance, if a couple were seen together there were advantages to the therapy, or if a sister or brother were seen by the same therapist the therapist would have more knowledge about the dynamics of the family. In this period it was commonplace for doctors to become friends with or socialize with their patients: university professors dated their students; and somatic practitioners treated all their friends and family members. As the helping field struggled to find a balanced approach with regard to multiple relationships, norms began to swing very far in the permissive direction.[2]

The dangers became apparent when evidence of sexual impropriety and misconduct between psychotherapists and patients became more widely known in the 1970s and '80s. Victims of sexual exploitation, supported by the women's movement, began to speak out publicly, lawsuits were filed, insurance companies came under legal pressure to pay out large judgments, and advocacy groups demanded accountability and change. In the field of psychiatry Nanette Gartrell, Chair of the Committee on Women for the American Psychiatric Association, along with Judith Herman (and many others), began researching the frequency of sexual inappropriateness within psychiatry.[3] Jean C. Holroyd and Annette M. Brodsky spearheaded research on sexual exploitation in the field of psychology.[4] These examinations of sexual misconduct cases prompted much thinking, research and writing to clarify why and how dual relationships shift from simple to complex and damaging.

Until the late 1980s, very little thought was given to the importance of understanding multiple relationships and how they might interfere with the therapeutic relationship in the somatic therapy field. The massage therapy industry was the first to consistently demonstrate concern about dual relationships.[5]

Throughout the 1990s and into the new century a more balanced view of dual relationships has emerged in many health care disciplines and educational institutions. Important wisdom will be gained when health care and educational providers realize that they have the responsibility of dealing with the issues surrounding dual relationships.

As complementary health care disciplines evolve, so does the understanding that somatic practitioners develop strong therapeutic relationships with their clients. They need to behave with the responsibility that comes along with the power of that position. There are still many practitioners who do not take the risks and dangers of dual relationships seriously. We hope that after reading this chapter that they exercise careful judgment when considering or engaging in dual relationships with clients.

> *No problem can be solved from the same consciousness that created it. We must learn to see the world anew.*
>
> —Albert Einstein

Sequential Relationships

Sometimes a relationship undergoes a change that is clearly acknowledged and publicly recognized: students graduate and are hired by their schools; classmates meet after graduation and form business partnerships; a former student joins the faculty and becomes a colleague; a former employee and employer marry. When one set of roles completely ends before a different set of roles begins, it is called a *sequential relationship*. Although the change in sequential relationships may be clearly one-way (e.g., the school employee never returns to being a student), the former relationship may still exert an influence. The influence may be problematic if there has been a significant shift in the power differential. For instance, when a student or employee who clearly has less power than the teacher or employer, begins to relate as a colleague of equal status, both parties need to transform their previous ways of relating. Therefore, people experiencing a relationship in transition must consider many of the same issues as those involved in dual relationships.

The Range of Dual Relationships

What follows are common circumstances in which professional relationships, including those between client/practitioner and student/school personnel, add new roles and thus become dual relationships.

Socializing

Socializing is defined as an unplanned personal interaction occurring outside of the therapy time. Socializing implies that neither party would have sought this more personal knowledge of the other if the interaction had not transpired. It may occur when a client and practitioner find themselves at the same social event, such as a concert, movie, lecture or party. In a school setting, socializing occurs at functions outside of classroom or office hours such as at workshops, retreats or celebrations. Meeting in a social setting expands an otherwise limited professional relationship to include the experience of the event itself and more personal knowledge of each other.

Group Affiliation

Group affiliation refers to the special case where a practitioner invites a client (or a client invites a practitioner) to attend an activity focused on a group with which he is personally involved. Various kinds of groups include: educational classes or workshops, political organization meetings, product marketing programs, religious group meetings, therapy groups, PTA meetings or recovery programs. In contrast to the more accidental meetings that take place in socializing, there is intention or purpose behind the invitation to attend a group and it may not be clear to the invitee at the time the invitation is extended.

Unexpected consequences may arise if a practitioner accepts an invitation to a group or invites a client to a group in which he is personally involved. For example, if the shared group experience turns negative either party could feel awkward continuing the professional relationship. This can be particularly problematic when the motive behind the invitation, or the nature of the group itself, is not made clear to the invitee at the time the invitation is extended. For example, if a client or practitioner accepts an invitation to a dinner meeting, only to find that it is a multi-level marketing recruitment meeting or religious group meeting this could create unexpected conflict depending on the beliefs and values of the persons involved. Also, if extremely personal information is revealed in this context, it could damage the trust and safety of the professional relationship.

Friendship

Friendship implies that two people have an intimate interaction based on personal sharing, mutual liking, and loyalty. Friends actively seek out one another's company in settings that often include other acquaintances and friends. Any power differential in the professional relationship must, in a friendship, yield to a greater equality of connection. In a friendship both parties want and expect their needs to be met equally in a give-and-take manner. Maintaining both a friendship and a professional relationship is usually very difficult and puts both at risk.

Dating

Dating involves a high level of interaction. When people date, their time together is more exclusive and generally is for the purpose of exploring each other as potential partners. As the couple's intimacy increases, the professional relationship takes a secondary role to the dating relationship and boundaries blur.

Sex

Sexual activity occurs as an isolated incident or as an extension of socializing, friendship, love or dating. Even when sexual activity occurs only once, its impact on the professional relationship can be devastating and far-reaching.

Family

Family relationships affect professional relationships when a family member becomes a client. While this can happen at any stage of a practitioner's career, students are especially susceptible to this type of dual relationship because in many school programs they are encouraged to practice their new skills and techniques on family members.

Financial Arrangements

Money adds an additional dimension to dual relationships. The most common types of financial dual relationships are: bartering; exchange of health care services; and employment.

BARTERING occurs when a practitioner and client exchange service for service rather than money for service. For example, a practitioner may offer sessions in exchange for laundry service, office cleaning, marketing assistance, or web site design. This type of arrangement illustrates how dual relationships may consist of trading professional roles.

EXCHANGE OF HEALTH CARE SERVICES involves two health care practitioners who exchange services. For example, a chiropractor and an acupuncturist agree to exchange sessions. The effects on the professional relationship of this specialized type of barter center on the reversal of roles each practitioner makes, from client to practitioner and back again.

EMPLOYMENT refers to cases where a practitioner or school hires a client or student to work for financial remuneration. The types of jobs may vary widely, from secretarial work to designing brochures to building a cabinet. Work-study employment, for example, is one way students afford their training. The multiple professional roles involved have varying levels of impact on one another.

Students

In addition to the kinds of dualities described above, students may experience other permutations in the professional relationship. For example, a student who is a public relations specialist may have as a client one of his teachers or administrators; a student with an injury may undertake long-term therapy with a teacher. Any duality can significantly influence the core relationship between student and school personnel.

The Risks of Dual Relationships

If dual relationships are common, why are they of such concern? This question generates a great deal of debate. When one of the interactions in a dual relationship is between a helping professional and a client, questions of concern include the following: To what extent does mutual and equal consent exist in making this relationship dual? Where does accountability lie? Will the therapeutic nature of the relationship be enhanced, hindered or unaffected by the dual relationship?

For example, the person who becomes a client of a physical therapist (who is her friend) is surprised when the therapist charges her for a missed appointment, believing the "friend" part of the relationship would understand and excuse a last-minute schedule change. This belief is particularly understandable if the "professional" part of the relationship had not clearly communicated different expectations. Misunderstandings such as this often lead to an estrangement and the end of a friendship. Therefore, when communication is lacking or cues are misread in a dual relationship, feelings get hurt, one or both parties in the relationship suffers, and the relationship itself in all its manifestations is endangered.

There are those who contend that any professional dual relationship is harmful while others perceive dual relationships as often benign or potentially beneficial. It is certain that ethical considerations enter the picture whenever a dual relationship occurs within the context of a helping relationship.

Many elements are involved in dual relationships, and these elements often interact in subtle ways. All practitioners should receive special training in recognizing, evaluating and communicating about dual relationship issues. In these ways, the risk in a dual relationship from a lack of understanding or poor communication is minimized. Furthermore, certain kinds of dual relationships are never ethical, when the risks are so high and the benefits so low that the relationship is unjustified.

If problems arise in a dual relationship, the relationship itself and the well-being of those involved suffer. What this means depends upon which human aspects are engaged (e.g., financial aspects, educational, social, romantic). Whatever issues are most prominent around the relationship are potentially vulnerable to harm if the relationship fails. Therefore, failed dual relationships can conceivably be related to failure in business, at school, or on a personal level.

Consider the following situations. In the first, a practitioner needs a web site and knows that one of her clients has the experience to design it. In the second, a practitioner needs a shelf built in her office and knows that one of her clients is a carpenter. The wise practitioner uncovers any potential for harm in either case by asking many questions of herself, her client, and her supervisor or peer group. How much professional experience does the client have in web design or shelf building? How successful has his other work been, and how similar were those jobs to what the practitioner envisions for herself? How invested is the *practitioner* in the outcome of the work—in other words, how much does the practitioner stand to gain from a successful web site or a sturdy shelf; and how much could she expect to lose from a job badly done? What is the potential impact of the outcome of the work on the *client*—will he gain significant exposure and referrals from a good job, or lose the goodwill of his therapist if his work is not up to her expectations? If the outcome proves to be negative and the therapeutic relationship ends, how much of a loss is this to the client and the practitioner? Does the potential for emotional harm to the client outweigh the potential benefit? Would it be better to just hire a carpenter or web designer recommended by a friend or found in the telephone book?

The most important factor to remember about professional helping relationships is that they deal directly with people's well-being. Issues regarding mental, emotional or physical health are near the core of the relationship and are therefore potentially vulnerable. For instance, a client with an injured shoulder invests his hopes for healing in a specific practitioner; or a client suffering from stress comes to rely on a hands-on session for relief. Will these clients lose therapeutic ground if a dual relationship with their practitioner goes awry?

Evaluating the Potential Risk in a Dual Relationship

The potential for risk may be seen along a continuum. Sometimes a single element in the relationship signals a high risk potential. A strong need or an emotional component signals that entering into a dual relationship with this client has a high risk factor. An illustration of this is a client who is in a great deal of pain and has come to rely on your expertise over many years. A number of factors work together to heighten or lessen the risk implied by any single factor. For instance, the risks are greatly multiplied if your client with chronic back pain is also the son of your friend, lives next door to you, and dates your daughter. In other cases the risks are probably very low, such as if your neighbor sends his daughter for a one-time birthday session. In addition, risks must be evaluated not just between clients and practitioners but also between two practitioners who have a dual relationship. Consider the following example:

> *The truth of the matter is that you always know the right thing to do, the hard part is doing it.*
>
> —Norman Schwarzkopf

> An acupuncturist who had been in private practice for just a year referred a client to a massage therapist who was a close friend and a seasoned professional. The client was so impressed after visiting the massage therapist once that he decided to pursue massage for his pain problem and decided to terminate the acupuncture treatments because of the expense.
>
> The acupuncturist was quite dismayed for several reasons. Foremost was his concern for his client's well-being because he felt this client needed more acupuncture treatments. He also he felt personal loss because he enjoyed working with this client, and his income would be diminished. He wondered if he should not refer more clients to this massage therapist until he felt more secure in his practice. He feared that if more referrals resulted in his loss of clients and income that it could create tension in the relationships between himself and the massage therapist. Yet he knew his potential income loss was a bad reason to stop referrals and might not be in his clients' best interest. At this point he realized he needed to get some supervision about this issue.

The following questions help you evaluate the risk potential of a dual relationship you are either engaged in or considering.

What is the Intimacy Level?

As the level of intimacy in dual relationship roles increases, so does the potential for harm if problems develop in the relationship. The levels of intimacy range from minimal (as in brief acquaintances or remote professional associations) to moderate (as in friendships or business partnerships) to high (as in sexual relationships and many therapeutic encounters—particularly over a long period of time).

Each role in the dual relationship must be evaluated, considering both social and professional intimacy. For example, occasional social acquaintances who also interact as professionals may have little concern about the duality of their relationship. At the other end of the spectrum, a sexual component in a professional dual relationship greatly increases the risk potential. Some professional roles also involve a high level of intimacy; massage therapists and other somatic practitioners often interact with clients on a deeply personal though not sexual level.

When a dual relationship combines an intimate professional role with a sexual role, the potential for harm is so great that it should never be entered into. Indeed, a sexual relationship with a client is a violation of most helping professional codes of ethics and in many states is illegal. One technique used by practitioners to foster an atmosphere of safety and clarity for their clients is publishing a straightforward policy statement about the inappropriateness of sexual contact between the practitioner and the client.

What Is the Power Differential Impact?

When a professional helping relationship shifts to a dual relationship, both parties need to be as aware as possible of the effects of the power differential in every facet of their interactions. In a relationship between a practitioner and client the power differential favors the practitioner. This is because the helping relationship is an authority relationship entered into because the client has a need and the practitioner has mastery, skill or knowledge that may help the client meet that need. The practitioner holds the authority. The client brings openness and some vulnerability to the relationship.

See Ethical Principles, pages 15-17, for details on the **power differential**.

And pages 14-15, for information on **fiduciary responsibility**.

Professional practitioners are expected to use the power differential to serve the client's needs, not their own. Practitioners must be well-trained to recognize the shifts transference and countertransference make in the power dynamics and assure that abuse of the power differential does not occur.

Two important factors within the authority relationship help determine whether duality in the relationship might work. First, can the person with more power be trusted to not abuse that power? Second, and of greater importance, is the person with less power capable of handling two different roles simultaneously with the authority figure?

Even an experienced practitioner cannot always judge a client's ability to handle a dual relationship. If the practitioner asks the client to engage in a new role with her, is that client capable of bringing equal consent to the new relationship? Or does the pre-existence of the power differential make the client's consent questionable? A new role may present a considerable and difficult challenge for the client. If the power differential looms large in the client's perception, that very perception prevents the client from communicating freely in the relationship. The key question to ask if a client wants a dual relationship is, "How clouded or clear is the client's judgment?"

Who Is Accountable for What in the Relationship?

Careful examination of all aspects of the relationship is needed to answer this question. Nevertheless, from an ethical—and often a legal—standpoint, whoever is acting in a professional role is held accountable for negative consequences of a dual relationship, whether those consequences are professional or social. The idea of accountability rests on several assumptions: the practitioner is aware of complexities and ethical considerations; the practitioner is trustworthy in maintaining the focus of the therapeutic relationship on the client; the client is in a position of greater vulnerability in the helping relationship.

Even if the client is the one who suggests adding a new role to the relationship, the professional is still the one to be held accountable. The decision to enter a dual relationship with a client demands integrity, consistency and authenticity in all roles—hopefully from both persons involved, but most assuredly from the one who holds the professional power.

What Is the Relative Maturity Level?

This question speaks to the issue of why some dual relationships work and why others fail. Psychological maturity enables a person to navigate the uneven terrain of dual relationships. The mature person shifts easily among changing levels of intimacy and changing power dynamics, distinguishes reality from transference/countertransference, and accepts responsibility for the consequences of her behavior. When this person is a professional, she acts ethically and in the best interests of the client at all times. When this person is a client, she uses the therapeutic relationship to maximize her well-being without compromising the practitioner. When this person engages in a personal relationship in addition to a professional one, she allows boundaries to adjust appropriately.

Such maturity is usually a function of age and experience. If both parties to a dual relationship exhibit such maturity, the relationship has a better chance of success. Difficulty arises when the ability to make intelligent judgments is compromised by desire. Most people are not good at making these kinds of judgments about themselves. Very few individuals say, "I am not mature enough to handle this complex dual relationship." Instead, the common internal thought is, "Maybe most other people couldn't handle this multi-layered relationship, but we can. No problem." If you think you are that rare individual, watch out! And if you find yourself talking to yourself in this way it is a good time to seek a professional consultation from someone who is thoroughly impartial and with whom you have no other relationship. If we are developed enough to think we can handle something that most people cannot, then we should be mature enough to tell it to a third party with the particular expertise to help us make that judgment.

What Are the Consequences of Non-Participation?

This final question is a litmus test when all other aspects of the potential dual relationship have been examined. If refusal to participate in a given aspect of a dual relationship brings negative consequences, it is likely that mutual and equal consent to the relationship does not exist. It is even possible that whoever suggests the dual relationship is attempting to manipulate or control the relationship to his advantage. In such cases, there may be tremendous pressure on one party to accept the proposed dual relationship.

Consider the possible consequences to a professional relationship if one person wants to initiate a more personal interaction and the other person refuses. Ideally, both the invitation and the refusal are dealt with maturely and the original professional relationship remains intact. However, in some circumstances the invitation carries with it a threat that refusal will damage the professional relationship.

If a practitioner asks a client to a social function, what happens in the mind of the client? Questions and alarms begin to sound. "What does this invitation mean? Is this a date? Is she interested in me? What happens if I say no? Will she be mad at me? Will it alter this great professional relationship I have with her? Well! I knew she was interested in me; I should've asked her out myself first."

If a client asks a practitioner to a social function or out to coffee, what happens inside the mind of the practitioner? "Is this casual or is this client asking me out? It's kind of flattering that he is interested in me. What will happen to our professional relationship if I say no? Will he be upset with me and never return for treatment? I shouldn't have accepted those gifts. I should've made this clear in my policy statement the way that book said I should. This is awkward, what should I do now?"

Accepting a dual relationship is often very enticing. It takes character strength to decline the travel agent client's offer of free tickets to your favorite getaway in return for keeping him company on his trip. It is very attractive to hire an A+ student who graduated last week to teach at your school when you are hiring new teachers: he may know the material, be a great person and understand the culture of your school, but it is usually too quick a transition from student to teacher without an intervening year or two to develop professional distance.

Skill and sometimes a great deal of courage are required in situations where refusing the dual relationship is the right course of action. When the invitation comes from a client, the practitioner needs to refuse even if doing so risks loss of income, loss of referrals or loss of a professional relationship. Similarly, when the invitation comes from a practitioner, the client needs to refuse even if doing so risks loss of the therapeutic relationship. Clear statements of professional ethics which every client reads before the beginning of the professional relationship support both practitioners and clients in finding the courage to do the right thing in difficult circumstances. This is helpful because the boundaries of the relationship have been laid out and stated beforehand.

Minimizing Concerns

For a dual relationship to work well both parties must share a clear understanding of the complexities involved. Furthermore, both parties must allocate equal responsibility for the establishment, continuation, and if necessary, termination of any part of the dual relationship. Mutual and equal consent to all aspects of the dual relationship is shared by both parties. Although this sounds reasonable, it is incredibly difficult to do. Even social relationships are often not equal nor mutual in power.

Practitioners should support clients' freedom of choice in undertaking dual relationships. The practitioner who educates the client about both potential positives and potential negatives of the duality provides the client with the tools he needs to make an informed decision. This education is important whether the suggestion for the dual relationship comes from the client or from the practitioner. If, for example, the client suggests attending a social event together, the practitioner helps the client recognize how adding personal dimensions affects an established professional relationship. The practitioner who offers to hire a client to do some work should encourage the client to think about the invitation and to discuss it with a trusted friend or colleague before responding. The client must consider the risks to the therapeutic relationship if the work relationship is unsuccessful. The risks of that loss are very real and should not be minimized.

" Any change, even a change for the better, is always accompanied by drawbacks and discomforts. "

—Arnold Bennett

A practitioner hired a longtime client to do some renovations to her kitchen. The practitioner found herself a bit uncomfortable with her client being in her private space and interacting with her family. Essentially everything went along fine until the kitchen caught on fire and was destroyed. The fire damaged the kitchen and many irreplaceable objects of sentimental value. After the fire the practitioner found herself feeling resentful toward the client wondering if the fire was caused by negligence or if it was just an accident. She was also upset with herself for entering into this exchange of services with the client. The client felt devastated, depressed and guilty. The practitioner felt she could no longer see him as a client and terminated the relationship.

A client approached her practitioner about walking his dog in exchange for treatment. This bartering arrangement continued for six months without any problems. The client and practitioner were very happy with the situation. It seemed ideal to the practitioner who never seemed to have enough time to walk his beloved dog. One day the dog pulled so strongly that the client lost her grip on the leash. The dog had seen another dog across the street and was running to visit and play with the other dog when it was hit by an oncoming car. The owner was grief-stricken and couldn't bring himself to continue seeing the client.

It is unethical for a practitioner to offer a client blanket assurance that the addition of other roles has no effect on their professional relationship. If it is of primary importance to either party that the professional relationship remain unchanged, then a dual relationship should not be initiated. Sometimes merely suggesting a dual relationship, much less entering into one, causes an immediate change in how two people relate.

When dual relationships develop more fully, such as in a friendship, the initial professional relationship may take on a lesser role and even perhaps end by mutual consent. It is impossible to know whether what can be gained is more valuable than what might be lost. The richness of our lives is often enhanced through our complex, growing and changing relationships. When both parties bring maturity and a sense of responsibility to the decision about developing a dual relationship, there is a good chance for each person to feel empowered and enriched by the experience no matter what may happen in the future to the relationship itself.

Seek Supervision

Professional supervision is invaluable if a practitioner is trying to decide about engaging in a dual relationship or working to evaluate one in which he already participates. The questions are often difficult to answer alone and many of the answers depend heavily on interactions of complex factors. Consulting someone else outside the relationship enables the practitioner to gain perspective and better see the whole picture, whereas it is easy to focus on only one aspect of the relationship when evaluating it alone.

Often the person in the power position of a dual relationship does not perceive the relationship doing any harm, while the person in the vulnerable position experiences negative consequences. No matter which role you find yourself in, supervision helps re-orient yourself to a position of responsibility and positive decision-making.

A client asked a practitioner to barter some artwork for treatment because he was low on cash and didn't want to stop treatment. The practitioner was aware that this client often had financial problems and wanted to help if he could. He told the client that he wanted a few days to think about it. The practitioner then took this issue to his supervisor to help him decide what to do. The supervisor had the practitioner explore how his desire to help others at his own expense, his issues with money, and the difficulties he had earlier in his career, all related to his desire to help this client at any level of risk. The client had said that the practitioner could view his work and decide what he wanted to pay for the paintings. The supervisor pointed out that this arrangement could lead to enormous problems if the practitioner didn't like the client's work or if he offered a price that was too low or even too high.

The practitioner and the supervisor came up with a plan that included informing the client of the risks to the relationship if he wasn't interested in any of his client's artwork and the dangers of the practitioner choosing a price. After this discussion with the client the practitioner would ask the client to take a few days to think about the risks and decide if he wanted to pursue this idea further. If he did he would have to set the prices for his artwork and understand that the practitioner might not be interested based on the type of art and the price.

Refer to the Supervision chapter, starting on page 241.

Supervision is even useful in analyzing dual relationships after when an error in judgment has already been made.

A practitioner treated a friend for a shoulder pain and the friend didn't like the service that she received. She felt physically hurt and in pain for a couple weeks after treatment and immediately stopped seeing the practitioner professionally and personally. Not only did the person lose a client, but also a friend. The practitioner and the friend were very upset about this turn of events. It seemed reasonable enough at the time; the friend had a need and the practitioner/friend seemed to have the expertise. The practitioner took this issue to supervision to understand what happened and what thinking errors she had made. She learned that she didn't fully appreciate or understand the risk she was taking by the following: treating her friend for a pain problem without informing the client/friend of the possibility that her treatment might not work; not acknowledging that the client/friend might not like her work; and forgetting the fact that the treatment might cause soreness for many days. She took it for granted that the friend would understand. It was a hard lesson to learn, but she never entered into a dual relationship lightly again.

The Special Case of Schools

For touch practitioners in training, the school setting is an important context in which to learn and practice the principles surrounding dual relationships. All the dynamics mentioned above can exist between teachers and students who consider adding social or other roles to their interactions. Indeed, one dual relationship in this setting often affects the dynamics of an entire class or faculty group, and may even affect the reputation of the school as a whole.[6]

Consider the example of a teacher and student who begin dating. Can the teacher remain objective when he has to evaluate and grade the student's work? How do other students in the class respond to their own evaluations if they feel the teacher is biased in one case? How does knowledge of the relationship affect the class's interactions in partner and group activities? If a different teacher has to fail or sanction the student, how does this influence the faculty relationship? If the social relationship ends badly, might the student bring charges against the school?

All of these examples have happened numerous times in many school settings, often with disastrous results for the student, the teacher and the school. A conservative stance is worthwhile in this setting, particularly given that the consequences can be far-reaching. Consider the following:

Precise, published policies are crucial in school environments to lay the groundwork for ethical behavior issues of dual relationships between students, teachers and administrators.

> A teacher tutoring a student after class made advances to the student. The student felt in awe of the teacher's knowledge and charisma. An intimate relationship followed and the other students became aware of it. Gossip was stimulated at the school and considerable tension in the class resulted because the student was called on frequently in class and received high grades. The relationship ended after a few months. The student was devastated and felt awkward about staying in school. She initiated a lawsuit against the school and the teacher, thus the school became embroiled in this controversy. The teacher was fired (and sued the school) and the school suffered for not having clear policies about relationships between students and teachers.

When boundaries about dual relationships between students and teachers are not clearly stated and enforced by a school there are often painful consequences that follow. In the above example, there were devastating effects on the students, the faculty and the reputation of the school. Everyone in this situation was upset and hurt for a long time. Sides were taken, students felt betrayed, angry and unsafe, faculty felt shamed, and there were severe financial consequences for the school.

> A female teacher and a male student became friends. The teacher needed to find someone she trusted to stay with her kids and the student needed to earn money, so she hired him to babysit her children. The student developed a close relationship with the teacher's children. He also had an unrecognized transference on the teacher and idolized her. This continued for a year until the student got upset with an interaction the teacher had with her children. The student felt betrayed and never saw the children or the family again. Everyone concerned experienced a great deal of pain in this situation: the student, the children and the teacher.

The point is that creating friendships between teachers and students can have negative consequences. The teacher should never have befriended the student in this manner. Although the student was fairly immature, the teacher was ultimately responsible for exercising very poor judgment in this situation. Bringing the student into the teacher's family was by far the biggest mistake in this situation.

A school director who was also a somatic practitioner had a client who expressed an interest in attending the school where she was the director. The client enrolled and for a short period of time he was a client and a student. After a few weeks, the practitioner/director discussed dual roles with the student/client. They mutually agreed to stop the client/practitioner relationship. A year later this same student asked to become a temporary office worker in the school. It was agreed that he could but that he wouldn't directly work for the school director. The student graduated from school and a year later became a teacher in the school. After several years the school director began seeing her former client/student/employee for occasional treatments. Their relationship lasted more than 10 years.

If this sounds complicated, that's because it was. Often the two would consciously and overtly state which roles they were in. They would not mix roles in their conversations and interactions. Although there were elements of a dual relationship along the way, it was also a sequential relationship where one role was left and another begun. What made this relationship work was clear, honest communication and deliberate acknowledgment of which roles they were in at the time.

In this last example both parties talked openly and communicated effectively about the transitions in their relationship. They moved quickly out of dual relationships and into sequential ones. Their ability to change roles and reverse positions of authority as well as the lasting nature of the relationship demonstrates how one can successfully navigate the complexities of human and professional relationships.

In Conclusion...

Dual relationships are a natural aspect of human interaction. They hold the potential to enrich our lives. They also hold the potential to cause great pain. A somatic practitioner must be especially aware of the dynamics of these complex relationships. With mature self-awareness and responsible choices, the ethical practitioner can safeguard the therapeutic relationship and enjoy appropriate overlapping connections with clients.

Chapter Highlights

- The term *dual relationships* describes the overlapping of professional and social roles and interactions between two people.
- A classic dual relationship occurs when two persons who interact professionally develop other roles socially.
- Potential benefits enrich dual relationships when both parties are emotionally developed and able to handle the multiple roles without confusion.
- In the health care setting it is the practitioner's responsibility to be educated and informed about the nature of dual relationships, and it is the practitioner who is accountable for informing the client about the parameters and possible impact of entering another dimension of the relationship.
- When one set of roles completely ends before a different set of roles begins, it is called a *sequential relationship*.
- The major conditions that prompt dual relationships are: socializing; group affiliation; friendship; dating; sexual activity; family; bartering; client/practitioner reversal; employment; and interactions between students and school personnel.
- Successful dual relationships may contribute fulfillment, growth and enjoyment to life.
- Ethical considerations enter the picture whenever a dual relationship includes the role of a helping professional.
- When communication is lacking or cues are misread in a dual relationship, feelings get hurt, one or both parties in the relationship suffers, and the relationship itself in all its manifestations is endangered.
- Issues to be considered before engaging in a dual relationship are: To what extent does mutual and equal consent exist? Where does accountability lie? Will the therapeutic nature of the relationship be enhanced, hindered or unaffected?
- To work well, both parties share a clear understanding of the complexities inherent in a dual relationship.
- Caution must be exercised when considering involvement in a dual relationship with a client—for there are many risks involved in a dual relationship.
- Failure in a dual relationship can affect financial, educational, professional, social or personal elements.
- Level of intimacy, the power dynamic, accountability, maturity and consequences of refusal to participate are indicators to use in evaluating the level of risk involved in a dual relationship.
- The practitioner who educates the client about both potential positives and potential negatives of the duality provides the client with the tools he needs to make an informed decision.
- When a dual relationship combines an intimate professional role with a sexual role, the potential for harm is so high that it should never be entered into.
- The professional involved is held accountable for negative consequences of a dual relationship.
- If refusal to participate in a given aspect of a dual relationship brings negative consequences, it's likely that mutual and equal consent to the relationship doesn't exist.
- Professional supervision is an important step when trying to decide whether to engage in a dual relationship or to evaluate one that already exists.
- School settings are a valuable context in which to learn and practice the principles surrounding dual relationships.

- How students interact with their teachers and their in-school clients sets the stage for their later professional interactions.
- Dual relationships are a normal outgrowth of human interaction.

Discussion Questions and Activities

- Make a list of the current and past dual relationships in your life.
- Which dual relationships have been successful? Why?
- Identify any negative outcomes from your dual relationship. In retrospect, do you think the negative outcome could have been avoided? If so, how?
- Discuss why it is always the health care practitioner's responsibility, rather than the client's, to ensure that dual relationship issues are discussed openly.
- Describe a sequential relationship you have experienced. What adjustments, if any, did you or the other person have to make when the relationship changed?
- Make a list of the most important relationships in your life. For each of these examine the following:
  1. Where do power differentials exist?
  2. In what ways do these power differentials influence the course of the relationship?
  3. What level(s) of intimacy exist in these relationships?
  4. How, if at all, have the maturity levels of the persons involved influenced the course of these relationships?
- Think of a time when a relationship you were involved in had the opportunity to become a dual relationship, but did not. Whose decision was it to refuse? What reasons were given for the refusal? What were the results of the refusal?
- In what situations might it be useful to have a written contract, however informal?
- Who are the people in your life who can give you clear, knowledgeable advice in the area of dual relationships?
- What relationships are so important to you that you would not risk them by entering into a dual relationship?
- What formal situations, such as a school or workplace, have you been in that had specific policies regarding dual relationships? How did that appear to affect relationships in that setting? Overall, was it a positive safe experience, or was it uncomfortable in anyway?
- Role-play with a partner; one of you is a practitioner, the other a client. In the first interaction, have the client suggest to the practitioner an added role to their relationship, and allow the practitioner to respond. Then in the same roles, have the practitioner suggest to the client an added role, and have the client respond. Switch roles and repeat the exercise. After the experience, discuss the following questions: What did you feel while playing each role? How easy or difficult was it to respond to the suggestion that the relationship change? How did your partner's reactions affect your perception of whether the dual relationship would work?
- The following scenarios are presented so that you may begin to apply some of the principles discussed in this chapter. Note that in some of these examples, the question is not so much "Should the dual relationship exist," but rather, "What pitfalls might occur and how might the relationship be handled to avoid negative consecuences?"

  You might find it helpful to confer about these examples with other students or practitioners, or with your supervision group. You may find that besides the details provided for each case, what is NOT known can have a large impact on any decision regarding appropriate action in the dual relationship.

- An old friend of yours has also been your client for several years. For the most part, your therapeutic encounters have been focused on enhancing a healthy life. Now, however, your friend is experiencing physical problems and you would like to take a firmer role in guiding him through some lifestyle changes that you believe would restore his health.

- You and your teacher at bodywork school both attended a school retreat. Your teacher has now asked you to attend a non-school related party with her.

- You are an acupuncturist who has treated several faculty members of a local bodywork school. You are considering taking some continuing education courses there and one or more of these faculty members may become your teachers.

- As a recent graduate, you have begun charging your clients a competitive fee for your services. One of your friends who was receiving your services for free during your schooling, fails to give you 24 hours notice and misses an appointment. Your policy is to charge for such missed appointments.

- You are a faculty member at a school where you also make private therapy appointments. One of your students comes to you for therapy. This student has been having difficulties in class and may fail.

- Your client is also your stockbroker. During her session with you, she gives you stock tips. You follow up on them and lose a significant amount of money.

- Your office assistant quits. You know that one of your clients is looking for employment of this type.

- You barter your services with one of your clients who has a laundering business.

- Your next-door neighbor comes to you for a session. That morning you discovered that his dog ripped up your new flower bed.

- A long-term client has become a friend. In one session you accidentally cause her an injury that lasts for six months.

- You and one of your teachers begin a sexual relationship. Two of your classmates confront you in the presence of the school administration.

- One of your family members comes to you for the first time for a treatment. Afterwards, he never speaks of the treatment and never makes another appointment.

5

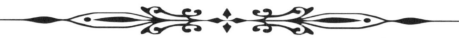

Sex, Touch and Intimacy

- ◆ A Psychosocial Overview
- ◆ Touch
- ◆ Intimacy
- ◆ Sex
- ◆ Sexuality
- ◆ Sex and Touch Therapy
- ◆ Sexual Misconduct
- ◆ Desexualizing the Touch Experience
- ◆ In Conclusion...
- ◆ Chapter Highlights
- ◆ Discussion Questions and Activities

EX. TOUCH. INTIMACY. What feelings and thoughts are conjured by these words? Excitement, shame, denial, ambivalence, pleasure? For humans these words describe experiences at the core of our being. As a somatic health care practitioner you might be asking yourself, "Why in the world do I need to think about these issues? What do they have to do with my work?" Clear boundaries around sex, touch and intimacy create the foundation for safety and trust which is the basis for healing in all therapeutic relationships, especially in somatic therapies.

This chapter focuses on sex, touch and intimacy issues in client/practitioner relationships. These three topics are profoundly present whenever a practitioner has physical contact with a client, yet they are rarely explored in educational training programs. These are the areas where clients state that they experience the most boundary violations from their practitioners. The two most common complaints clients make about health care professionals are: the practitioner did not listen to the client; and the client felt violated by the practitioner, most often from unwanted or insensitive touch or in personal remarks made to the client.[1] Unfortunately, most clients opt to find a new practitioner rather than discuss their concerns.

As part of this chapter's exploration, we examine cultural and personal beliefs about sex, touch and intimacy, and how these may relate to both the client's and practitioner's experience during an actual session. We also focus on practical, ethical steps for practitioners to take regarding sex, touch and intimacy issues to create a safe environment for both client and practitioner.

A Psychosocial Overview

We are born as sexual beings with a need for touch and intimacy. We require a healthy environment that supports our natural development in these areas to thrive as organisms. However, each of our uniquely personal experiences is culturally bound by unconscious, embedded beliefs. How our beliefs develop is more often a product of cultural values than a natural unfolding of one's own biology and identity and the interplay with our environment. This cultural overlay is influenced by religion, family, social mores and the larger social fabric of the time. Our "unique" selves would most likely look different if we were raised in another place and time.

A society influences the type and volume of information available to its members. Examples from United States history illustrate the problem of getting information about human sexuality. In the 1800s, several "health reformers" (including Sylvester Graham of Graham Cracker fame and John Harvey Kellogg of Kellogg's breakfast cereal) believed sexual feelings, thoughts and activity debilitated the body. Although these sentiments were based on opinions largely influenced by religious beliefs, they were presented as fact. In that same century federal laws that made it illegal to send sexual literature through the mail were applied to the mailing of birth control information. In the mid-20th century, during the political era of McCarthyism, "one Congressman insisted that studying human sexual behavior was paving the way for a Communist takeover of the United States."[2]

Though we live in a society that considers itself the most accomplished and sophisticated in the world, more recent examples show that we are still struggling with these issues. The editor of the *Journal of the American Medical Association* was fired by the AMA for publishing an article that reported on a 1991 Kinsey Institute study asking students to define sex. This kind of cultural legacy makes it difficult to obtain sensitive, accurate, complete information about sexuality that might actually help us to become more responsible, respectful, happier human beings.

Psychosexual Effects on the Individual

Why might there be confusion between sex, touch and intimacy? Did you receive a good sex education? Before you answer that question for yourself, consider this definition. A good sex education is one where:

- the information you received was developmentally appropriate for your age at the time;
- the learning was ongoing throughout your childhood, and you clearly received all the necessary facts;
- the teaching was sensitive to your feelings and needs;
- you were given a model for decision-making rather than a finite set of rules about how to behave;
- you and your body were treated with respect.

How good was your sex education? Did you receive a good touch education or a good intimacy education based on the above criteria? It is just as crucial for us as humans to be "fluent" in discussing touch and intimacy needs, but rarely do any of us get direct education and experience regarding the issues of touch and intimacy.

Most people find it extremely difficult to talk about sexuality. Even if practitioners are comfortable with sexuality, touching and intimacy themselves, they might still find it difficult to talk to clients about these issues. This is true for several reasons. First, cultural experience tells them that it is usually improper to talk about these topics. Second, if those conversations occurred they were most likely only with sexual partner(s) or in an impersonal, clinical setting. Third, if as youngsters they did not have role models for open communication then it is often difficult to comfortably discuss sex, touch and intimacy. And finally, to complicate the matter further, if they were not respected and if their bodies were violated in any way, their ability to deal with these topics in an open manner is usually severely compromised unless they resolve the effects of those experiences.

The Distinction Between Sex, Touch and Intimacy

By definition, sex, touch and intimacy are three distinct behaviors and experiences. The fact that they overlap at times is what creates confusion. Most people would concur that good sex includes all three. A person who only feels intimate with someone when sex is involved might start to believe that intimacy and sex are the same thing. Men are more susceptible than women because most cultures assert that men are not supposed to express feelings (a form of intimacy) except during sex.

How is all this related to health care or somatic therapy? Unfortunately, personal and cultural perceptions of sexuality, touch and intimacy histories also influence how individuals experience health care. As an example, for many years in the United States massage was a euphemism for illegal sex through prostitution. In the 1980s many people made sexual innuendoes or were genuinely taken aback when someone said they were making a legitimate career choice to be a massage therapist. More than 20 years later, although there is much more mainstream acceptance and understanding about the benefits of massage and other bodywork therapies, there is still a profound cultural legacy and taboo in certain segments of the population.

The general public, clients and somatic practitioners share in the confusion about how touch therapies and sexuality are and are not related. The intentional misuse of language (e.g., massage as a euphemism for prostitution) has had a profound impact on the public's understanding of touch modalities. The misuse of words is not just a cognitive problem; it is a personal and cultural issue about how people relate to certain parts of the body and human experience.

Touch

Touch is a basic human need and a sensory process that also communicates. However, as with any communication, the intended message may be misunderstood by the receiver. Many countries such as the United States are "low-touch" cultures. The kind of touch given to children tends to be more for caretaking, retrieving and punishing, and less so for nurturing and affection. For example, modern media such as advertising, magazines, newspapers, movies, music videos and comics most often displays most touch as either romantic, sexual or violent.

Exploring Touch and Culture

Humans need touch. We crave it, we hunger for it, we get sick and can even die for the lack of it. But we still do not know where touch belongs in our lives. In fact we are often actively discouraged from touching each other. This conditioning begins early: kindergartners are taught to keep their hands strictly to themselves and are chastised for unnecessary and inappropriate touching. Many children learn early on that touching is bad. We lose our childlike innocence and after a while non-sexual touch, the most basic form of communication between humans, seems strange and uncomfortable. Only in a few settings is giving and receiving this vital nourishment acceptable: ritual greetings and leave-takings; contact sports; physical aggression; grooming; and professional touching by hands-on practitioners.

> "Sight and all the other senses are only modes of touch."
> —Samuel Butler

This is not as true, however, outside of the United States. Psychologist Sidney Jourard made a study of couples' behavior in public situations in a variety of different cultures. In a comparison of touching in cafés he observed that in San Juan couples touched each other 180 times per hour. In Paris they touched 110 times per hour. In Gainesville, Florida it was two times per hour and in London it was not at all.[3]

By the time we reach adulthood many of us have actually forgotten *how* to touch. We have lived through years of "hands off" indoctrination. Naturally we are confused. We have been told all our lives that the only "right" ways to satisfy this intense physical need is through sex, violence or contact sports. Touch between parents and their children even becomes strained and confused. In the book, *touch*, Tiffany Field, PH.D., quotes Ashley Montagu, "Such alarm is understandable in a society that has so confounded love, sex, affection and touch. The genuinely loving parents have nothing to fear from their demonstrative acts of affection for the children or anyone else."[4]

What do we do, then, if we just want to be comforted? As often as not we do not even identify the need as such. We misinterpret the need for touch as sexual desire, or hunger, or depression. We may seek out sexual relationships less out of love than out of a need for contact. Or in the absence of someone to hug our outer skin, we hug our *inner* skin by overeating. There are many ways we try to satisfy our need for comfort when all we really need is to be touched. We do not just have "skin hunger;" we often have skin *starvation*.[5]

Knowing Where Touch Begins

The sensation of touch actually begins in the womb. The skin, derived from the same cells as the nervous system, is a perfect instrument for collecting information about our surrounding environment long before birth. A fetus withdraws from the touch of a probe at less than eight weeks of gestation, showing that the link between touch and survival is one of the first and most important protective mechanisms to develop.

All human babies are born too soon. Our heads are so big that we cannot afford to gestate any longer than we do, so we are born *before* we are physiologically ready. Most other mammals can move around, at least in a limited way, very soon after they are born. Think of newborn foals or deer, which are up and walking a few moments after birth. Humans, on the other hand, are incredibly slow. In fact, the average time between birth and crawling is identical to the average time between conception and birth, nine months. What does all this have to do with touch? Simply this, newborn human infants are not fully developed. They cannot see clearly or differentiate sounds. They communicate with the world almost entirely through their skin. Virtually all mammals, particularly the young, show behaviors of snuggling. Montagu asserts that touch is a basic behavioral need and that the absence of it causes abnormal behavior[6] and abnormal physical development as well.[7]

Consider a newborn baby. One moment it is supremely comfortable in a snug, climate-controlled, perfectly shaped uterus. The next moment it is painfully squeezed into a bright, noisy, cold, wall-less world. All babies benefit from regular touch—perfectly healthy ones and those who suffer from colic, cocaine exposure, AIDS or abuse. Touch reduces stress (as measured by chemicals in the blood). Babies cry less, sleep more and are generally easier to soothe when touched. The messages we receive through our skin, particularly about our safety and well-being, have resonating effects on our behavior for the rest of our lives. Research findings document evidence that the cause of failure to thrive or to mature psychologically can be linked to the lack of demonstrative love.[8]

Even older babies who are not yet crawling use their skin as a way to get information about the world. Watch a baby explore a new toy: the first place it goes is into the baby's mouth. This baby is not really interested in how the rattle tastes. It happens that a huge number of sensory neurons are located in the skin of the lips and tongue and this is where a baby gets information. A baby puts a new toy into his mouth to find out what it *feels* like!

Many other cultural statistics show that children who are welcomed with lots of physical touch and tactile stimulation usually grow into well-adjusted, capable and loving adults. Children who are touch-deprived in infancy show tendencies toward aggressiveness and violent behavior. This has been well-documented in cultures throughout the world.[9]

Naturally, there are countless other variables that influence human behavior besides how we are touched as babies. It makes sense that during this most vulnerable time of our lives we form patterns and expectations about how the world works, specifically about how *safe* and *valued* we are in the world, through our skins. Numerous studies show that for lower and higher mammals, receiving touch that is pleasurable, safe and appropriate reduces sickness, depression and aggressive behaviors. In fact as we learn more about this everyday, yet miraculous phenomenon, we may find that touch holds more answers than we ever imagined.[10]

Babies are not the only people who suffer from touch deprivation; nor are they the only ones who benefit from adequate touch in their lives. Touch in infancy aids all areas of development: physical; mental; and psychological. Touch in adulthood is equally beneficial. It stimulates immune system function, reduces stress and keeps us literally

Sex, Touch
and Intimacy

"connected" to our community. That sense of connectedness turns out to be a major factor in long-term health. Research shows that adults who have a life-partner live longer, healthier lives than people who live in isolation. For both genders and all races in the United States, people who live alone have death rates anywhere from one to five times higher than their partnered peers. This is true for lifelong singles, divorced and widowed people. Rates for all forms of heart disease and a wide variety of cancers, stroke, pneumonia, diabetes, cirrhosis and suicide are higher across the board for people who live alone.[11] Touch is essential in infancy; it is vital in adulthood.

The Dynamics of Touch

What really happens when one person touches another? How does a hand on your head or your shoulder translate into better health for you? Human touch can completely change the way the body functions. Welcome touch can make the body work better from heart rate to blood pressure to digestive system efficiency. In a 1998 study, the *Journal of Applied Gerontology* reports that elders received benefits from giving massage to infants. The elders did not receive massage, yet they benefited from the touch.[12] In another study, reported in *Massage Therapy: The Evidence for Practice*, "agitated" or aggressive elders, decreased the number of agitated behaviors with the implementation of a 10-minute massage. These behaviors continued to decrease with the number of treatments.[13]

When we receive human touch or any stimulus to the skin, information races to the brain. The brain receives that information and creates a response in the body (depending on the interpretation). This response is a relaxing, pleasurable one (*parasympathetic nervous system response*) if the stimulus is soothing and welcome, or an anxiety-provoking, upsetting one (*sympathetic nervous system response*), if the stimulus is perceived as threatening. A parasympathetic nervous system response from being touched lowers blood pressure, increases digestion, slows breathing and generally makes us feel more relaxed and at ease.

Generally, studies indicate that touch is essentially a positive experience for the person receiving it as long as the touch does not impose more intimacy than the person desires or communicate a negative message.[14] Therein lies the challenge: How do you know if your touch is too intimate or sends a negative message for any specific person? You must train yourself to attune to clients' verbal and nonverbal feedback and be willing to discuss sensitive issues with them.

How touch is interpreted is a complex matter. When people receive touch they go through an analytical process (often largely unconscious) to determine the meaning of that specific touch. According to research done by Heslin and Alper,[15] individuals consider the following aspects in this process:

- what part of the other person's body touched me;
- what part of my body is touched;
- how long the touch lasts;
- how much pressure is used;
- whether there is movement after contact is made;
- if anyone else is present to witness the touch, and if so, who;
- the relationship between myself and the person who touched me;
- our situation.

In addition to Heslin's and Alper's findings, other components should be considered as well:

- the verbal exchange that accompanies the touch;
- any nonverbal behaviors present;
- prior touch experiences in my life or with the person who has touched me.

We like to be touched by some people and not by others. While one person's touch makes us feel cared for, warm and safe, another's may make us feel threatened, cold and queasy. This holds true whether the touch is from friends, partners, co-workers, acquaintances or health care practitioners.

It is a complicated process that humans go through to determine if touch is a positive or negative, wanted or unwanted experience! Add to this equation the familial, ethnic and even regional differences in norms regarding touch and then combine prevailing cultural and gender differences, and it is easy to see how "touchy" this experience is for us.

Gender and Touch

There are also gender differences around touch. Girls are touched more frequently and less roughly than boys. As boys reach puberty, non-sexual touch decreases just as sexual experiences increase. So for many men, touch and sex become synonymous. Consider the following scenario:

> After receiving weekly bodywork therapy for a few months a client expressed a change he experienced since he was receiving massage therapy on a weekly basis. One day, he said that he wasn't "jumping into bed" with women he was dating since he had been receiving massage regularly. He said, "I realize in retrospect that one of the main reasons for choosing to be sexual with someone was to experience touch." Since he was now receiving touch regularly through massage, he better understands his needs.

His experience demonstrates the profound confusion most of us experience in differentiating these very primal, human and necessary needs, as well as how best to get them met. The confusion is not limited to men. Women confuse touch and sex as well.

Much fear and misunderstanding about sexual orientation abounds. The prevailing attitude has been that heterosexual sexuality is normal and homosexual or bisexual sexuality is not. Consequently we become acculturated not only to deny same gender feelings but to avoid anything that would remotely look like same gender intimacy and sexual activity. Touch has now become suspect. Who is touching whom? And why? Men are socialized to be more wary in this regard than females. Same gender touch for men is virtually taboo because it is automatically assumed to indicate homosexual desire which is culturally unacceptable. For women there is much less stigma to touching one another.

Women are usually less concerned with the gender of a person who touches them but they want to know that person. Given this, in a touch therapy setting some female clients might not choose a male practitioner if they do not know him. Some men may especially avoid male practitioners because they cannot imagine being touched so intimately by another male. On the other hand, some men prefer male practitioners because they mistakenly assume that a man is automatically stronger than a female. Some clients choose same-sex practitioners to avoid possible cross-gender sexual tension.

Unfortunately, there are few images of men as nurturers in this society. Related to this phenomenon is an interesting and confusing paradox at play in terms of health care practitioners. Men traditionally have been given the power to do things, know things and fix things. For this reason health care has predominantly been male-dominated except in direct interaction fields such as nursing, physical therapy and massage. Consciously, the culture automatically views men as having the information and techniques necessary for healing. Yet the cultural unconscious says that men are not necessarily a source of comfort or trust. This is exacerbated by a picture of males as perpetrators of violence. Male practitioners might be seen as both powerful and fearsome. This does not make for an easy therapeutic relationship.

Female practitioners may need to do more to prove their competency, but they are more easily accepted as someone safe and nurturing. Male practitioners must work harder regarding their professional image but are successful as long as they are attentive to possible touch and gender concerns.

Honoring The Power of Touch

Healthy people seek hands-on therapy because it feels good. Beyond satisfying the need for touch, it strengthens responses to mental and physical stressors. For instance, a good massage, in addition to lowering blood pressure, increasing immune system activity and helping the body to get rid of wastes, makes the client more alert, emotionally calmer and more capable of dealing with everyday challenges.

But somatic work can do even more than that. Helen Colton, author of *Touch Therapy*, suggests that people recovering from accident or trauma have greater than normal need for touch and comfort. "Touch may even be *the* basic need of patients, more vital than medication, so that, when their touch need is satisfied, patients can direct their energies toward dealing with problems and traumas that they have."[16]

> A client driving a small truck was rear-ended by a city bus. In her words, "the accident turned her long-bed truck into a short-bed truck." When she began somatic treatment she was a mass of bruises and her pain threshold was very low. But as the treatments slowly proceeded, she realized that what she valued most was the opportunity to feel how much of her body *didn't* hurt from her accident. This helped her to maintain a good attitude — which was a key factor in her recovery process.

Physical and sexual violence are prevalent in our society: abusive touch occurs between family members, acquaintances, friends and strangers. As a culture we are numbed to the effects of such violations. As individuals we may interpret all touch to be a hurtful, powerful tool used against us and therefore avoided. These "accepted" touch taboos and behaviors are reinforced by painful experience. Personal touch histories are very complex and not obvious to others. It is safe to assume that for most people touch has been a mixed experience.

Practitioners need to pay attention to the verbal and nonverbal communication clients give regarding touch. Let clients know why, when and how you will touch them. When possible, give clients a choice about this. In training you may have been taught a specific way to do a procedure or treatment and assume you must do it that way. Demonstrate respect to clients by being creative and finding other ways to work that better suits their needs if necessary. The variety and innovation will also help you stay interested in your work.

A client can experience sexual confusion when receiving touch therapy or a medical modality—even where there are not overt sexual cues. Touch in and of itself is a sexual cue for some people.

> An acupuncturist found that three male clients started to communicate with her in ways that felt too personal: one wanted to meet for coffee; another hinted about his openness for a date; the third kept asking her personal questions. She decided to ask for feedback from several trusted female friends who had also received treatments from her. The behavior that each noted was how much this practitioner casually touched each of them above and beyond the necessary medical techniques. For the practitioner the amount of touch was normal given her high-touch family background and her intent was to use touch as a reassuring gesture for her clients. But her frequent touch was suggestive to her male clients.

One way to address the touch component in the client-practitioner relationship is to talk about it directly as part of the first appointment. Let your clients know what kind of touch to expect during each treatment and ask permission to proceed with the kind of touch described. Clients need to have the option of saying no. Keep in mind that clients in the less powerful position can find saying no difficult.

High-touch practitioners such as the acupuncturist might incorporate a clarifying tool with her clients to avoid confusion and mixed messages: add a "touch education" component to her intake interview either verbally or in a written statement; describe her use of touch while letting clients know that it is optional; and limit her touch with clients while they are not directly receiving treatments.

For client comfort and safety practitioners must be willing to modify behaviors. More importantly, you must also be sure that you are not touching a client in hurtful ways based on your own history.

> A massage therapist found that clients weren't feeling his presence or depth in touch. Since he had been physically abused as a child, he was afraid of hurting others which prevented him from making real connection and contact.

> A shiatsu practitioner who had been physically abused as a child was criticized as being too hurtful in her work. She honestly thought that touch was supposed to feel like this since she had no other somatic experience to the contrary.

By addressing the personal trauma, each of these practitioners successfully learned healthy, contact-full touch.

Receiving touch is a learned response. The more often your clients do it, the better they receive it. They get to know and understand their body through the medium of touch, and learn to accept and integrate all the benefits it has to offer for a better and healthier life.

See Ethical Principles, pages 15-17, for details on the **power differential**.

Refer to Ethical Practice Management, pages 165-167, for **informed consent**.

Intimacy

Our cultural confusion about the meaning of intimacy is revealed through dictionary definitions and how we use these words. "Intimate" is described as: "very personal, private, indicative of one's deepest nature, marked by close association." When you turn to the definition of "intimacy" new meanings are revealed: "having sexual relations" and "illicit sexual relations."[17] Surprisingly, "intimate" and "intimacy" have come to mean very different things and the original meaning of "intimate" transforms to a sexual connotation when the term "intimacy" is used. Culturally we seldom talk about sex in a direct, honest way, so we must create euphemisms for sexual activity and intercourse. Take a moment to think of all the slang words you have heard or use to talk about sex as well as the slang used for sexual body parts. How many people give their elbow or knee a nickname?

Betsy Tolstedt and Joseph Stokes from the University of Illinois used three measures of intimacy for a study they conducted regarding marital satisfaction.[18] Intimacy was assessed in terms of physical, emotional and verbal factors:

- Physical intimacy entails affectionate and sexual touch
- Emotional intimacy refers to feelings of closeness, tolerance and support
- Verbal intimacy involves disclosure of emotions, feelings and opinions

Many people experience sexual encounters without emotional or verbal intimacy. People often complain about the lack of intimacy in their lives, but it is important to consider what the complaints are actually about. Upon examination, a person might feel satisfied with the amount and kind of affectionate touch received from a partner but wants more sexual interaction. Or the person may feel supported and respected by a partner, but finds the partner uncomfortable talking about her feelings and concerns. It becomes clearer that some intimacy needs are being met in this particular relationship while others are not. When we feel dissatisfied about the level of intimacy in our lives it is helpful to look at each of these three areas and apply them to various relationships including partner, friends, family and colleagues. The results illuminate not only others' comfort levels with the different types of intimacy but also our own.

Establishing Appropriate Intimacy

The distinctions between physical, emotional and verbal intimacy also shed new light on therapeutic intimacy for somatic practitioners. In a therapeutic relationship that involves the client's body as the focus of treatment, concerns about intimacy take on greater importance. The appropriate intimacy for any therapeutic relationship is a one-way intimacy. Practitioners physically touch their clients, allow them to disclose thoughts and feelings, and offer both verbal and physical support. The therapeutic relationship's function is not for the clients to do the same for the practitioner. This seemingly clear-cut protocol is often challenging in practice.

One difficulty with establishing appropriate intimacy in therapeutic touch relationships arises simply from to the presence of touch. Touching the client means that the practitioner has automatically violated a cultural taboo. Even if the client is voluntarily present and consents to touch, cultural meanings of touch still exert a strong influence on one's immediate experience. This cultural violation may make both client and practitioner uncomfortable and nervous, especially if clear boundaries haven't been discussed and established.

This context sets the stage for the following possible sequence of events. Once the cultural taboo concerning physical intimacy is overridden, the client needs to quickly create safety. She may therefore attempt to find out as much as possible (and as quickly as possible), about the person doing the touching by asking questions, sometimes more personal than professional. In other words, the movement is from increased physical intimacy to increased verbal intimacy. If the practitioner is not savvy to the safety or comfort needs of the client, it is easy to fall into answering all the questions even if they are not appropriate or relevant to the treatment at hand. The focus can then shift from the client's relevant concerns to the practitioner's personal life.

Conversely, a practitioner who feels anxious (often unconsciously) about violating the touch taboo might be the one to initiate chit-chat with the client and either ask questions of the client or reveal personal information unnecessary or inappropriate for the relationship. Once this dynamic is set in motion it is easy for the client or practitioner to think that, given the physical and verbal intimacy, greater emotional intimacy is now expected or required. This is the point where confusion often abounds about the expectations and boundaries of the relationship: are we now friends, do we socialize, do I act on romantic feelings?

Another factor in this confusion relates to practitioner self-care. As stated earlier, therapeutic relationships entail a one-way intimacy. The appropriate focus is client-centered, meaning the concerns and needs of the client are the focus of the work together. Practitioners who spend their days listening to, helping and facilitating change in others need a strong support system wherein they receive the same nurturing. Those with a support system who are actively intimate with others usually do not want nor need to solicit intimacy from their clients. Practitioners who do not experience intimacy elsewhere in their lives are vulnerable to using their clients to fulfill personal needs.

Practitioners who are unable to create avenues for intimacy in their personal lives often jeopardize their professional relationships. Perhaps these practitioners are shy, tired, busy, vulnerable or in a crisis. Maybe they lack self-confidence or feel uncomfortable with intimacy. A practitioner on the giving end of one-way intimacy occupies a powerful, safe place since it does not entail any real risk-taking on the practitioner's part. Being actively involved in relationships with two-way intimacy in one's personal life is a challenge and can feel like a loss of control of self. A common boundary crossing occurs when a practitioner devotes the entire session to discussing his personal problems with the client and essentially uses the client as a sounding board. A seriously problematic situation occurs when a somatic practitioner uses the session as a seduction to become intimate with a client.

> At a social event, a practitioner becomes attracted to someone and offers a complimentary session. In that session the client talks while the practitioner appears nurturing and emotionally available. The practitioner touches the client physically without any risk of returned touch. The practitioner is in control of the situation since the client is in a more vulnerable position.

Aside from the fact that this is not a way to start a healthy, equal relationship, it is certainly manipulative, unethical and undermines one's professional integrity.

To mature is in part to realize that while complete intimacy and omniscience and power cannot be had, self-transcendence, growth, and closeness to others are nevertheless within one's reach.

—Sissela Bok

Sex

Of the three concepts "sex" is the most culturally taboo to discuss and the most fraught with anxiety. As a culture, we are most comfortable thinking about sex in regard to gender, biology, reproduction and heterosexual activity. "Sex" in common usage has come to mean heterosexual intercourse. Many people deny sexual feelings, erotic sensations and a complete range of sexual behaviors that are not intercourse or heterosexual.

Sexual behavior occurs on a continuum. The starting point on the continuum differs from person to person and varies from day to day and year to year. Sexual behaviors involve overt acts as well as emotional feelings and physiological changes. This means that behaviors such as talking, holding hands, kissing, or even exchanging a look are sexual if an accompanying sexual feeling or sensation is present.

Historically, a limited definition of sex was a problem in identifying sexual abuse and incest. Prior to the late 1970s, many women who had been sexually violated did not identify their experience as sexual abuse because intercourse had not occurred. Though they knew their boundaries had been violated, and though they experienced bodily shame and felt sexually guilty, they did not make the direct link to sexual abuse. Men are also sexual abuse survivors. Women are used as the example because the first time incest and sexual abuse were taken seriously in the United States was in 1978 with the publication of Susan Forward's book, *Betrayal of Innocence: Incest and Its Devastation*, which focused on girls as victims.[19]

In recent decades, society has witnessed a sexual exploitation rampage. Sex appeal is promoted, advocated and revered. We are deluged with sex, sexuality and sex appeal. Michael V. Reitano, M.D., Editor in Chief of *Sexual Health Magazine*, says, "Virtually every advertisement, movie, television show, magazine or book has either at its core or as part of its appeal issues of sex: how to achieve it, maintain it, enjoy it, remain safe from it, embrace it, abolish it, prohibit it, exploit it."[20] Even animated characters in children's movies possess sex appeal. Skewed views on sexuality perpetuate the association of sex with the touch professions in the minds of the consumer, despite a growing respect and appreciation for the holistic health benefits of somatic work.

The sex industry has used massage therapy as a front for prostitution, and the word "massage" still summons questionable associations for some consumers. The association between massage and the sex industry is not only perpetuated by advertisements, movies and television. Many telephone Yellow Pages as well as the Internet have inappropriate listing policies. When the average person opens up the Yellow Pages or searches the Internet for a legitimate massage therapist and is inundated with suggestive photos and words with sexual overtones inviting him to call, it reflects badly on the entire industry of professional therapists of integrity. The attitude of sex for sale and exploitive sex versus healthy sexuality reflects the attitudes of the society.

Examining Cultural Values

Sex is also laden with cultural values. These values may serve a positive purpose: providing group cohesion, group functionality and group security. Problems arise when cultural myths, which often arise from values, are treated as facts. The following beliefs are not "true" in and of themselves, but their repetition has given them the aura of fact:

- Boys should get experience.
- Girls need to abstain from sex until in a committed relationship (preferably marriage).
- Girls are passive and boys are aggressive (this appears to be changing).
- Sex and love are the same.
- Same-sex attractions are abnormal and to be avoided.
- Older people are asexual.

Many people believe our sexually permissive culture has created problems such as child abuse and pornography. In fact, pervasive sexual repression in many cultures has produced a sexual-obsession backlash. This obsession occurs in the societal context of sex repression, where even sex education is opposed in schools. For example, Jocelyn Elders, the U. S. Surgeon General, was fired in 1994 for advocating that masturbation should be taught as an alternative to intercourse in an "abstinence-only" curricula. When people are uncomfortable and feel shame about their own sexuality, they can become focused on the sexuality of others to an obsessive degree. Why? Perhaps they are trying to deflect their own discomfort with sex, or are trying to determine if they are "normal," or attempting to gain some knowledge about sex. Unclear social boundaries, mixed messages, fear and lack of access to truthful information make frank discussions about sex rare.

The Sexual Response Cycle

Prior to the 1950s we did not have information about the physiological aspects of the sexual response, mainly because the technology necessary to obtain this information was not available. In 1954 gynecologist and researcher Dr. William Masters, with his assistant Virginia Johnson, began studies of the human sexual response. With 694 volunteers, they observed and recorded physiological responses during sexual behavior. Results of this research were first reported in 1959 and later published in the groundbreaking *Human Sexual Response* in 1966.[21]

Masters and Johnson identified a "Sexual Response Cycle" in men and women that consists of four phases:

1. An excitement/arousal phase (lasting several minutes to hours);
2. a plateau phase (30 seconds to 3 minutes);
3. an orgasmic phase (3-15 seconds); and
4. a resolution (with orgasm—10 to 25 minutes; without orgasm—several hours).

Distinct, gender-specific physiological changes occur in each phase. The most relevant information from this research for all health care practitioners who touch clients is the "excitement phase," because touch and other environmental cues can automatically trigger the sexual response cycle. As humans, sexual response starts with any stimulus an individual perceives as erotic, and involves the senses or cognitive processes. Being in a familiar place or setting, seeing someone attractive, hearing music, having a memory or fantasy, or receiving touch may stimulate a sexual response.

Isolating the physiological or anatomic functioning aspect is key to understanding the physical associations between the somatic treatment and the sexual response. There are three significant physiological connections, all of which stem from the body's nervous system: the sensory aspect; the parasympathetic nervous system; and the limbic system. The primary sensory aspect is touch. The tactile stimulation of hands-on work provides a central and peripheral nervous system tune-up of sorts, and the client's whole sensory mechanism is stimulated.

Sex, Touch and Intimacy

Touching certain areas of the body further complicates the matter. For instance the areas of the abdomen, lower extremities and buttocks share the same two nerve plexuses as the genitals—the lumbar and sacral plexuses. Stimulation of these nerve plexuses, as may occur in treatments such as massage to the abdominals, gluteals or thighs, are not confined to local perception but instead are diffused throughout the area, and therefore the genital nerves can be affected.[22]

The parasympathetic nervous system provides the second vital link between touch and the sexual response. This aspect of the autonomic nervous system is responsible for the body's regulation of the "rest and digest," or the restorative responses. It also counterbalances the effects of the sympathetic division, which regulates the "fight or flight" dynamic. Furthermore, parasympathetic influences regulate both the relaxation response induced by hands-on treatments as well as the physiological changes that occur during sexual arousal. When methods such as slow, rhythmic, repetitive stroking, passive movement, slow, broad compressions, reflexology and acupressure are used, the relaxation response, under parasympathetic control, is induced. The parasympathetic nervous system also controls the primary and secondary bodily responses that occur during sexual arousal. These are vasocongestion, or the increase of blood supply to the genitals, and myotonia, which is the increase in muscle tension that is the result of sexual stimulation.[23]

The third link is the limbic system. The limbic system is a group of structures that form a curved border around the brain's core. This complex aspect of the brain controls emotional and sexual experiences.[24] Stimulation of the body by therapeutic touch influences the limbic response. This not only serves to be another physiological connection between sex and touch, it may also explain why emotional responses occur during or after a treatment.

Sexuality

What is sexuality? Some think that sex and sexuality are synonymous. Because sex is most obviously biological and physiological, oftentimes sexuality is viewed solely as a physical process. However, most sources agree that sexuality is greater than the sum of its parts—that sexuality encompasses biological (anatomy and physiology), psychological (thoughts, feelings and values) and cultural (family, society and religious) influences.

According to THE SEXUAL HEALTH NETWORK, "Sexuality spans the biological, psychological, social, emotional and spiritual dimensions of our lives. It begins with us and our relationship with ourselves and extends to our relationships with others. Our relationship with ourselves includes how we feel about ourselves as a person, as sexual beings, as men and women, and how we feel about our body, and how we feel about sexual activities and behaviors."[25]

The ways in which we express our sexual nature are as different as the number of human beings on this planet. How we integrate our sexual nature into our personality is greatly influenced by genetics, upbringing, health status, and cultural, social and religious influences. While we do not have control over possessing a sexual nature, we can learn to control when and how we express it.

Sexuality is innate. Human sexual-erotic functioning begins immediately after birth and continues until death. Contrary to popular belief, those who choose to not act sexually still possess sexuality. Although sexual feelings can be ignored or we can decide not to act on them, sexuality is not something we can excise from our being. There are people who have chosen a religiously celibate lifestyle who celebrate their sexuality as a vehicle for personally connecting with their god(s). Sexuality is complex because it includes the multiple meanings we give it; it is a uniquely subjective experience for each of us.

Three specific aspects of sexuality are essential to consider: sexual orientation; sexual identity; and sexual behavior:

- Sexual orientation refers to which gender(s) we are attracted to sexually.
- Sexual identity is how we *label* ourselves and is usually the same as how we understand our sexual orientation: If a female is attracted to a male then she identifies herself as heterosexual. If she is attracted to a female then she identifies herself as homosexual or lesbian, but because of cultural stigma she might more readily act, appear and identify as heterosexual rather than risk identifying herself, internally and externally, as a lesbian.
- Sexual behavior is what we actually do sexually.

Healthy sexuality assumes that sexual orientation, identity and behavior are congruent in an individual. However, for many this congruency is difficult to attain. Because of stigma, sometimes people who know that their orientation is for same-gender partners, and who identify themselves as gay, have not yet engaged in same-sex sexual behavior due to fear, shame or other reasons.

Sexual orientation is misunderstood and feared because of cultural beliefs that say there are two orientations, heterosexual and homosexual. These same beliefs place a value on each, most commonly that heterosexuality is "good" and homosexuality is "bad." In the 1940s, research by Alfred Kinsey shed light on sexual orientation and the reality of human sexual experience.[26]

Kinsey's researchers asked people about their sexual orientation in two ways: what were the psychological responses (attractions, fantasies) they had to others and what were the overt sexual behaviors in which they participated. The research results (later known as the Kinsey Scale) showed that sexual orientation actually falls on a continuum rather than on extreme ends of an exclusively heterosexual or homosexual scale. Not only was bisexuality a viable orientation, but when both psychological responses and overt behaviors were considered, most people fell within a range on the continuum. Making this concept even more interesting is the fact that it is "impossible to determine the number of persons who are 'homosexual or heterosexual.' It is only possible to determine how many persons belong at any particular time to each of the classifications on the scale."[27]

In other words sexual orientation can shift; it is not necessarily a permanent or fixed reality. In fact, other studies show that in cultures where variations in sexual orientation are acceptable, more people act within a wider sexual range.

Touch practitioners and all health care providers need to attune to sexual orientation in several ways. First and foremost is the issue of making assumptions about the sexual orientation of clients and colleagues. Such assumptions do not create safety for clients and peers, and, if assumptions cause clients to leave a core part of themselves out of the therapeutic experience, practitioners miss the opportunity to facilitate the client's healing. Secondly, if practitioners are uncomfortable with orientations other than their own, it is their professional responsibility to look at their biases so that they do not inadvertently cause harm to clients. Given the cultural legacy, initial discomfort about other orientations is inevitable. People who are comfortable with this issue have examined their inherited fears and beliefs and learned new ways to respond appropriately and with care.

" I was brought up to believe that how I saw myself was more important than how others saw me. "

—Anwar el-Sadat

Recognizing The Family as Sex Educator

How do people learn all these sexual myths and scripts? Books, friends, religion, subgroups and experience are all part of sex education. In this century the media bombards us with sexual messages. Recent research of sexual content on television in the United States revealed that more than half to two-thirds of prime-time shows contain sexual content, yet less than 10 percent refer to risks or responsibilities of sex. In one week 88 scenes of intercourse were depicted with almost half (47 percent) of these interactions between characters with no prior romantic relationship.[28] However, despite these other factors the most influential teacher of sexual concepts and attitudes is the family.

Although many people report that sex was never discussed in their family, the family still conveyed many beliefs and messages about sex and sexuality through example and by what was left unsaid. Authors Miriam and Otto Ehrenberg describe four family sex types that illuminate the sex education styles predominant in American culture.[29] In reading the descriptions, keep in mind that there are few "pure" nuclear families, so the definition of family can expand to include all those people who influence a child's upbringing. Also in any given family system there might be a combination of influences including parents, step-parents and perhaps grandparents.

What many people find when working with these models is that although different types might be represented in their family, usually one parent had more influence than the other and therefore shaped the predominant experience. Another common experience is that the family type shifted at different points in the family's life cycle or at different stages of a child's development.

> **Sex Repressive:** In this family type sex is seen by parents as inherently immoral, dirty and evil, so the family actively squelches sexuality in their children. Ironically, research has shown that children from these families are more likely to become sexually active than their peers but are less likely to use birth control and take other precautions since they feel ashamed and guilty.
>
> **Sex Obsessive:** This family type focuses on sex as a main issue to discuss, flaunt and emphasize. Rather than letting their child's sexuality unfold naturally there is a tendency to propel children into precocious sexual behavior. This family does not respect children's boundaries, rationalizes uninhibited behavior and projects adult needs into the parent/child relationship.
>
> **Sex Avoidant:** This family type is intellectually accepting of sex as a positive life experience, but emotionally uncomfortable with sex and sexuality. Generally, negative input is not present but neither is any real discussion. Typically, children may be given reading materials or permission to attend sex education class in school but parents do not follow up with their own input. As a result their children receive a double message about sex: it is okay but probably dangerous since no one wants to talk about it, and they are left to their own devices regarding decision-making.
>
> **Sex Expressive:** This family type understands sex as a life-enhancing force that is neither ignored nor emphasized. Parents are willing to talk openly about sex and set reasonable limits around their children's behavior. These children gain respect for their bodies and their sexuality, and because of this they tend to be sexually responsible.

The Impact of Family Patterns In A Therapeutic Setting

The categories above described by the Ehrenbergs are useful in making connections between practitioners' behaviors and their own family system patterns. Practitioners must

To put the world in order, we must first put the nation in order; to put the nation in order, we must put the family in order; to put the family in order, we must cultivate our personal life; and to cultivate our personal life, we must first set our hearts right.

—Confucius

understand how sex education affects the ways in which they relate to others, especially clients. Conversely, a client's background and history directly affects how she understands, communicates about and feels about the therapeutic experience.

Family patterns are important to recognize as a factor influencing the practitioner and client. Knowing the possible impact of family patterns can be useful in understanding the sexual dynamics in the therapeutic relationship. Consider the following possibilities:

> Practitioners from sexually obsessed family environments might be overly focused on sexuality and engage clients sexually. Those from sexually repressed backgrounds might judge sexual feelings they experience while giving or receiving treatments to be unacceptable and shameful; or, they might project, needlessly shaming a client who has legitimate sexuality concerns that need to be discussed. Practitioners from sex-avoidant backgrounds might notice, but choose to ignore, sexual aggression from clients and put themselves at risk. Sex-expressive backgrounds might help practitioners feel comfortable talking about a client's bodily responses to touch and set appropriate boundaries.

Through an awareness of family patterns, practitioners can respond consciously, professionally and ethically concerning sexuality in the treatment setting.

Sex and Touch Therapy

All humans are, by nature, sexual beings, therefore it is not possible to entirely keep sex and sexuality out of the treatment room. Biology equips people with a sexual nature to preserve and propagate the species. Every client and every practitioner brings their sexual nature and background with them into the therapeutic setting. The ultimate ethical challenge is to acknowledge the role of inherent sexuality in a milieu where sex is absolutely inappropriate. In other words, practitioners must allow sexuality and at the same time, de-sexualize the experiences of both giving and receiving hands-on therapy.

Cultural beliefs and personal experiences manifest in somatic therapy. By its nature, it breaks the cultural and personal taboos of touch. An ethical touch therapy treatment could be misinterpreted by a client because of her prior touch history. Physical intimacy may be confused as a prelude to sexual activity. If touch has been experienced only in sexual situations for a client, then touch therapy may mean sex to that person.

The location and atmosphere of a touch therapy session holds many potential cues. Depending on the treatment the specific factors that could allude to sex include: degrees of nudity; the manner of draping; the positioning of the client; the type of touch; lubricants such as oils and creams; and certain lighting. As one student aptly noted, the kind of smile on the practitioner's face can make a client aroused or scared or both.

Typically, the sexual nature of the client or practitioner is regarded only if something sexually inappropriate happens that requires ethical intervention. A reactive stance is insufficient. Diligence in ethical efforts, requires that practitioners be proactive in understanding human sexuality (both their own and that of their clients) and acting appropriately. Practitioners must always appreciate the impact that treatments can have on the sexual response, take full responsibility for how they are affected when performing their work, and remain keenly aware of the potential effects of touch on clients.

What we see depends
mainly on what we look
for.

—John Lubbock

Male somatic therapists are sometimes avoided by both men and women clients because of perceived danger or homosexual fears. Additionally, male therapists may be susceptible to subtle and overt seduction from female clients and may find themselves inappropriately responding to these clients. One reason for this stems from the cultural myth that women are not sexually aggressive so their overtures should be discounted and ignored. Another reason has to do with the socialization that men and women have received about how they relate. In a culture that assumes everyone is heterosexual, many of us were raised to see the other gender only in terms of romantic and sexual potential instead of as human beings. This dynamic pervades many daily non-sexual interactions. Women have also been told that their sexuality should be hidden and indirect and that flirting is permissible to express both interest and power. Men often unconsciously feel they must respond to a woman's flirting because otherwise their masculinity and sexuality might be questioned. Given all this, it is very possible for a male practitioner to discount a female client's sexual behavior as part of the cultural norm, neglect to set appropriate boundaries with her and then find himself in a compromising situation.

Female practitioners report having to deal with sexual innuendos, provocative jokes and aggression from their male clients. This may be due to sexual scripts men are taught. The social pressure to "act like a man" is interpreted by some men to mean they must project a secure, aggressive and sexual image. One way for men to assert a semblance of power is to appear sexually powerful whether or not they actually feel this way. Joking and bringing up sexual topics is for some men a form of flirting and an enactment of a cultural script. Male clients who have no harmful intent often use sexual jesting as an attempt to tolerate the intimacy of the therapeutic relationship, and to garner some control in a vulnerable setting. Because humor is often used socially to diffuse tension, in a situation where the tension is sexual, the humor often becomes sexualized.

Consider these situations: in most massage sessions, the client is nude (underneath the sheets/towel) or partially naked; in a shiatsu or acupressure session the client is fully clothed but is often lying on the floor rather than on a table, and the practitioner leans over and even straddles the client's body during the session; in acupuncture the client may be wearing varying degrees of clothing with the practitioner sticking needles into vulnerable places; in a physical therapy session the client is usually partially unclothed and in a vulnerable position; in some energy treatments there is more than one practitioner involved at a time; in an osteopathic session, the client may be fully clothed or asked to don an open-backed hospital gown; and many chiropractors set up their clinics with several tables in one room and the client receives a treatment in full view of others waiting for their appointments.

Many clients are surprised at and unprepared for the high level of intimacy (physical, emotional and verbal) that occurs in the therapeutic setting. Practitioners must be aware of the impact of the setting itself on the client. They must also consider reactive behaviors in that context.

Sexual Feelings During Treatment Sessions

Consider the following three observations:

- Clients often experience sexual feelings when receiving treatments.
- Practitioners often have sexual feelings when giving treatments.
- Many clients and practitioners are confused, ashamed, embarrassed and sometimes behave inappropriately in response to these feelings.

Many types of touch therapy provide a sensual experience. Unfortunately, while sensual originally meant "connection with the senses as opposed to the intellect," the concept has become associated with indulgence in the baser pleasures of the senses, licentiousness, brutishness and grossness.[30] Sensuality incorporates the awareness of bodily sensation, taking pleasure in sensation and utilizing sensation to be more fully present in our bodies. However, because of the family, cultural and religious beliefs discussed earlier, most people learn to tune out their body's sensations. Touch therapy often reawakens this awareness in clients and practitioners.

Sensuality and sexuality are not the same although they can occur on the same continuum. Sensual and sexual feelings are part of being a vital human being and are normal. Denial of sensual and sexual feelings is pervasive and dangerous. Staying personally (and culturally) unconscious, individuals are more likely to act in ways that are harmful to themselves and others. Ethical behavior, however, includes the ability to distinguish between feelings and actions. Experiencing a sensual or sexual feeling does not mean that a sexual behavior will or must automatically follow.

Given the nature of the sexual response, some clients experience sexual arousal regardless of the practitioner's behavior. Sexual arousal is in some ways distinct from attraction. Arousal is at times disembodied—not related to the particular individual a person is with at the moment but more as a result of other cues. At other times the arousal is based on a specific attraction to the other individual. Sorting out this distinction is helpful in understanding what is happening in the moment with a client. The practitioner's ethical responsibility is to respond non-sexually to the client and to eliminate any misunderstanding on the client's part as to the intent of the practitioner.

A practitioner is also likely to experience sexual arousal because of the personal nature of the work. Sometimes practitioners are personally more in tune with their physical responses.

Sexual talk, sexual relations, sexual acts and activities, sexual pleasures, sexual intercourse, or being involved in a sexual manner, is always unethical and must never occur in the professional relationship.

> One practitioner in supervision shared that he had experienced several attractions in one week: one with a client, one with his doctor and another with a salesperson. He was concerned about his lustiness. As he talked it was clear that none of his behavior was unethical and the feeling was probably in response to his ending a relationship in which he had felt sexually shutdown.

A sexual response can be completely bypassed under most circumstances. Or if a sexual response does occur, as long as the erotic energy is not entertained it is short-lived and the treatment continues with ethical safety. Regardless of the situation or circumstances, if sexual arousal does occur, on the part of either the practitioner or the client, it is always the practitioner's responsibility to establish and maintain appropriate boundaries.

Sexual Attraction to Clients

It is normal for sexual feelings to arise during a session or for practitioners to feel attracted to a client. The most ethical response at such a time is to acknowledge the feeling(s) to yourself, refocus on the client's needs, and after the session process the feelings by yourself or with a trusted colleague or supervisor. Unfortunately, many professionals react to the feelings with fear, shame, judgment, guilt and projection.

Others might indulge in fantasizing about the client during a session, which objectifies the client and results in being out of relationship with the client in that moment. If this happens, not only is the practitioner using the client for personal gratification, but he is also at risk for unethical behavior. Once the practitioner stops relating to the client as a person, it is easy to see the client as someone who can take care of the practitioner. If as a practitioner, you start to fantasize during a session, do not panic, just begin the refocusing steps described below.

One reason most practitioners avoid acknowledging sexual arousal and attraction is that it leads them into unfamiliar territory that the culture presents as dangerous and not to be explored. But it is more dangerous for both the client and practitioner to avoid these feelings. If sexual feelings or attractions occur, it is critical to distinguish what underlies the attraction and how to respond. These are some questions to ask yourself:

1. **WHAT IS THE QUALITY OF THE FEELING I'M HAVING?**
   Is it a fleeting, temporary feeling? Perhaps you were reminded of someone, or you like your client's hair. Often these initial responses are just part of being human and are nothing to worry about. They are not necessarily about the other person and do not need to be addressed with the client. What does matter is the extent you let yourself become distracted during the sessions as well as your ability to refocus on the client's needs.

   Is the attraction enduring or intense? Do you fantasize about a client? Is there a client with whom you want to have sex? Do you experience certain kinds or patterns of attractions to clients? For example, you find you always like middle-aged businessmen, or for the past six months you have been attracted to every married female client. These attractions may indicate personal needs or countertransference issues which should be dealt with in supervision. These are the situations which breed unethical behavior.

2. **DO I TREAT THIS CLIENT DIFFERENTLY IN SESSION THAN OTHER CLIENTS?**
   Feelings in themselves are not unethical, behaviors are. Changes in behavior can be as subtle as lingering with your hand or slipping past a normal boundary on a body part, or as blatant as engaging in sexual activity with the client. Practitioners rationalize their behavior by saying that the client initiated the behavior or propositioned the practitioner. In a therapeutic relationship the practitioner is ultimately responsible for all interaction with the client no matter who was the initiator. The practitioner is paid to know what behaviors and actions are beneficial or detrimental to a client whether that concerns giving a particular treatment or hugging and kissing a client.

3. **IS THIS ATTRACTION SO STRONG THAT I WANT TO PURSUE A RELATIONSHIP?**
   The complexity of this question requires time to thoughtfully consider all issues. Generally, this is a boundary practitioners should not break, especially if they are in a pattern of wanting to date clients. However, there may be the rare instance that the attraction is so strong that a therapeutic relationship is not feasible. First, you need to know if there are any laws in your state restricting practitioners in your field from dating former clients. If none exist, for ethical reasons it is useful to talk about the attraction to a trusted colleague or supervisor to assess the quality of the attraction and the underlying motivation.

Assuming that you and the client are free to pursue a relationship and you decide to do so, know that you first need to discontinue the client-practitioner relationship. A lapse of time is recommended between the last session and the first social activity. Practitioners have been reported by clients for sexual abuse in situations where a date occurred immediately after a session.

Never ask a client for a date during a session when he is vulnerable and you are in the power position. Be prepared that he may like you better as his practitioner and is not interested in dating you. You then must decide if it is possible to continue as his practitioner. And if you do continue, what will you do about the attraction and possible feelings of disappointment, rejection, anger or sadness that you might experience? The attraction may be so strong that it interferes with your role as a practitioner, or you may just feel awkward continuing in that role.

Erections In The Treatment Setting

Is there any other bodily function that is so misunderstood, revered or feared? While an erection is one of the most obvious indicators of physiological arousal, it does not necessarily mean that emotional or sexual desire is also present.

Men experience erections even when they are not necessarily emotionally desirous of sex (when they are afraid or need to urinate). Touch, itself, on any part of the body can stimulate a physiological response that results in a partial or complete erection. In a therapeutic setting spontaneous erections are often uncomfortable for practitioners and clients. The difficulty lies in that many practitioners are uncomfortable or fearful when a client has an erection response during a session.

Several realities shape female therapists' perceptions of erections. Many were raised with pervasive myths about erections: If you are with a man and he has an erection a) you have caused it and b) you are responsible for taking care of it. Additionally, having grown up in a culture rampant with sexual abuse and rape, erections are often associated with sexual violence. Intellectually, most women know this is not true but the cultural message may be powerful enough to derail rationality.

If a male therapist notices a male client having an erection, several issues should be considered. A man is not necessarily fearful of another man's erection unless he is being threatened or if it is perceived as a sexual come-on. Sometimes erections are even more disturbing to a male therapist if he responds by feeling aroused because then he may question his own orientation. Both male and female practitioners often either ignore erectile response or overreact, becoming passive or aggressive with the client in discussing the condition. Each of these responses puts the practitioner in a vulnerable position.

Ensure safety by obtaining sufficient information to discern the "intent" of the client's erection—whether it is merely a physiological response to touch or part of sexual desire. If a practitioner is verbally aggressive about the erection or hurts the client physically to quell the erection, the practitioner is abusing the client. Many practitioners learn in school to discourage erections by "pressing hard on certain points." There are more respectful, clear and safe ways to deal with erections in men and arousal in women.

Arousal in Women

It is difficult to know when female clients are sexually aroused. Early signs of sexual arousal include changes to the clitoris, labia and vaginal walls, but these are not obvious to a practitioner. Other changes such as nipple erection and skin flush could be non-sexual reactions to cold, soft tissue manipulation (increased blood flow to the skin) and nerve enervation. Besides, client arousal does not mean sexual intent.

Practitioners whose female clients had an orgasmic response on the table usually say they had no clue that the client was aroused until she made verbal comments (e.g., direct communication, moaning) or displayed nonverbal behaviors (e.g., breathing changes, muscular rigidity, strange movements) that alerted the practitioner to the arousal.

If you view all the things that happen to you, both good and bad, as opportunities, then you operate out of a higher level of consciousness.

—Les Brown

Remember that because of socialization practitioners are less suspect, thus less alert, to women who are sexually inappropriate within the context of a therapeutic relationship.

As well as being difficult to observe, female sexuality is often expressed much less directly than male sexuality. Be aware of female clients repeatedly exposing themselves during the treatment. One or two episodes may be an accident, poor boundaries or a lapse in judgement. It may be helpful to distinguish the context surrounding the behavior. What were the client's verbal cues? Did the client watch to see your reaction? With a sexually inappropriate client the number and intensity of behaviors usually escalate. Regardless of the reason, the practitioner needs to verbalize the physical boundary of draping at this time. A person with poor boundaries may seem like a well-adjusted individual comfortable with nudity while in actuality her lack of boundaries comes from a history of sexual abuse. You will probably never know. Taking a chance breaches the tenets of professional ethics.

Sometimes clients with an inappropriate attraction to the practitioner may sublimate or redirect those feelings by pumping the practitioner for personal information or giving gifts to the practitioner.[31] In this case the client is not aware of the attraction, which emphasizes the argument against accepting any gifts from clients. The client may also leave valuables and insist on seeing the practitioner when the valuables are retrieved. Some clients do know they are attracted to the practitioner and use the same above techniques to attract the attention of the practitioner. While all these examples of behaviors are inappropriate on some level, a more serious type of arousal expression during a treatment session is when a female client talks about her own sexuality or the practitioner's sexuality. This type of talk combined with other verbal or nonverbal requests or innuendos should not be ignored.

When To Address Erections and Arousal with Clients

When do practitioners need to talk to their clients about erections or arousal? The answer is simple: whenever the client or practitioner is uncomfortable. Once one party is uncomfortable the session is not going to be truly beneficial because the attention is diverted. There are several simple things to assess whenever an erection occurs:

- If a man has a partial or full erection, shows no signs of discomfort or embarrassment through verbal or nonverbal cues, and you are comfortable, it is not necessary to talk about it at the time.
- If a man has a partial or full erection and acts uncomfortable via nonverbal cues (body tension, flushed face), and although he has not been inappropriate in any way during the treatment (and even if you feel comfortable), then it is wise to talk with him to assuage his discomfort.
- If a man has a partial or full erection and has displayed other verbal and nonverbal behaviors during the session that seem to indicate sexual intent, then you are ethically obligated to talk with him immediately (using the Intervention Model described in the next section).

This is also the case for sexual arousal in women. It is of ethical importance to immediately talk with the client if she indicates sexual intent in verbal or nonverbal behaviors.

There is no recipe for dealing with the sexual arousal of a client. The action a practitioner takes depends on the client and circumstances. In any situation where a client indicates that arousal has occurred, the practitioner must determine, at that moment, the best way to handle the incident. When first aware of the situation, the practitioner must change what she is doing. The antidote to the parasympathetic response is activation of the sympathetic response. Actions such as changing tempo to a quicker pace and moderately increasing the pressure and depth of touch encourages sympathetic nervous system involvement. Move to a less risky area of the body, such as the upper extremity or the face and head. As long as the client does not indicate further sexual interest, give the client a minute or two to pass through this phase, since the arousal will likely subside, and she could continue without further arousal. In these cases it is often more appropriate not to discuss the situation at that time. Whether it is discussed after the session depends on the situation and the practitioner's sense that it is fitting and necessary. Discussing it may simply mean informing the client that arousal can be a short-lived physiological response that may occur, and that while it would never be acceptable to act on it, the incident was not interpreted by you as improper or unethical.

Both male and female practitioners need to be prepared for sexual arousal from both sexes and all sexual orientations. One proactive way to address the possibility of arousal and erection with clients is to include some basic written information in your client intake. If you model a healthy comfort level talking about all physiological changes a client might experience during a session, you have provided several things: an opening for the client to express concerns; an education for a client about how the body works; good boundaries; and a safe environment.

The Intervention Model

The Intervention Model is a communication model developed by Daphne Chellos,[32] for practitioners to use when verbal or nonverbal communication from a client is unclear or when practitioners feel their boundaries are being violated. For instance, a situation in which the client expresses sexual interest requires a clear, unequivocal response that this is an inappropriate interest. This model also applies when a client is having emotional reaction or release during a session, such as crying or expressing anger. The goal is to empower you as you use these steps as a guide (combined with your intuition), to assess situations and make decisions.

> *Important principles may, and must, be inflexible.*
>
> —Abraham Lincoln

The Intervention Model is based on basic, sound communication skills. Many practitioners already possess these skills and will find this model quite familiar. However, most practitioners are generally unprepared to address sexual issues in a somatic setting even if they have had counseling experience, sex education training and extensive professional training. Most do not practice discussing such complex, sensitive issues in the somatic setting. Role-playing situations in a school setting or with other practitioners is vital to prepare yourself so that you can feel confident when a questionable situation occurs.

The Intervention Model is a gender-free, orientation-free model. The same responses are utilized with both male and female clients. Sometimes this is a difficult concept to practice because people are socialized to communicate in different styles based on gender and other perceived differences.

Depending on the situation you may need to go through all the steps or stop after step one. Typically, steps one and two follow in that order but steps three through eight might be addressed in a different order, and some steps may not be included at all. Learn them all and then use your intuition and good judgment.

1. STOP THE TREATMENT USING ASSERTIVE BEHAVIOR:
Assertive behavior means that you address the client with body language congruent with what you say verbally. Make eye contact if possible (by doing this, you are both reminded

that you are dealing with a human being), stand in a relaxed yet grounded manner and use a firm voice. Do not shrink and get quiet (passive) or violate your client through yelling or touching inappropriately (aggressive).

Make sure the client is properly covered (i.e., redrape the body part being attended, adjust client's clothing/gown). This provides a literal boundary that reassures both client and practitioner. Additionally, if touch has contributed to a sexually aroused state, this ensures that you are stopping a cause of the stimulation.

Maintain safety. If the client's behavior feels intimidating do not stay too close to the table and position yourself so that you have easy access to your exit door. Leave immediately if the client actively threatens you.

2. **DESCRIBE THE BEHAVIOR(S):**
Respond directly to the client's verbal or nonverbal communication by stating the obvious. This sounds so simple that it borders on the ridiculous, but is actually difficult to do. When we see a behavior, our first impulse is to interpret it rather than describe it. Describing a behavior lets the client know you are paying attention without judging the behavior. Examples of this kind of communication are:
- "I notice you're tightening your muscle and grimacing when I pass over this area."
- "I am aware that you made a comment about my appearance, then made a sexual joke, and now you have an erection."

3. **CLARIFY THE CLIENT'S INTENT:**
Once you state the obvious, ask the client a direct question as a follow-up. Something simple like, "Tell me what's happening?" or "What are you experiencing?" allows the client to tell you what the behavior means. Some clients respond in a more straightforward manner about this than others depending on many factors, including their comfort level or their intent in receiving treatment.

Two cautionary reminders: resist answering for the client and wait for a clear answer. Often, when we are uncomfortable we tell someone what his experience is even if we asked him to tell us. Or we accept any answer even if the response does not give us any information, so that we stop having to talk about it. Either way, if the practitioner does not clarify the client's intent, she cannot accurately assess the situation and might put the client or herself in a difficult position.

4. **EDUCATE THE CLIENT:**
Some clients experience unexpected, disturbing emotional and physiological responses during a hands-on treatment. When this happens and we become aware of their concern, we can share information. For instance, an educative statement for a client who has an erection and has expressed embarrassment is, "Sometimes clients become aroused as a physiological response to touch. It is a normal body response."

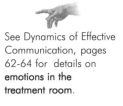

See Dynamics of Effective
Communication, pages
62-64 for details on
**emotions in the
treatment room**.

5. **RE-STATE YOUR INTENT:**
This statement addresses and clarifies the therapeutic contract so that client and practitioner feel safe. After an education statement (as in step #4) you might add, "It is never my intent to create sexual arousal during a session. If it happens and I am clear that your intent isn't for sexual inappropriateness either, then I'm comfortable in continuing the session if you are."

6. **CONTINUE OR DISCONTINUE THE SESSION AS APPROPRIATE:**
You should terminate the session of any client who has sexual intent or is behaving inappropriately. Remember, you do not need to go through all the above steps to exercise this option!

Set conditions if necessary and get the client to agree to them. Sometimes after going through all the above steps, a client's intent is still unclear to you. Perhaps she gave an answer that sounded good but felt incongruous to you and you are left uncertain. Let the client know that you will continue this session but will stop if she behaves in any way that does not work for you.

7. **REFER CLIENT TO OTHER PROFESSIONALS AS APPROPRIATE:**

This step is usually done after the session is complete. If it becomes obvious that a client could benefit by receiving other professional help such as a psychotherapist, counselor, or other medical practitioner, give this information to the client when he is fully dressed and alert.

8. **DOCUMENT THE SITUATION:**

After the client leaves, document the occurrence and obtain supervision or peer support. Difficult communication with a client often evokes ethical questions and safety concerns. An objective person provides a reality check, or needed emotional support. Remember that client confidentiality must be honored unless you fear for the safety of yourself or someone else. Documenting the situation and what you did to address the matter is vital should a client decide to lodge a complaint against you. Showing that you also sought out supervision to address the issue indicates your commitment to ethics and professionalism.

Sexual Misconduct

The problem of sexual misconduct has been with us for millennia. The topic was addressed by the Greek physician Hippocrates in 400 B.C.E.: the Hippocratic Oath that members of the medical profession continue to use today. The key section as it pertains to sexual misconduct is: "Whatever house I may visit, I will come for the benefit of the sick, remaining free of all intentional injustice, of all mischief, and in particular, of sexual relationships with both female and male persons."[36] Similar admonishments to doctors, warning them against inappropriate sexual behavior toward their clients, are found in European medical texts dating from the Middle Ages and Renaissance.

Sexual misconduct is not limited to sexual relations with a client. Sexual misconduct occurs when the fiduciary aspect of the therapeutic relationship is compromised. A continuum of behavior exists from sexual impropriety to sexual violation. This continuum goes all the way from: looking at a client in a seductive way; making subtle comments; engaging in obvious verbal and physical flirtatious behavior; to inappropriate touching and sexually-related behavior. Allegations of sexual misconduct create casualties on all sides: practitioners lose their licenses, practices or reputations; clients are traumatized by inappropriate or abusive behavior, or behavior that they perceive as abusive; and health care professions are publicly humiliated or singled out for unflattering media attention. This impacts all somatic practitioners, whether you work in the service industry, health profession or spa industry. Sexual misconduct complaints apply to employers, employees, practitioners, consumers, co-workers, teachers and students. A comprehensive, even exhaustive, exploration of this and related topics is presented in the book *Sexual Abuse by Professionals: A Legal Guide*.[33]

Statistics on the subject reveal that 70 percent of sexual misconduct complaints against health practitioners are filed by female clients against male practitioners. Approximately 20 percent are from female clients complaining about female practitioners. Of the remaining 10 percent of complaints, roughly five percent are from male clients bringing

See Ethical Principles, pages 14-15, for details on **fiduciary responsibility**.

See Business Ethics, pages 196-207, for information on **legal issues**.

allegations against women. Females, therefore, make up about 90 percent of the victims of sexual misconduct and 25 percent of the perpetrators. Many of those working in the field "have speculated that male victims of practitioners of either gender are underrepresented across the board because of particular male characteristics inhibiting both recognition and reporting [of abuse]."[37]

Examining The Roots of Sexual Misconduct

Sexual misconduct is a very complex problem, encompassing issues of sex, gender, power and communication. Sexual misconduct is the result of the blatant disregard of ethics, boundaries and genuine care for the client. Perpetrators of such behavior may do so because of psychopathology, ignorance or a period of weakness brought on by unusual circumstances. Although most reported sexual misconduct is committed by males, female practitioners also commit acts of sexual misconduct.

Sociopaths prey on others to satisfy their own needs; they are not inconvenienced by social, ethical or legal considerations. Such a person could be involved in multiple cases of sexual misconduct or other inappropriate behavior throughout their lives. Sexual predators in the health care field are known to have had sexual contact with many of their clients throughout their careers, often with several individuals during the same time span. Reason, education or peer pressure have little or no effect on the sexual predator.

Most practitioners cannot imagine themselves or their colleagues being sexually inappropriate with a client. Unfortunately documented legal proceedings prove otherwise. For instance consider the following cases taken from court transcripts.

A male massage therapist in the process of performing a full-body massage on a 20 year-old female client pulled down the client's bra and proceeded to massage her breasts and nipples. He asked her if she enjoyed his massaging her breasts and nipples to which she responded "no." He started to massage her legs and worked his way upward. Without her consent he removed her underwear and massaged her vagina. The client attempted to turn over on her stomach to stop the therapist from massaging her vagina. The respondent penetrated her vaginally and anally with his finger while alternately massaging her back, shoulders and buttocks. During the session, the client was covered from the waist up by a sheet. However, the massage therapist continually adjusted the sheet that was to cover her from the waist down so that it was "half on, half off." The massage therapist claimed that he touched the clients' breasts and genitals because she had not specifically indicated those body parts on his intake form on which he specifically asked, "What areas of your body would you prefer not to be worked on." The recommendation of the hearing was that his license to practice massage therapy be revoked and a $1,000 fine be imposed.[34]

Ignorance is another root of sexual misconduct. Slowly progress is being made through the increase of knowledge and education. Many individuals have no idea that casual sex with their clients or students is wrong. They did not receive the education to lead them to an understanding of ethics, boundaries and appropriate conduct with those in their care. These individuals may have engaged in sexual relationships with their teachers, supervisors or health care providers in the past and are repeating learned behaviors. In other cases these individuals were in environment(s) where this type of behavior was commonplace.

> A patient, his wife and daughter went to a chiropractor for treatments. The patient and his wife had difficulty in their marriage because of his wife's severe back injuries which interfered with sexual activity. The chiropractor began having an affair with the wife during scheduled treatment sessions for which he issued bills and was paid. The chiropractor was sued for malpractice by the wife's husband.[35]

It is possible the chiropractor realized that an affair with a client was unethical, but he chose to take the risk with the wife, never dreaming that the husband would file suit. Unethical behavior often leads to other unforeseen complications. In general when given the proper education and training, practitioners learn that sexual relationships with clients are destructive and inappropriate and in the future refrain from acting upon sexual urges.

Practitioners who find themselves in a period of weakness brought on by unusual circumstances may know what is the right thing to do but have difficulty behaving appropriately anyway. For example, an individual who has suddenly lost his spouse through an accidental death may be so distraught, confused and vulnerable that rational behavior becomes nearly impossible. Many people have experienced times in their lives when for one reason or another all rationality was gone and satisfying one's immediate needs was all that mattered. This is not to excuse inappropriate behavior on the part of such practitioners, only to view it in context. These individuals may have inappropriate sexual contact with clients once or twice over their entire lifetime at these particular times of crisis. They need strong personal and professional support systems. If these practitioners receive the appropriate assistance at the time of crisis, they are less likely to inflict pain on others.

The Sexual Misconduct Continuum

As stated, the boundary violations that constitute sexual misconduct do not necessarily involve sexual intercourse between the practitioner and the client. The more common improprieties are: gestures or expressions that are seductive or sexually demeaning to a client; failure to ensure a client's privacy (e.g., improper draping, not providing a gown); sexual comments about a client's body or clothing; sexualized or sexually demeaning comments to a client; off-color jokes; strong interest in or disapproval of the client's sexual orientation; comments made during a treatment or consultation about sexual performance; conversation initiated by the practitioner about sexual problems, preferences or fantasies of the practitioner or client; unnecessary examinations or treatments; the practitioner not obtaining informed consent to work on the breast or pelvic area; and inappropriate touching.

Sexual violations often involve actual sexual contact: encouraging the client to masturbate in the presence of the practitioner or masturbation by the practitioner while the client is present; intercourse; doing inappropriate work (e.g., touching breasts for any purpose other than therapeutic treatment; performing intra-anal coccygeal adjustments without gloves); or in the most extreme case — rape. Regarding sexual contact or intercourse, it does not matter whether initiated by the client or the practitioner. It is ultimately the practitioner's responsibility.

Analyzing Risk Factors

The following questionnaire was developed by Ben Benjamin, PH.D. and Angelica Redleaf, D.C.[39] This questionnaire informs you about the clarity of your professional/sexual boundaries. If you answer these questions as honestly as you can, you get an accurate risk factor assessment. No one need see this but you.

> " You never find yourself until you face the truth. "
> —Pearl Bailey

Risk Factors Questionaire

Place a check next to the number (1, 2, or 3) of the statement that applies to you. When you have completed the questionnaire, add up all of the numbers that are the same.

1 ____ I want a particular client to like me.
1 ____ I like it when my clients find me attractive, but I keep this to myself.
2 ____ Sometimes I schedule the clients that I really like last so that I can spend more time with them.
2 ____ I tend to accept gifts or favors from a specific client without examining why the gift was given.
2 ____ I have a barter arrangement with a client that is sometimes a source of tension for me.
3 ____ I engaged in sexual contact with one or more of my clients.
1 ____ I attended professional or social events at which I knew that a client would be present.
2 ____ A specific client often invites me to social events and I don't feel comfortable saying yes or no.
2 ____ Sometimes when I'm working on clients, I feel like the contact is sexualized for myself and maybe for the clients.
2 ____ There's something I like about being alone in the office with specific clients when no one else is around.
3 ____ A client is very seductive and I often don't know how to handle it.
2 ____ I invited clients to public or social events.
1 ____ I find myself cajoling, teasing and joking a lot with clients.
3 ____ I allow clients to comfort me.
3 ____ Sometimes I feel like I'm in over my head with a particular client.
2 ____ I feel overly protective of some clients.
3 ____ I sometimes drink or use recreational drugs with clients.
3 ____ I do more for a specific client than I would for any other client.
2 ____ I find it difficult to keep from talking about certain clients with people close to me.
2 ____ I find myself saying a lot about myself with some clients—telling stories, engaging in peer-like conversation.
3 ____ I call a specific client a lot and go out of my way to meet with him/her in locations convenient to him/her.
2 ____ I invite clients to my home.
3 ____ I often tell my personal problems to clients.
3 ____ I enjoy exercising my power over some of my clients.
3 ____ I am going through a crisis at this point in my life.
3 ____ If a client consents to sex, it's okay.
2 ____ I am surprised by how much I anticipate a particular client's visit.
2 ____ I frequently think about a particular client.
1 ____ I haven't been in a relationship in a long time.
1 ____ I feel lonely much of the time, unless I'm working.
2 ____ I have trouble asking certain clients to pay my full fee.
1 ____ I talk about my personal life to my clients.
2 ____ I find myself working weekends to accommodate a few clients whom I like.
1 ____ I notice that some of my clients are very dependent on me.
2 ____ I feel under tremendous personal/professional pressure and I'm afraid I might burn out.
1 ____ I like it when my clients look up to me.
2 ____ I feel like I've very little to give lately.
2 ____ My relationship with my significant other isn't meeting my needs.
3 ____ I've touched clients in inappropriate ways at times.
3 ____ I've had sex with clients.
3 ____ I've had sex with clients in the office.
2 ____ I dress exceptionally well when I know a particular client has an appointment that day.
2 ____ I fantasize about what it would be like to have sex with some of my clients.
2 ____ I'm not charging one or more of the clients to whom I'm attracted.
2 ____ I have some of my clients take off more of their clothes than needed.
2 ____ I sometimes sneak looks as clients are undressing.
2 ____ I feel it's okay to date clients.
2 ____ I sometimes tell dirty jokes to my clients.
2 ____ I like doing work on those areas of clients' bodies that are close to their erogenous zones.
1 ____ I feel totally comfortable socializing with clients.
2 ____ I compliment clients when I think they look nice.
1 ____ Some clients feel more like friends.
2 ____ I often tell my personal problems to one or more of my clients.
2 ____ I feel sexually aroused by one or more of my clients.
3 ____ I'm waiting to dismiss a particular client so that we can become romantically involved.
2 ____ To be honest, I think that goodbye hugs last too long with one or more of my clients.
2 ____ The appointments with one or more of my clients regularly last longer than with others.

Totals: 1 ____   2 ____   3 ____

If you have checked off one or more Number 3, you are at the highest risk level. You are in danger of violating professional boundaries. Not only can this damage clients, but could also damage your career. Asking for professional help from a psychotherapist or a consultant would be a good idea. You may also benefit from attending professional trainings in the area of personal and professional boundaries. Ignoring such a high risk level can result in serious consequences.

If you checked off more than three Number 2, you have the potential to move into a higher risk category at any time, especially when stressed.

If you checked off between four and eight Number 2, you have entered a risk factor that is heading toward possible danger. You could use some help getting yourself on track concerning professional boundaries.

If you checked off more than five Number 1, you could be overstepping your professional boundaries. You may not be in danger of crossing a sexual boundary, but you may be crossing other boundaries in your professional relationships.

Breaking the Silence

Health care recipients used to keep silent about improper behavior. Today they are speaking out in record numbers. Until very recently, the complaint process has been little-known, little-used and far from impartial. To quote the organizers of the Third International Conference on Sexual Exploitation by Health Professionals, Psychotherapists and Clergy, "The tendency is to shoot the messenger, blame the victim, and coddle the man."[38] However, the number of complaints are expected to increase as clients become less afraid of complaining, as awareness of the complaint process rises, and as the process itself becomes fairer and less humiliating for the person filing charges.

In reality, clients' complaints serve as the major factor in monitoring the behavior and regulation of practitioners. Women, especially, are increasingly sensitive to inappropriate behavior on the part of either male or female practitioners. In the treatment setting, as in greater society, they have taken the lead in the fight against abuse, misconduct and harassment.

Marshaling evidence to prove sexual misconduct malpractice is difficult because the actions often occur behind closed doors and proof becomes a matter of the word of the victim against that of the alleged perpetrator. Tangible evidence of the boundary violation can include cards, letters, diaries, journals, gifts, receipts for meals, phone records, answering machine tapes, photos, videotapes, appointment books and self-disclosures by the victim to friends and relatives.

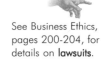

See Business Ethics, pages 200-204, for details on **lawsuits**.

Widespread education about ethical behavior is necessary to prevent the next generation of health practitioners from compromising their clients' welfare and the public trust. That training already has begun in some schools. As for the current practitioners whose education included no substantive training in sexuality, ethics, communication and other important skills—it is never too late to learn.

The health care market is an increasingly consumer-driven health care market. Practitioners who develop a strong sense of awareness of their own attitudes and behavior cultivate a wide range of skills in interpersonal communication, and adopt office procedures with their clients (especially their female clients) in mind, are far more likely to become or remain successful—as well as to prevent unnecessary difficulties for themselves and their clients.

Sexual Harassment

Somatic practitioners often work in group practices or other health care offices. They must not only be aware of sexual misconduct in the treatment setting, they must be aware of sexual harassment in the work environment as well. Both sexual misconduct and sexual harassment create significant problems in a health care practice. The two issues are not identical, but they are closely related; each is a boundary violation occurring when one person's "safe space" is invaded by another. The laws and professional regulations regarding sexual misconduct are still in a state of flux. For a hint as to where they are likely headed, we examine the more fully evolved body of law and regulations relating to sexual harassment.

Sexual harassment generally involves the behavior of a supervisor, manager, employer, or employee toward staff at the same or a lower level of power. An understanding of this issue is vital to all health care practitioners.

Sexual harassment is an issue arising in a workplace or an educational institution. It generally involves one person having power over another's employment, money, grades or advancement and abusing that power though sometimes it instead involves harassment by a co-worker. There are two recognized forms of sexual harassment:

1. *Quid pro quo* (Latin term meaning an equal exchange or substitution, "this for that"): a demand for sexual favors in exchange for job benefits;
2. Hostile work environment: unwelcome acts such as physical or verbal conduct, or visual displays, that make the individual's job difficult.

The U.S. Equal Employment Opportunity Commission (EEOC) defines sexual harassment as "unwelcome sexual advances, requests for sexual favors and other verbal or physical conduct of a sexual nature" when:

- submission to such conduct is made a term or condition of an individual's employment, either implicitly or explicitly;
- submission to or rejection of such conduct is used as a basis for employment decisions affecting such individual;
- such conduct has the purpose or effect of unreasonably interfering with an individual's work performance or creating an intimidating, offensive or hostile work environment.

Sexual harassment can be in the form of physical contact, such as touching, hugging and stroking. Verbal sexual harassment includes inappropriate ways of addressing a person, use of sexually explicit language, or use of words that refer to an individual's body parts. It can also be visual, such as displaying "girlie" or "hunk" calendars or other visually explicit material, regardless of whether that material is intended to offend. The intent of these actions is difficult to determine. A determination of intent is not necessary to a finding of sexual harassment. Heavier penalties are usually exacted in cases where the intent to offend is established.

A finding of quid pro quo sexual harassment requires that a plaintiff prove that receiving job benefits or protection from job detriments was dependent upon his or her submission to a supervisor's unwelcome sexual demands.

A hostile work environment claim generally requires that a plaintiff prove a pattern of offensive behavior—unless the one incident was especially outrageous. A single use of offensive language, or a single hug or bump in the hallway, is not sufficient. A hostile work environment claim must prove two things: 1) subjectively, the individual had to regard the behavior as sexual harassment; and 2) another reasonable person would also regard this incident or behavior as sexual harassment.

The "reasonable person" measure has been modified in recent years in recognition of the fact that some material, speech or behavior that is considered outrageous by most women is regarded as acceptable by many men. Instead of a "reasonable person," therefore, a "reasonable woman" standard has been substituted by the courts in some male-female harassment cases.

An institution's liability is established when the employer has had direct or legal notice of any of these types of sexual harassment and failed to take immediate and appropriate action. The major factors courts and enforcement agencies consider in determining liability are: the nature of the conduct; the frequency and openness of the conduct; and whether it could easily have been avoided by the victim.

Sexual harassment is perpetrated by the same gender as well as cross-gender. In a March 4, 1998, decision, the U.S. Supreme Court unanimously ruled that "federal law protects employees from being sexually harassed in the workplace by the same sex."[40]

Comparing Similarities Between Misconduct and Harassment

ABUSE OF POWER

Sexual misconduct and sexual harassment are similar in that each generally involves a person of greater power taking advantage of a person of lesser power. "Sexual harassment is particularly volatile because it often fuses two levels of power: the power of employers over employees and the power of men over women....It is the confusion of public and private, bringing together two arenas of men's power over women. Not only are men in positions of power in the workplace, but we are socialized to be the sexual initiators and to see sexual prowess as a confirmation of masculinity," writes Michael Kimmel of SUNY Stonybrook, a sociologist and leader in men's studies.[41] His words about male-female sexual harassment apply just as well to sexual misconduct in the therapeutic relationship because the practitioner holds greater power in the dynamic etween the practitioner and client.

See Ethical Principles, pages 15-17, for details on the **power differential**.

POSSIBLE ABSENCE OF INTENT

Sexual misconduct and harassment also are similar in that each often arises out of a lack of awareness of what kinds of behavior are offensive or even harmful. In other words, the intent to harass may be absent from the perpetrator's conduct. As a result preventive measures for sexual misconduct and sexual harassment also are quite similar: Both practitioners and consumers need to learn ways of prevention that safeguards those people with whom we work and those with whom we are involved in health care relationships.

Prevention Strategies

Strategies for preventing sexual harassment or sexual misconduct include the following:

- Obtain training to facilitate an understanding of the power of roles.
- Gain an understanding of the impact of one's own sexuality and the sexuality of those with whom one interacts professionally.
- Learn appropriate ways of behaving around and of communicating with both genders.
- Discover what behaviors are considered unacceptable.
- Determine the types of situations that may lead to such transgressions.
- Ascertain the effects of abuse and harassment.
- Understand the potential legal and financial consequences of unacceptable behavior.

Experience is a good teacher, but her fees are very high.

—W.R. Inge

Steps to take to help prevent sexual harassment by supervisors or co-workers are:

- Develop and post a policy against harassment.
- Teach employees what constitutes harassment.
- Improve morale and productivity.
- Address complaints before they develop into litigation.
- Establish an effective and confidential complaint process.

Desexualizing the Touch Experience

Health care professionals are responsible for creating and maintaining a safe environment for clients and themselves. Practitioners benefit from extensive training in the physical and emotional effects and ramifications of touch. Many practitioners are often painstaking in their efforts to cultivate and enrich their clients' physical well-being, being ever mindful of the indications, precautions and contraindications for treatment. In some cases practitioners are also conscientious about their clients' emotional condition and spiritual well-being as well as the client's physical status. Although these measures help keep treatments physically and emotionally safe, they do not address ethical safety.

Practitioners must ensure that the touch experience is not sexualized. A sexually safe treatment environment provides much more than the assurance that a practitioner does not flirt with, attempt to date, or sleep with a client.

The term DESEXUALIZE is best defined by examining its opposite, SEXUALIZE. **Sexualizing** means making an event, procedure, conversation or experience into something that is sexual or could be interpreted as sexual.[42] Desexualizing, then, means ensuring that the treatment is **not** in any way turned into a sexual experience for either the practitioner or the client. While the terms **sex** and **sexuality** share a common root in their meanings, as discussed earlier, their differences are significant in the therapeutic setting.

Practitioners are naive if they believe that correct intentions and acting professionally guarantee the absence of inappropriate expressions of sexuality in treatment sessions. The ethically safe touch experience does not just happen; it must be created, structured and sustained. Structuring safety means at all times proactively demonstrating absolute professionalism in all practice aspects, particularly around the connections between sex and touch. It also means being prepared to deal with the physiological reactions of arousal if they occur. The following suggestions apply to practitioners of both gender.

- Observe and know yourself. Be aware of your own tendencies toward flirtation and notice the times and places where you sexualize an event or conversation. Consider how you come across and the messages you transmit to others, especially clients. Take time to think about your work environment and your approach with clients. Ask yourself, "Is there anything about me or my work space, or that I say or do, that is likely to be sexualized?" For instance, your client is experiencing tension and is holding her breath. As you coach your client to breathe more fully you begin to make slight sighing sounds with your mouth close to the client's ear. The client may misconstrue this as a sexual overture.
- Be clear about your own intentions toward your clients. Your clients are not candidates for your romantic interest or sexual pursuits, and you must be steadfast in this rule. Sexual contact with a client before, during or after a treatment session or during the course of treatments is never appropriate. If you want to date a client and the feeling is mutual, realize this is a very precarious situation and that you are inviting potential

problems, the very least of which is the development of unethical patterns in your client interactions. Always seek guidance for this issue with a mentor, supervisor or professional consultant so that you can make decisions responsibly and with full recognition of the possible ramifications. If a romantic relationship is pursued, first terminate the professional relationship. Never be in the position of being a client's therapist as well as his new suitor. Being clear about and adhering to your own boundaries sets limits for your clients and diffuses the erotic energy. Create guidelines under which you enter into dual relationships with a client. If you wish to engage in a romantic relationship, specify the minimum time between terminating the therapeutic relationship and beginning a social relationship. Some disciplines cover this in their conduct codes.

- Establish ethical touch safety at the initial contact. Do not wait until new clients arrive for their appointments to discover if they are ethically appropriate. Determine their intentions and goals for the treatment when you first talk with them to set up the appointment (either on the phone or in person). Assess them by their demeanor, language and approach as to whether they are seeking non-sexual treatment. Ask questions such as, "Why are you seeking this course of treatment?" and "What are your goals for this session?" If they remain vague and obscure, inform them directly that the treatment you offer is "therapeutic and non-sexual." This is especially critical in the massage and bodywork professions and particularly so when doing out-call or residential massage for a new, unknown client, either at a hotel or the client's home. (Telephone screening is more difficult when a receptionist answers calls.) Beyond determining that they are not seeking sexual services, it is wise to ensure your own ethical and physical safety. For instance, in the client's presence, place a telephone call to a friend (or the concierge if at a hotel) and tell that person where you are, when you expect to be done, and that you will call back when the session is over. If possible, avoid setting up your treatment table in a bedroom unless you are working with an injured or ill client.

- Maintain a professional appearance and demeanor. Dress appropriately when you give treatments, avoiding provocative or revealing attire.

- Establish a professional treatment space. Sight, sound, smell, touch and imagination all have the potential to arouse. Desexualize your work space by providing a professional atmosphere that communicates clear boundaries in all regards. If the area you use for sessions is a spare bedroom in your home, remove all bedroom furniture. Declare your treatment table a sacred healing space and do not pursue sexual interests with anyone, even your mate, on your table. Clarity about your role during a session, regardless of who is the recipient of your work, allows you to secure your professional boundaries, making you less likely to give mixed signals to clients. This also fosters your mate's trust and appreciation of the professional nature of your work.

- Choose appropriate music. If the use of music is customary in your particular discipline, make certain it is soothing, without being sensual or romantic. Music containing lyrics about lovemaking or instrumental music that sounds seductive give mixed messages about the intention of the session.

- Establish a pre-treatment thinking process. Ask yourself the following questions before working with a client: Is this course of treatment necessary? Am I the right person to do this? Should someone else be in the room? Would I do this if this client wasn't attractive to me?

The value of an idea lies in the using of it.
—Thomas A. Edison

See Ethical Practice
Management, pages
165-167, for details on
informed consent.

- Provide Informed Consent. Before the first treatment begins, always inform the client about what you intend to do for the treatment protocol so she knows what to expect. Take her into the treatment space and discuss the session scenario. Explain whether you will begin prone or supine, the anticipated sequence of where you will work, how she will be draped and any other pertinent details. Repeat this process whenever there's a major change in the treatment procedure or the areas you work on. Invite the client to have a third party present, particularly during sensitive procedures, when working on minors or if the client has any history of abuse.

- Allow privacy. Regardless of how well you know the person, always allow him complete privacy while changing. Some clients begin undressing before you have a chance to leave the room. In these instances ask them to wait and leave promptly. Remember, they are not responsible for setting professional boundaries, you are.

- Use appropriate language. Strive for professional ways to communicate about your work. Realize that what you say may be interpreted differently from what you mean, and avoid language that could be sexualized. For instance, acupuncturists might want to refrain from using a phrase such as "sticking in a needle" and instead say something with less emotional charge like "gently apply a needle." In a massage therapy setting instead of using misleading and suggestive terms such as "full-body massage," describe it as a "full-hour relxation treatment," or use other terminology which accurately explains the treatment. Also, consider using the phrase "residential treatment" when talking about "house calls." All practitioners need to be thoughtful when referring to certain anatomical parts avoiding suggestive terms. Obvious examples of this are using clinical terminology such as "gluteal area" versus "butt," and "inguinal area" or "groin" instead of "crotch." Less obvious, though, are phrases that can be suggestive. For example, direct clients to "move your feet apart," versus "move your legs apart" or "open your legs." When making comments to a client about his body, avoid statements containing sexual innuendo (e.g., Wow! You really look great!) or statements that refer to anything other than what is related to the treatment.

- While it is essential to report objective findings that are related to physical well-being, refrain from commenting about matters such as weight gain or loss and other appearance issues, especially when a client is on the table (unless that is part of your agreed-upon treatment). When you make such comments, it fosters the notion that you are observing his body in a judgmental way, and can make a client feel like a bug under a microscope. Also, comments that sound like compliments are commonly misinterpreted as flirtation. If a client thinks you are flirting and he happens to become sexually aroused during the treatment, he may become confused about the intentions of the treatment and be inclined to pursue sexual interest. Awareness of cultural language helps you to avoid colloquialisms. For instance, in some areas, calling people "honey" is commonplace and rather endearing, yet many find the expression demeaning.

- If your treatment requires clients to partially or fully disrobe, always use proper draping techniques. While clients have clear choice about what to wear under the draping linen so they are comfortable (e.g., underclothes, shorts, swimwear), proper draping is not optional. If a client insists on forgoing the draping linen, explain that you are more comfortable when draping is used, and that in the interest of your professionalism, draping techniques are used with all clients. Offer to adjust the room temperature, turn on a fan, or uncover her feet if she claims to feel too warm. Ensure that draping is secure and doesn't allow "drafts" or partial exposure of areas intended to be draped.

- Be mindful of body contact during the session. Beyond using proper body mechanics, pay attention to how you brace, support and lean. Be conscious of where your body may contact the client's body during your strokes, manipulation, stretches and other techniques. Avoid contacting the client with areas other than your extremities. Maintain a professional posture and stance throughout the session. Even accidentally allowing your genital or breast to touch or brush against a client can be quite unnerving. Consider the following example of how a client can perceive an action as a subtle sexual contact: A chiropractor performs a manipulation on a client's back. While standing at the client's head, the practitioner unconsciously leans over allowing her pelvis to come in contact with the top of the client's head.

- Prevent straying strokes or movements. When working areas such as the medial thigh, ischial tuberosity, the sacrum, or the subclavicular/pectoral area, strokes must not stray, even accidentally. The slightest "slip" in these areas is invasive and inappropriate, and could give the client the wrong message about your intentions.

- Diffuse any hints or signs of sexual arousal immediately. Teach yourself and your staff what behaviors are unacceptable. You should know what to do if you find yourself becoming sexually stimulated when a client is on your table.

- Be aware and in control. Honor your clients' boundaries as well as your boundaries. Pay attention to where your mind and eyes are wandering. Honest awareness of your state is the first step in this process if you are experiencing sexual arousal. Conscious recognition, along with an ethical self-pep-talk, may be enough to distract you and interrupt the response. Put the client's welfare ahead of your personal needs. Regain focus and control by: changing the approach; moving to a less risky body region; and directing thoughts to the clinical perspective of the work. If this happens with more than one client, or repeatedly with the same client, seek support for the issue by consulting with a mentor, supervisor or professional consultant.

- Keep accurate records. Document whenever a client does anything questionable (e.g., flirts, sends inappropriate correspondence, gives you improper gifts). Write a summary of the impropriety as though it were to be read in court or before a board. Include the basic details, how you handled it, and the names, dates and telephone numbers of other professionals with whom you discussed this (such as a peer supervision group).

- Participate in ongoing supervision. Seek help immediately from a supervisor, colleague or other professional if you find yourself overly attracted to a client or are in a vulnerable situation.

- Inform your clients of their rights. Develop and post a Policy Statement. Address client complaints and dissatisfaction promptly, before they develop into litigation.

- Treat all clients equally, regardless of age, gender or attractiveness. Be particularly careful of extending special considerations or expressions of endearment that you wouldn't ordinarily give to anyone else. For example, a physical therapist was treating a client who disclosed personal information about a recent death of a loved one. At the conclusion of a treatment session, touched by the client's disclosure, the therapist gently kissed the client's forehead. While the kiss was well-meaning, the gesture could easily be misinterpreted and the therapist could be charged with sexual misconduct.

- Commit to continued education, particularly in the areas of ethics, boundaries and communications skills.

See Appendix A, pages 257-262, for a **Client Bill of Rights** and sample **Policy Statements**.

In Conclusion...

Sexuality is a natural part of the human experience. By recognizing this fact, somatic practitioners can consciously choose to create a professional treatment space, to maintain clear boundaries, and to deal ethically and compassionately with unintended sexual responses. They can also protect themselves and their clients from sexually inappropriate or damaging behavior. Through an awareness of the physical, social and cultural dynamics and a knowledge of behavioral strategies, practitioners can enhance their effectiveness as a safe, healing presence in the treatment setting.

Chapter Highlights

- The differences between sex, touch and intimacy are often confused.
- Touch is a basic human need and a sensory process that also communicates.
- By the time we reach adulthood many of us have actually forgotten *how* to touch, after having lived through years of "hands off" indoctrination.
- The sensation of touch begins in the womb.
- Many cultural statistics show that children who are welcomed with lots of physical touch and tactile stimulation tend to grow into well-adjusted, capable and loving adults.
- Numerous studies show that for lower and higher mammals, receiving touch that is pleasurable, safe and appropriate reduces sickness, depression and aggressive behaviors.
- Touch is a relaxing and pleasurable experience (*parasympathetic nervous system response*) if the stimulus is soothing and welcome, or an anxiety-provoking and upsetting one (*sympathetic nervous system response*), if the stimulus is perceived as threatening.
- Many factors contribute to a client's interpretation of the meaning of a specific touch during a treatment. They include: what parts of the body were involved; the duration and pressure of touch; whether an observer was present; whether there was movement after contact was made; and how well the practitioner is known and trusted.
- A practitioner needs to be attuned to the verbal and nonverbal communication a client gives regarding touch. They may reveal important information about a client's prior experiences with touch.
- There are many gender differences around touch.
- There is much fear and misunderstanding about sexual orientation in many cultures.
- The gender of the practitioner and the client can influence how touch is interpreted.
- Let your clients know what kind of touch to expect during each treatment and ask permission to proceed with the kind of touch described.
- Clients always need to be given the option of saying "no" to a touch.
- The three different types of intimacy are physical (affectionate and sexual touch), emotional (feelings of closeness, tolerance and support) and verbal (disclosure of emotions, feelings and opinions).
- Appropriate intimacy for any therapeutic relationship is a one-way intimacy: somatic practitioners touch clients and offer them support both verbally and physically. However, the personal life and the feelings of the professional shouldn't be discussed.
- The association of sex and the touch professions in the mind of the consumer is perpetrated by the media. Awareness of this social construct assists practitioners in de-sexualizing the therapeutic session.
- The term "sexuality" encompasses biological (anatomy and physiology), psychological (thoughts, feelings and values) and cultural (family, society and religious) influences.
- The three aspects of sexuality are: sexual orientation (referring to the gender(s) to which we're sexually attracted); sexual identity (how we label ourselves and understand our orientation); and sexual behavior (what we actually do sexually).
- Practitioners shouldn't make assumptions concerning a client's sexual orientation. Doing so may cause clients to leave a core part of themselves out of the therapeutic experience and the practitioner misses an opportunity to facilitate healing.
- A person's sex education is largely determined by how his family regarded sex.
- The four family sex types are: sex repressive (sex is seen by parents as immoral); sex obsessive (sex is regarded as a main issue and overemphasized); sex avoidant (intellectually sex is accepted as a positive life experience, but emotionally the family

is uncomfortable with it); and sex expressive (the family is comfortable talking about sex openly and setting reasonable limits around their children's behavior).

- Practitioners and clients often experience sexual feelings during a treatment session.
- Having sexual feelings during a session is normal; acting in a sexually inappropriate manner in response to these feelings is not.
- Practitioners must allow sexuality and, at the same time, de-sexualize the experiences of both giving and receiving hands-on therapy.
- The Sexual Response Cycle consists of four phases: an excitement/arousal phase ; a plateau phase; an orgasmic phase; and a resolution phase.
- Health care practitioners who touch clients may automatically trigger the excitement phase in the sexual response cycle.
- Touching certain areas of the body such as the abdomen, lower extremities and buttocks may stimulate nerve pathways that lead to the genitals and thereby induce a sexual response.
- Touch may trigger the parasympathetic nervous system that controls the sexual response including vasocongestion, the increase of blood supply to the genitals, and myotonia.
- Touch may stimulate the limbic system, causing an emotional response and physiologic sexual response to occur during or after a treatment.
- Regardless of the situation or circumstances, if sexual arousal does occur, on the part of either the practitioner or the client, it is always the practitioner's responsibility to establish and maintain appropriate boundaries.
- The practitioner is responsible for responding non-sexually to the client and eliminating any misunderstanding on the client's part as to the intent of the treatment.
- Sex, sexual talk, sexual relations, sexual acts and activities, sexual pleasures, sexual intercourse, or being any way involved in a sexual manner with clients is always unethical and must never occur in the professional relationship.
- If you experience a sexual feeling toward a client, you must assess the quality of that feeling so that you can continue to monitor your actions and act ethically as a professional.
- If your attraction to a client is so strong that you wish to pursue a relationship, you need to first discontinue the client-practitioner relationship and wait a reasonable amount of time before dating that person. Consult a supervisor for advice.
- Client arousal doesn't always equate to sexual intent.
- If you model a healthy comfort level talking about all physiological changes a client might experience during a session, you have provided several things: an opening for the client to express concerns; an education for a client about how the body works; good boundaries; and a safe environment.
- The eight steps in the Intervention Model are:
    Step 1. Stop the treatment using assertive behavior.
    Step 2. Describe the behavior(s).
    Step 3. Clarify the client's intent.
    Step 4. Educate the client.
    Step 5. Re-state your intent.
    Step 6. Continue or discontinue the session as appropriate.
    Step 7. Refer client to other professionals as appropriate.
    Step 8. Document the situation.
- The Intervention Model is a communication model for practitioners to use when verbal or nonverbal communication from a client is unclear or when practitioners feel their boundaries are being violated.
- Sexual misconduct isn't limited to having sex with a client.

- Sexual misconduct is the result of a disregard of ethics, boundaries and genuine care for the client.
- The Risk Factor Analysis is a questionnaire to assess professional/sexual boundaries.
- Sexual harassment generally involves one person having power over another's employment, money, grades or advancement, and abusing that power.
- Two forms of sexual harassment involve: a demand for sexual favors in exchange for job benefits; unwelcome acts such as physical or verbal conduct or visual displays that create a hostile environment, making the individual's job difficult.
- Provide a safe experience for your clients by: observing and knowing yourself; clarifying about your own intentions toward your clients; establishing ethical safety at initial contact; maintaining a professional appearance and demeanor; establishing a professional treatment space; providing informed consent; choosing appropriate music; establishing a pre-treatment thinking process; allowing privacy for the client while changing; using appropriate language; using proper draping techniques; being mindful of body contact during the session; preventing straying strokes or movements; diffusing any hints or signs of sexual arousal; staying aware and in control; keeping accurate records of questionable events; participating in ongoing supervision; informing your clients of their rights; treating all clients equally regardless of age, gender or attractiveness; committing to continued education, particularly in the area of ethics, boundaries and communication skills.

Discussion Questions and Activities

- Describe the healthy sexual images in your culture.
- Define healthy sex.
- Describe the difference between sex, touch and intimacy.
- What are your earliest memories of sexuality?
- Describe the experience of the senses of your earliest sexuality memories.
- Experience touching as many different textures as possible. What kinds of thoughts and feelings occur with each texture?
- When you receive touch, what aspects do you consider to determine the meaning of that specific touch?
- Consider the differences between touching a newborn baby, a lover, an elderly person and a stranger.
- Touch exercise: Find a person with whom you are comfortable and vice versa. Touch that person at various depths with intent. Perhaps use the forearm. First, just barely touch. Then touch the skin. Next, distinguish between the skin and the muscle. Continue to the comfort level of each and discuss the experience.
- Identify an experience in which the meaning of a touch was misinterpreted.
- List some gender differences surrounding touch.
- Why might a male or female client choose a male or female practitioner?
- List the three different types of intimacy and what each one entails.
- How might the presence of sexual myths and sexual scripts add to mixed gender client/ professional misunderstandings?
- Describe your reaction to a time when a client experienced sexual arousal during a treatment. What will you do differently if this happens again?

- Portray how a client's family style regarding sex types exhibits itself during a session.
- Clarify the similarities between sexual misconduct and sexual harassment.
- Consider the following scenario: A new client of yours tells you that she received a very uncomfortable session from a female practitioner in town. She said the woman's fingers kept touching her pubic area and the practitioner's body contacted the client in ways that felt intrusive. What do you do?
- How would this scenario differ if the practitioner was a male?
- How would this scenario differ if the client was a male?
- If a professor is discovered having sex with a student, should the professor be suspended from teaching duties?
- What messages did you get in your family about sex and sexuality?
- What role does sex play in your life?
- What is the relationship for you between sex, touch, intimacy and love?
- Have you had periods of celibacy (either intentional or unintentional)? What was that like for you?
- When you were young what rules did you learn about sex?
- What are the differences and similarities in sex for men and for women?
- What kinds of stress might cause you to make an unwise decision?
- Interview other professionals about their experiences with sexually inappropriate clients and discuss how those situations were handled or mishandled.
- How might you gracefully respond to a sexual comment made to you by a person of the sex opposite to your own sexual orientation? How does that response differ between the context of your personal life and the context of your professional life?
- If you already see areas in your sexuality that may cause ethical dilemmas or uncomfortable situations, how will you prepare yourself to avoid those situations?
- What are the important sex, touch and intimacy issues for you in relation to your profession?
- Designate one page for each of the following statements. Write down your responses, spending approximately five minutes on each page.

    A lover is someone who...

    How I want my sexuality expressed in my life is...

    What things block sexual expression?

    What is my present relationship with my own sexuality?

    What would I like it to be?

6

Ethical Practice Management

- ✦ Professionalism
- ✦ Scope of Practice
- ✦ Standards of Practice
- ✦ Policy Statements
- ✦ Working with Minors
- ✦ Informed Consent
- ✦ Declining Potential New Clients
- ✦ Dismissing a Client
- ✦ The Team Approach
- ✦ Spa and Salon Issues
- ✦ In Conclusion...
- ✦ Chapter Highlights
- ✦ Discussion Questions and Activities

The business and practice management systems a practitioner develops and implements set the tone for an ethically run practice. How you manage your business impacts how your clients feel about you and your practice. You may do wonderful work and be a caring and compassionate person, but your clients will not hold the same level of trust in you and your abilities if the foundation of your business is poorly considered. Ethical practice management involves the art and skill of managing daily working affairs with others from a base of honesty, integrity and forthrightness. This chapter focuses on: attitudes, policies and procedures relating to your conduct with clients; maintaining client records; honoring confidentiality; building alliances with other health care providers; working within the appropriate scope of practice; and accurately representing abilities. The business management issues that relate to the topics of finances, marketing, negotiating contracts, legalities, employees and insurance claims are covered in the next chapter.

Professionalism

The root of the word professional is "profess" which means to declare, claim or openly affirm a belief or an opinion. Webster's Dictionary[1] defines a professional as a person who conforms to the standards of a profession; has or shows great skill; engages in a given activity as a source of livelihood; follows a learned profession. Professionalism stems from your attitudes and is manifested through your technical competency, your communication skills, your ability to manage boundaries, your respect for yourself and clients, and your business practices. In the article, *What Is a Professional?* Jerry Buley, PH.D.,[2] identifies six major factors of a professional: gives high quality performance; is predictable and consistent; is self-motivated, self-reliant and takes responsibility; works well under pressure; is always willing to learn; and understands her interconnectedness with humanity.

The term professionalism also relates to ethical behavior. High standards of action with clients result in both ethical and professional behavior. Obviously, ethical violations are unprofessional, although not all unprofessional behavior is an ethical violation. For example, a messy waiting room with visible dust bunnies is unprofessional but certainly not unethical.

The basis for true professionalism lies in integrity. Someone may talk, walk and look the part, but if that person does not come from a base of integrity, the facade wears thin quickly, ultimately resulting in the loss of clientele. The dictionary[3] defines integrity as the quality or state of being complete; unbroken condition; wholeness; honesty; and sincerity. Integrity is an essential quality for a true healing professional. People who possess integrity behave ethically, honor confidences and keep their word. Integrity can be divided into three major levels: the first level is keeping one's agreements; the second is being true to one's principles; and the highest level is being true to oneself.

It is rare to find somatic practitioners who value professionalism without the integrity behind it. More often they love what they do and are genuinely concerned about the well-being of their clients, yet neglect to develop a professional demeanor. A truly effective practitioner combines outward professionalism with internal integrity.

Scope of Practice

More than 2,500 years ago Hippocrates proclaimed this primary warning to physicians: *do no harm*.[4] This decree is the basis for the enduring responsibility of all helping professions to define, clarify and regulate what they do. Scope of practice (Scope) regulations are an extension of this mission. Many of the hands-on professions are still developing consistent standards, mainly due to varying educational requirements and outdated regulations. Most professions' Scope evolves over time. For instance, in the fairly recent past physical therapists needed a prescription from a medical doctor to provide services; now in many states they do not. All things considered it may be difficult for individual practitioners to discern the parameters of their scope of practice. This section defines Scope and introduces the four key factors which shape and change it.

Many practitioners enter a wellness career because of their experience with the results of that particular modality. Their enthusiasm often leads to the misconception (and often arrogance) that this particular technique helps almost anything. Exactly what is Scope and who determines its parameters? What determines whether a practitioner is functioning within her Scope? Is a practitioner qualified to teach a client to do stretches at home, perform passive stretches on a client during a treatment or sell nutritional supplements in the waiting room?

Sandy Fritz, author of *Mosby's Fundamentals of Therapeutic Massage* defines Scope as, "The where, when, and how a professional may provide their service or function as a professional."[5] As succinct and simple as this sounds, the *where, when,* and *how* can be quite complicated, and they vary greatly throughout geographic regions. Despite its broad diversity, however, Scope is consistently influenced by four key factors: the law, educational training, competency, and personal accountability. Together, these factors circumscribe and ultimately define one's Scope.

Key Factor One: The Law

The law is a pivotal factor in determining Scope, yet it is often the most difficult to decipher. Four levels of government make laws that affect practitioners: federal, state, county and local municipalities (city and town). The federal government, besides imposing taxes, authorizes the accreditation of schools and regulates financial aid. The subordinate governing bodies, state, county and municipal, exert a more tangible influence on Scope, offering three regulatory methods known as *licensure, certification* and *registration*. Each method has its particular requirements and provisions.

Licensure requires practitioners to obtain a license to perform their services; unlicensed persons who practice, break the law. *Certification* is not to be confused with private group certification such as given by the National Certification Board for Therapeutic Massage and Bodywork (NCBTMB) which is a voluntary option offering the use of vocational titles to identify professional services. *Registration* is the means by which a government agency keeps track of practitioners by informational record keeping.

Because this can be complicated and confusing, many competent, conscientious practitioners are unclear about the regulatory laws that apply to them. For example, although a practitioner was licensed many years ago, she may not have received notification of updated revisions. Even recently licensed practitioners with current awareness of the applicable law may find it difficult to understand the vague and tedious terminology. A myriad of inconsistencies further complicates matters including the delivery of the information. Some governing agencies issue thick booklets that attempt to define

> *Laws should be interpreted in a liberal sense so that their intention may be preserved.*
>
> —Marcus Tullius Cicero

everything from the wording used in advertising to legal hours of operation; others offer little clarification. The process for researching pertinent regulations is greatly simplified by utilizing the Internet.

Professional Titles

Legal names and professional titles cited in the law are numerous and varied. License titles are not necessarily the same as professional certification titles. The examples below are accurate at the time of publication of this book, but check with your local licensing board and/or professional association for current status.

For instance, the assortment of titles is abundant in the area of massage. The laws of Adams County, Colorado use the term 'massagists' to define persons who offer massage for a fee. A bit more updated is Rhode Island which maintains its outdated reference to "masseuse" and "masseur," but redeems itself by including a revision which uses the term "massage therapist." Worcester, Massachusetts, calls a licensee a "massage/muscle therapist," while Connecticut commissions their licensees to specify that they are a "Connecticut licensed massage therapist." Maine allows non-licensed persons to perform massage but the law prohibits them from using the terms "massage therapist" or "massage practitioner" which are reserved for licensed individuals.

Titles for acupuncturists also vary. The two most common are: L.AC. (Licensed Acupuncturist) and C.A. (Certified Acupuncturist). Florida recently changed from C.A. to A.P. (Acupuncture Physician) which allows acupuncturists to order and interpret lab tests. Both titles can be used in Florida. Two states give the title "doctor" as a matter of statute. New Mexico authorizes D.O.M. (Doctor of Oriental Medicine) and Rhode Island is D.AC. (Doctor of Acupuncture).

Two major approaches to titles exist in the acupuncture field. The American Association of Oriental Medicine was the first professional group in the United States for acupuncturists. It believes acupuncturists should hold the doctorate designation rather than master. The Alliance for Acupuncture and Oriental Medicine postulates that many professionals are capable of practicing acupuncture at different levels. Now toss certification into this mix. The National Certification Commission for Acupuncture and Oriental Medicine (NCCAOM) is the certifying body for Acupuncture, Asian Bodywork and Chinese Herbology. The board certification titles are: DIPL.AC. (Board Certified Acupuncturist); DIPL.CH (Board Certified Chinese Herbalist); and DIPL.ABT (Board Certified Asian Bodywork Therapist). A twist to this is that chiropractors can claim board certification in acupuncture with as few as 50 hours, but this designation is from the Chiropractic Board, not the NCCAOM. Traditional Chinese Medicine consists of five branches; however in the United States, most people are captivated by the concept of needles and that is what they think of as Oriental Medicine. Currently no state license provides a standard for herbs. As an example, acupuncturists in Massachusetts cannot use herbs unless they pass the National Certifying Exam in herbology.

Procedures, Techniques and Other Regulations

The law can permit or forbid any number of activities so it is wise for practitioners to consult laws and regulations in their state, province, or locality regarding Scope. Some of these laws are straightforward and others vague. Many seem frivolous. These laws typically restrict practitioners from performing services or procedures that require a different license (e.g., M.D.) or limit activities which could be linked with sex or sexual enterprise.

Assessment and Diagnosis:

For somatic practitioners who are not considered primary care providers the areas of assessment and diagnosis can be of concern. While diagnosis is generally restricted to the Scope of primary care providers, assessment is an integral part of most practitioners' work. There is often significant misunderstanding about the definition and role of assessment. Many people confuse the concepts of assessment and diagnosis, and for that reason they shy away from learning about them. Whitney Lowe, L.M.T. provides the following definitions.[6]

ASSESSMENT skills are a systematic method for gathering information to make informed decisions about if and how treatments should proceed. Since assessment is really information gathering, you cannot do any kind of treatment without performing some level of assessment. For instance, when your hands feel a tight area in your client's muscle tissue, you naturally focus your attention on reducing the tension in that area. You performed assessment through palpation and chose a particular course of action as a result of your assessment of the client's tissue state. Gathering information about someone's condition to determine if you should proceed with a given treatment is assessment, not diagnosis.

DIAGNOSIS, on the other hand, is assigning a name or label to a certain group of signs or symptoms. To arrive at a diagnosis the practitioner (usually a physician) performs some type of assessment and based on the findings, assigns a name or a label to the problem. When you assign a name or label to the problem and state to the person they have "x" condition, you have given him a diagnosis.

> A client comes to a somatic practitioner complaining of neck pain accompanied with bouts of dizziness. During the intake/assessment phase the practitioner realizes he doesn't understand the cause of the client's pain or the dizziness associated with it. Nevertheless, the practitioner has been trained in a variety of techniques and feels competent in proceeding with treatment. This action is out of the scope of practice because this practitioner doesn't have the training to assess what is actually occurring. These symptoms could indicate a brain tumor, pressure on the intervertebral artery, cancer or a disk injury. While the treatment may not harm the client it could delay the client in seeking appropriate treatment.

Technique Restrictions:

On occasion a Scope rule may also refer to rarely heard-of procedures. An example is the term *"heliotherapy."* New Jersey law permits massage practitioners to do this procedure and Rhode Island law prohibits it, further specifying that it can only be performed by physical therapists. *Taber's Cyclopedic Medical Dictionary*[7] defines heliotherapy as, "Exposure to sunlight for therapeutic purposes." One is left to wonder if that means using heat lamps, tanning lights, or working on a client under a skylight with the sun shining in.

Each profession has certain proscriptions against treating certain parts of a client's body. For example in most places in the United States where there is licensure, massage/ bodyworker therapists are not permitted to work directly on breast tissue. In some states breast massage is permitted as long as there is informed consent. In other countries such as Canada it is an integral part of the training and the therapy.

Ethical
Practice
Management

Sexual Enterprise:

Government officials (particularly in the United States) enacted laws and regulations in the attempt to hinder sexual enterprise. Examples include limiting hours of operation, placing physical restrictions (e.g., treatment room doors to remain unlocked, treatment rooms must have a window), not allowing practitioners to work out of their homes or do out-calls, requiring annual fingerprinting and making cross-gender treatments illegal.

These examples demonstrate that state regulation is hardly a cure-all to a profession's problems. While state regulation is often perceived as the remedy to the problems caused by a hodge-podge of local laws, state laws can be as irrelevant and outdated. Such restrictions tend to anger legitimate practitioners. If practitioners want to influence the laws that govern them, they must do more than vote in elections. They must know their laws and become active in changing them.

Getting Involved

Ethical practitioners are concerned about the quality of the overall profession. This quality is affected by both good and bad laws. Therefore, it is important for practitioners to work in their communities to increase the understanding and acceptance of their services as a valuable wellness modality. It is equally important to abide by all laws governing their practice and work for the repeal or revision of detrimental or specious laws. In brief; practitioners must get involved. Individually and collectively practitioners make a difference by helping shape and change the laws that govern them. Here is where to start if you want to find out about your laws, clarify what a law means, or if you disagree with a law and want to change it:

1. If you have state licensure, call the state office that issues your license. If you do not have state licensure but have municipal regulations, call your city or town hall and ask for the department that issues licenses for your profession.
2. Ask for the person who answers specific questions about practice laws. Find out if a professional board exists. Ideally, a governing body has an appointed advisory board consisting of both licensed, experienced practitioners and lay persons. A board serves to oversee the relevance and implementation of the laws.
3. Ask for a copy of applicable laws to be sent to you. Read these laws.
4. If a board doesn't exist, ask what must be done to create one.
5. In the event that a bill must be passed to create a regulatory board, contact your local senators and representatives. Be prepared because they are likely to ask you for specific, documented ideas. Find ideas of what you want by researching other states' laws.
6. If no laws govern where you practice, contact your professional organization's local chapter for information on action that has been taken toward legislation.

> " Never doubt that a small group of committed people can change the world. Indeed, it's very often the only thing that does. "
>
> —Margaret Meade

Key Factor Two: Educational Training

One definition of Scope is "the knowledge base and practice parameters of a profession."[8] Use of the term "practice parameters" implies there's a collective Scope for a profession. However, defining these practice parameters is not always an easy task. The phrase "knowledge base" suggests that there's a common framework of fundamental information provided by the educational training process in a particular field.

Training in many of the somatic modalities is unlike training in the branches of chiropractic, acupuncture and physical therapy. In these more standardized professions, basic training programs throughout the country are fairly consistent in what they teach the students to know and do. Educational offerings in massage and bodywork training programs are as diverse and inconsistent as the local laws that govern them; it is difficult to define a comprehensive, consistent, common knowledge base.

Ultimately, if local licensing laws exist where you practice, they govern your Scope and determine what you can and cannot do. Even if laws exist, however, many of them are very general and make no mention of specific modalities. So, while the laws serve as a guide, two practitioners governed by the same laws may have significant differences in their scopes of practice based on their education and unique knowledge base. Beyond the law's watchful eye, educational training individualizes Scope and it becomes a personal issue rather than a collective one. Ethical practitioners must be mindful about the limitations of their training, regardless of what they are lawfully permitted to do.

Key Factor Three: Competency

As surely as educational training and the laws which govern practitioners influence Scope, so do ability and proficiency. This brings forth the questions, "What determines competency?" and "Who is the ultimate judge of competency?" In many localities the law states that competency is presumed once the required number of hours of formal education is complete. Growing numbers of city and state laws require practitioners to pass a written exam as a method to verify competency requirements. Unfortunately, written exams vary in degree of difficulty and efficacy, which is why many licensing boards defer to tests developed by national certification boards such as NCBTMB and NCCAOM.

> *It is not what you say you believe that is important, but what you model, encourage, reward and let happen.*
>
> —Patricia Fripp

Beyond basic training, offerings for advanced studies abound. Once again the ethical concern of competency brings more questions. Does a practitioner need credentials from a week-long course, or does it suffice to attend a two-hour seminar to become adept in a new method? Is watching a video on the subject, or reading a book adequate to claim proper training and competency? How much and what type of training is adequate?

A client comes to a practitioner complaining of fatigue and achiness throughout the body. With little more than a weekend's training in nutrition the practitioner recommends various dietary supplements and change in diet for the client. Over the next several weeks the client's condition deteriorates and he ends up in the hospital.

Patricia J. Benjamin, PH.D., former national director of education for the American Massage Therapy Association (AMTA), warns against "paper tiger" credentials: credentials, titles or certifications which may sound impressive, but which lack teeth. She says, "A disturbing number of practitioners are claiming credentials in various disciplines or specialties only after an introductory workshop or a few hours on the subject. If a credential is to mean something of value, it must represent meeting a certain standard of quality or the significant mastery of a particular area, and not just a passing familiarity."[9]

In an evolving profession, determining competence requires self-accountability on the practitioner's part. In addition to meeting all legal and educational requirements, the ethical practitioner must seriously evaluate her training, experience and confidence before offering treatment to clients as a professional.

Referrals

One of the great mistakes practitioners make is to believe that they can do it all. Knowing when and how to refer clients to a more appropriate professional is as important as anything you do in a professional practice. Awareness of your scope of practice, the limits of your training and knowledge, your personal and professional limitations, your areas of weakness and your blind spots is an asset to your professional work.

In the beginning phases of practice (the first five to 10 years), some practitioners believe their work accomplishes almost anything if applied correctly. The saying "When all someone has is a hammer, everything looks like a nail" is an apt one for this professional practice phase. A seasoned practitioner in any field knows, or at least suspects, the limits of her work and regularly refers clients to other practitioners.

Consider the following examples: a seemingly simple neck and headache pain might turn out to be a brain tumor; a case of headaches could be meningeal irritation (meningitis) or even a bleeding from one of the vessels in the brain (a stroke); pain in the low back at L1 and L2 may indicate cancer spreading to the spine; the sudden appearance of pain in the front thigh after a strenuous activity could indicate a blood clot in the femoral artery; and difficulty raising the arm above the head because of a protective pectoral spasm can indicate cancer in the lung.

Your motto should be, "When in doubt, refer out." Develop a network of professionals whose work you know to be of the highest quality. In the best of circumstances you cultivate ongoing professional relationships with these individuals and communicate with them directly. Your clients and colleagues act as resources for the development of this network. Keep track of how your clients are treated and how they feel about the services they receive. Over time you accumulate a list of reliable referral sources.

Key Factor Four: Self-Accountability

Scope of practice is a very individual thing. Self-accountability is the most decisive factor that keeps you functioning within your individual scope of practice. When you are self-accountable you are answerable to and responsible for what you say and do, even when there's no external authority present. Unless you have internalized the laws and guidelines that define the limits of your practice you are at a high risk of violating your professional scope of practice and ethical responsibilities.

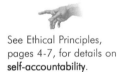

See Ethical Principles, pages 4-7, for details on **self-accountability**.

In the seclusion of your private practice and behind the closed doors of your treatment rooms, you are often left with no one but yourself to hold you accountable and you could conceivably transgress the scope of your practice without anyone ever knowing. Governing laws, education and training and competency influence your Scope only when you obey the laws, carry out what you have learned and been trained to do and perform your work competently. No matter what code of ethics you outwardly subscribe to, and regardless of your proclaimed litany of beliefs, it is self-accountability that creates and sustains your personal and professional ethics and keeps you functioning within the parameters of your scope of practice. Self-accountability enforces scope of practice.

Personalize Your Scope

Governing laws in your locality, an individually acquired knowledge base and a capacity to apply and practice responsibly and well, are what personalize the Scope. These steps assist in clarifying your Scope:

1. Update your resume. This is a very effective way to outline what you know about the breadth and width of your acquired knowledge base. List education, training and work experience, including what you did before you became a practitioner. Everything you know and have done contributes to who you are as a person. In some cases the work may actually enrich your Scope. For example, a practitioner who was a physical therapist before becoming a massage therapist has a knowledge base and experience that makes her personal Scope different from a chiropractor

who becomes an acupuncturist. She would most likely have very different approaches to working with a client who sees her for low back pain.

2. Define your personal strengths. List techniques, procedures and modalities that you do regularly and in which you feel competent.

3. Reread your local licensing laws. Become familiar with what is permitted and prohibited by the law and stay current with legislative changes that affect you. Function honestly within your legal limits.

4. Retire the techniques and modalities you know but seldom do. As in all skills, "Practice makes permanent" (not necessarily perfect) and, "Use it, or lose it." If, for example, you haven't performed foot reflexology since your course in school three years ago, serve the client who requests a reflexology treatment by referring him to a colleague who does it regularly. Do not list reflexology on your business card. If your list reminds you of aspirations you have long forgotten, decide if you want to pursue them at this time.

5. Network with other professionals. Talk with them about their Scopes and see how yours is different from theirs. The contrast helps you better identify your own parameters, strengths and limitations. Also, knowing what others do and their specialties offers you referral options for clients whose needs exceed your abilities.

6. Represent yourself honestly. Be realistic about what you were officially and properly trained in, versus information you acquired in your travels through life. Being self-taught is a valuable attribute but there are substantial differences between working in a field or researching it for years and watching one or two videos on a subject.

7. Be attentive to high risk areas. These situations tempt you to go beyond your qualifications. Prepared responses for these situations such as, "That isn't within my scope of practice; I can refer you to someone for that."

When I do good, I feel good; when I do bad, I feel bad. That's my religion.

—Abraham Lincoln

Standards of Practice

While Scope of Practice mainly covers the limits of a practitioner's service, Standards of Practice describe the underlying principles of a given field, the expectations of professional conduct and the quality of care provided to clients. Standards of Practice often elaborate upon the items in a Code of Ethics. The contents of Standards of Practice, Scope of Practice and Codes of Ethics frequently overlap.

The broad categories covered in Standards of Practice are: professionalism, competence, professional excellence; legal and ethical requirements; protecting the public and profession; responsibility to the client; confidentiality; business practices; professional relationships, roles and boundaries; prevention of sexual misconduct; professional conduct; educating the public; research; fees; accurate representation of Scope; professional appearance; continued education; courtesy; and integrity. Some Standards of Practice list a broad statement for each category while others elaborate in great detail. The specific requirements vary greatly in the different professions. Check with professional associations (most associations post this information on their web sites) to find the most current standards. The following list contains common statements in most Standards of Practice:

- Conduct practice in a professional manner.
- Dress appropriately.
- Respect the rights and dignity of all clients.

- Provide accurate information to the client about the profession and services provided.
- Maintain high standards and give highest regard to the clients' welfare.
- Communicate clearly using appropriate terminology.
- Provide services within the profession's Scope of Practice and in accordance with extant laws.
- Abide by the profession's Code of Ethics.
- Accurately represent your level of competence, education, training and experience.
- Make judgments that are commensurate with qualifications and accept responsibility for the exercise of sound judgment.
- Perform appropriate assessment.
- Refer to other practitioners.
- Seek professional advice when needed.
- Act with due regard for the needs, special competencies and obligations of colleagues.
- Refrain from falsely impugning the reputation of any colleague.
- Remain in good standing with professional associations.
- Maintain accurate records and store them properly.
- Protect clients' confidentiality.
- Provide a safe physical environment.
- Maintain adequate and customary insurance.
- Promote business in an honest and dignified manner.
- Recognize the psychological principles involved in working with clients.
- Avoid dual relationships that could exploit or harm clients, employees or co-workers.
- Refrain from practicing when your judgment or competence is impaired by intake of drugs/alcohol or physical/mental incapacity.
- Refrain from participating in sexual conduct, sexual activities or sexualizing behavior with clients.
- Maintain and promote high standards of practice, education and research.
- Seek remuneration for services that is deserved and reasonable.
- Protect the public and profession from unethical, incompetent or illegal acts.
- Report to the proper authorities any other practitioner's alleged violations of the law, Code of Ethics, Scope or Standards of Practice.
- Participate in activities that contribute to the health and well-being of the public.

Policy Statements

A policy statement is a useful vehicle for creating boundaries that encourage trust, safety and comfort. Policies explicitly define the expectations for both clients and practitioners. They make managing a practice easier, circumvent potentially awkward situations, provide means for conflict resolution and demonstrate professionalism. The policy statement also embodies the salient points from a practitioner's Code of Ethics, Scope of Practice and Standards of Practice documents. Ultimately a policy statement increases the chances for a successful outcome of the services provided.

Policy statements can be designed in various formats: resembling a letter, a page with bulleted items or a combination of the two. Eight major areas to cover are: type of service; training and experience; appointment policies; finances; client/practitioner expectations; personal relationships; confidentiality; and recourse policy. Some of these sections may

Standing in the middle of the road is very dangerous; you get knocked down by traffic from both sides.

—Margaret Thatcher

only be a line or two on the finished policy statement. Written policy statements set a professional tone, even if you do not have specific policies stated for every situation.

Periodically review your policies, delete ones that are no longer appropriate and add ones to further clarify your requirements. The main caveat with policies is: Do not have a policy you will not or cannot enforce. If you alter a policy for a client either on a one-time basis or if you change that specific policy permanently, make it very clear to the client what you are doing and that all other policies still hold.

Refer to the sample **policy statements** in Appendix A, pages 260-262, for ideas.

1: Type of Service

Provide a clear definition of services, including benefits as well as limitations. This section might include: areas of expertise; specialization; specific conditions your work addresses, such as headaches and back pain; target populations served, such as seniors or athletes; special equipment or products used; certain people with whom you do not work such as pregnant women or people with certain medical conditions; and a description of the referral network of related professionals that you utilize.

Discuss your specific policies with colleagues before printing your updated policy statement.

2: Training and Experience

Describe your training and experience to increase the client's sense of safety and confidence. This section includes educational experience, organizational memberships, additional training, years of experience, specialty study and licensure status. Although it may seem unnecessary for some professionals to provide this information, clients feel safer when they know the practitioner's experience with a particular problem or modality.

3: Appointments

Clarification of appointment policies is particularly important at the beginning of the treatment process. Establishing a time frame for your interactions with a client creates a boundary. The structure and expectation about treatment time and your availability is determined by the specific situation. Since different disciplines (as well as individual practitioners) have varying time policies, clients may easily make inaccurate assumptions about your policies.

Punctuality on the part of the practitioner connotes respect for both parties. While being late under certain circumstances is understandable, tardiness is usually perceived as annoying and disrespectful. Written, straightforward communication about these policies is a way of establishing clear boundaries. A policy statement should include the length of initial and follow-up appointments as well as guidelines for scheduling changes, lateness, cancellations and emergencies.

Start and End On Time

Starting and ending a session on time establishes a clear boundary. Practitioners who run professional practices are generally on time. Every practitioner may be late occasionally but if the practitioner consistently runs a little late, this is a significant signal that he has difficulty with the boundaries of time and has possibly set up his schedule without enough space to respect the client's time. For instance, if a practitioner needs 45 minutes of actual treatment time for each appointment and schedules clients at 45 minute intervals, there's no leeway for the unexpected. If this practitioner finds it difficult to keep this schedule and run on time, it makes sense to change the interval to an hour. Schedule appointments with 10 or 15 minutes of leeway to make calls between sessions, take notes, enjoy a snack or accommodate clients who need a little extra time to get ready.

Another type of time problem occurs when a practitioner keeps a client significantly beyond the ending time of the appointment without asking the client's permission. The client may have other commitments after the appointment with this practitioner. Blatant disregard for the client's time is as much a boundary violation as any other.

The concept of time varies for different cultures. In certain cultures time is not very important or it may even be a non-issue. Time is often a precious commodity in Western culture and usually holds great significance to clients. If the boundary of time is consistently violated a client may draw several conclusions: the practitioner does not care; the practitioner is too busy to really listen; the practitioner is unprofessional; the practitioner is inattentive; the practitioner is irresponsible; the practitioner is overwhelmed; the practitioner has poor time management skills; or the practitioner has no respect for time.

Cancellations

Cancellations can be disconcerting for both parties, particularly if they happen frequently and at the last minute. A clear cancellation policy reduces this problem. Some practitioners require a 24-hour cancellation notice or the client is billed (either in part or full) for the session. Other practitioners whose practices consist of last-minute or walk-in clientele often only require a four-hour or eight-hour cancellation policy. Along with this policy some practitioners stipulate that the client is **not** billed if the appointment slot is filled. A simple statement often suffices, such as; "If cancellation is necessary, please give 24-hour notice or you are charged for the appointment unless it can be filled. Emergency cancellations are determined at the practitioner's discretion."

Turnabout is fair play. Consider including a statement like this: "If I need to cancel an appointment, I do so within 24 hours whenever possible. If an emergency arises and I can't keep an appointment, I provide a 50 percent discount with a client's next session. For non-emergency cancellations of less than 24 hours, your next session is at no charge."

See Business Ethics, pages 182-191, for specifics on **finances**.

4: Finances

The exchange of money serves to solidify the professional contract between the practitioner and the client as it clearly indicates that the practitioner is providing a service to the client in exchange for a fee. Charging a fee helps clarify the distinction between personal time and work time. At the beginning of the professional relationship clear communication about your fee policies is vital because many people have strong emotional responses to issues involving money. Financial policies should include the following: fee structure; sliding scale schedules; package plans; credit terms; insurance reimbursement; product guarantees and returns; bounced checks; gift certificates; and barter.

See page 162 for details on **recourse policies**.

5: Client/Practitioner Expectations

This section provides an overview of the procedural structure of a typical session, draping, communication guidelines, attitude, the level of interaction outside of the actual treatment, illness and etiquette expectations.

Procedures

Ease the anxiety some people feel about seeing a practitioner for the first time by giving new clients a description of what occurs during the first and subsequent sessions. Address these questions: Do you start with an intake interview and a history? If so, how much time is allotted and does this take away from the "hands-on" portion of the session? Does the length of sessions vary? Will the client need to disrobe or wear specific clothing? What safety measures are observed? What happens if something occurs that makes the client uncomfortable? Should a client refrain from eating prior to sessions? Do you allow interruptions (e.g., telephone calls)? If so, how are they handled? Are there any unusual reactions the client might experience during or after the first (or subsequent) session?

Draping

Appropriate draping is crucial if clients need to remove some or all of their clothing to receive your treatment. Draping or covering a client fosters a sense of safety and emphasizes your professionalism. Instruct clients about your standard procedure: tell them to undress to their level of comfort; direct them as to which articles of clothing to leave on; or ask them to put on a smock. Tell them how to position and cover themselves on the table (e.g., lie on the table and cover yourself with the top sheet or towel). Inform clients that you leave the room while they change in private and you knock before entering.

Draping concerns are not limited to the initial covering of the client: they also include draping for privacy throughout the session. Sometimes it is necessary to add more draping in the course of the treatment if your work entails some type of movement, positioning or work that exposes another part of the body. Also it is best to only uncover the area that is directly receiving work and never work under the drape.

Communication

Describe the verbal and non-verbal communication a client can expect from you and you expect from the client. Carefully choose the language and terminology you use with clients as they convey your attitudes. Your policy statement might include a description of the depth of information and self-disclosure you require.

Attitudes

Your attitudes toward your work and people greatly impact the therapeutic outcome. Ethical health care professionals demonstrate respect for all clients regardless of their age, gender, race, national origin, sexual orientation, religion, socio-economic status, body type, political affiliation, state of health and personal habits. Unfortunately, not everyone has reached this point of maturity. Nina McIntosh states in her book, *The Educated Heart*, "We owe clients our care and attention. We may not connect with a person right away, but if we cannot imagine ever having a caring attitude toward a particular client, we shouldn't work with him/her. We need to be on the alert for anything that interferes with our abilities to touch a client in a respectful, non-judgmental way. We are not just touching bodies—we're touching spirits."[10]

Interaction

Clarify the level of your availability to clients: your hours (including parameters for extended hours); location (e.g., do you also work with clients at their business or home?); how quickly you return telephone calls and e-mail; the time allotted before and after sessions to answer questions or offer support; and terminating the professional relationship.

Follow-up tends to be a weak area in most practices. While it is a good idea to place appointment reminder calls, first find out if your clients want you to do it, when they want it and where they want to receive the calls. Some practitioners call new clients within 48 hours after their first session just to check in. Others also like to call clients who have experienced a major shift or event during the session. Regardless of the type and frequency of follow-up, always discuss the policy first with your clients.

See pages 168-170 for details on **terminating a client relationship**.

Etiquette

Etiquette concerns behaviors that fall under the heading of good manners: cancellation notification and being punctual (see above); hygiene (e.g., bathing prior to a session and refraining from wearing strong perfume); and personal habits such as smoking on the premises or arriving in an altered state.

Illness

An ethical question arises whenever a practitioner is at risk of infecting a client. If a practitioner has a condition that is clearly infectious, the decision to cancel an appointment is easily made. More difficult is the case of the common cold. When a practitioner has a cold or symptoms which may indicate the onset of a cold, there is a tendency to ignore the situation or dismiss it as inconsequential. This avoidance of clear decision-making can be exacerbated if the practitioner is experiencing financial pressure. Nevertheless, the practitioner's responsibility to the client should take precedence ("Do no harm"). The practitioner is obligated to notify the client prior to the appointment to discuss it.

This becomes even more important if the client is immunologically compromised. Two of the most common clients in this category are those receiving cancer treatment, especially chemotherapy and those with HIV. These clients are most susceptible to all infections. Their cases are clear-cut but only if the practitioner is aware of the client's condition. If there's ever any question of compromising a client's health, the ethical action is to call and cancel the session or offer the client the option of canceling the session.

The same expectations apply to clients. Include in your policy statement that if a client is sick and may be infectious, he should either postpone his appointment or at least call you to discuss the situation.

6: Personal Relationships

Engaging in personal or social relationships with clients outside of the therapeutic relationship is difficult at best, and often leads to undue discomfort or even pain and suffering by the client. Dual relationships require enormous attention, maturity and excellent communication.

The ethics of dual relationships varies to some degree among the professions. In psychotherapy there is almost universal acceptance that dual relationships of any kind are unethical. While not deemed unethical in other professions, they are certainly discouraged. Any exceptions to keeping the relationship limited to one domain must be carefully justified and defined.

Some people have very stringent policies about working with friends or family members. There is no right or wrong here although it is easier if you do not need to accommodate dual relationships. You are the only one who can gauge your ability to keep clear boundaries. Even if you can work effectively in a dual relationship, there is the question if the other person is capable of managing multiple roles. Another aspect of working with family and friends is that they are more likely to test your policies and limits—although not always intentionally. Clear policies makes enforcement less awkward.

Sexual relations with clients is a blatant violation of most professional Codes of Ethics and in many places is against the law. Policies that include a straightforward statement about the inappropriateness of sexual contact between the practitioner and the client contribute to an atmosphere of safety. The practitioner is responsible to see that sexual misconduct does not occur.

The ability to calmly reflect may be one of the most underdeveloped of professional skills. Reflection helps us work smarter; reflection helps bring our values into our actions; reflection brings our private self into our professional self; reflection helps us gain perspective on our priorities.

—Susan R. Komives

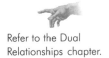

Refer to the Dual Relationships chapter.

7: Confidentiality

Confidentiality can be defined as the client's guarantee that what occurs in the therapeutic setting remains private and protected. First and foremost, the issue of confidentiality concerns the client's rights to privacy and safety. These rights belong equally to every client you see regardless of age, status or relationship to you or another client. These same rights apply to both verbal and written interactions you have with anyone other than the client.

As a model for confidentiality in the somatic professions, we turn to the profession of psychotherapy where these issues have been examined and developed over many years.[11] The ethical guidelines of most helping professions include a statement about confidentiality (with the goal of helping practitioners make ethical decisions regarding confidentiality). Nevertheless, these ethical statements often fall short of satisfactorily defining the parameters of the client's right to confidentiality. As with other ethical questions throughout the book, practitioners may find it challenging to apply confidentiality guidelines in complex situations.

Most people are clear about major confidentiality breaches such as sharing important personal information about a client with a third party, yet subtle situations occur where boundaries are easy to cross. Consider the following scenarios:

> A well-known politician comes to you for treatment. Do you think twice about sharing this exciting news with your friends?

> Your best friend sends his wife to you for a session. Do you stop and consider if it is appropriate to answer his questions about her session?

> You schedule a session with a 13-year-old boy who will be accompanied by his mother. Prior to the session do you think about whether to work with the boy alone or with the mother present?

If you answered "yes" to any of the questions posed in the scenarios, you have already begun to deal ethically with the issue of confidentiality in your work.

Maintaining Confidentiality

Confidentiality guidelines for somatic professions generally state that information shared between client and practitioner during a session remains private. These guidelines are usually further interpreted to mean that client names, details of treatment and information shared by clients during sessions are not discussed by the practitioner with anyone else.

Behind confidentiality issues are two assumptions: that an important and personal relationship exists between client and practitioner, and that trust is an essential element in this relationship. The client who knows that his right to privacy is honored is more likely to develop the trust necessary for a successful, healthy outcome of the therapeutic encounter. For example, it may be very tempting to tell your friends about the well-known politician/athlete/musician/film star who is your client, or to do a little name-dropping at a social function. You might even be tempted to use this client's name or title in your advertising (e.g., "acupuncturist to the mayor!") All of these actions, however, cross the ethical boundary of confidentiality. The mayor, like every client, has the right to privacy about her sessions with you.

The closer and more confidential our relationship with someone, the less we are entitled to ask about what we are not voluntarily told.

—Louis Kronenberger

If the mayor chooses to tell others that she knows your work, you have gained a valuable referral. You, however, are still bound by the ethics of confidentiality. Her reference to you does not give you permission to discuss her case with others. If you break this ethical policy, even in casual conversation, it looks as though you are trading on a well-known name and you always run the chance that what you have said could get back to your client. If the situation turns out negatively, you may lose not only the client but professional respect as well. If you work with celebrities or public figures and you want to let others know, obtain disclosure permission (preferably in writing) from the client.

All your clients deserve the same confidential treatment you would give the mayor. In the introductory scenarios the spouse asking about his wife is, hopefully unknowingly, asking you to cross an ethical boundary. And though a number of your friends may know you treat each of them, you are not implicitly authorized to say anything about another's session. You can avoid unethical behavior by saying in a light-hearted manner, "You know it's against my policies to discuss anything that happens within a session to anyone. I'm sure [Terry] would enjoy talking with you about her session." Finally, if you trade sessions or otherwise treat a fellow health professional, he too benefits more from your work together if you maintain his privacy and safety.

Limits of Ethical Confidentiality

The limits of confidentiality can be an area of confusion and misinformation on the part of both practitioners and clients. Not all health care relationships are held to be "privileged" relationships. Unlike a psychotherapist, medical or psychological information about the client is not necessarily legally held in confidence by the practitioner. Therefore it is vital that a well-researched and clear policy statement regarding confidentiality be presented and the practitioner discloses any exceptions to absolute confidentiality.

Two major considerations underlie the limits of professional confidentiality: the practitioner's obligations to the law; and the practitioner's obligations to others.

Regarding your obligations to the law: the legal system may have the right to subpoena your client lists or even your client records. Client files contain information so that you can properly work with any given client. Although you want your files to contain accurate and thorough information, your actual treatment records should only include information as it relates to the treatment and not superfluous notes (e.g., refrain from inscribing details about a client's eccentricities or personal relationships).

Some reasons for breaking confidentiality include: there's a clear and imminent danger to the client or another individual; a client discloses an intention to commit a crime; you suspect abuse or neglect of a child, an elderly person, or an incapacitated individual.

Confidentiality and its limits do not exist in black and white terms. When making ethical decisions, practitioners choose among various levels of thinking and functioning. From one vantage, abiding by the law may seem clear-cut; from another vantage, doing what is best for your client may mean questioning the law; from still another vantage, protecting a third party may mean breaking the client's trust. The practitioner must combine knowledge of the situation with a clear understanding of the ethics involved, and temper these with wisdom and experience.

Practitioners may also reveal details of therapy encounters to their supervisors or supervision groups. In these discussions the names of clients are withheld although other pertinent information and treatment particulars may be shared.

Actions That Minimize Confidentiality Problems

When you tell your clients up front about the limits to the confidentiality of your work together, they are much better able to give informed consent regarding treatment from you. Therefore, early in your professional relationships let your clients know that you hold your work together as confidential, and that you may discuss your work with your supervisor and that legal or ethical obligations may require you to break confidentiality in extreme circumstances.

The practitioner should avoid making unilateral decisions about breaking confidentiality. Even in some of the legal instances described above, if you must make the decision to break confidentiality, you should discuss your decision with the client beforehand. In this way, while the client may not agree with your decision, she is informed of your reasons.

When you want permission to discuss the professional relationship elsewhere, you should have a specific reason for doing so. This reason should be discussed with the client, and the client needs to give specific written consent. For example, you may wish to correspond about the client with another health care provider, or to use details about the client's condition, treatment and outcome in an article or presentation. The client's permission should specify exactly what details, such as name, dates of visit and treatment records he is authorizing you to share, as well as any specific limitations on where, when and how you may share the information.

In general, as soon as you perceive a potential problem surrounding confidentiality, the situation should be discussed with the client. When the 13-year-old boy and his mother are in your treatment room together, whatever one shares the other hears and confidentiality between the two of them is implicitly set aside. At the first session these clients should be informed about whether you will work or speak with either of them privately; if so, specify whether you keep what one says to you confidential from the other and what limits you may put on this confidentiality. In this way both son and mother utilize the therapeutic encounter more successfully.

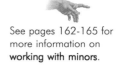

See pages 162-165 for more information on **working with minors**.

Health Insurance Portability and Accountability Act

Significant changes have been made regarding how health care practitioners protect their clients' privacy. The right to privacy is mentioned in many places in American law (and probably many other countries). The Fourth Amendment to the U.S. Constitution in particular guarantees that "the right of the people to be secure in their persons, houses, papers and effects, against unreasonable searches and seizures shall not be violated."

This all has to do with every client's right to privacy, or client confidentiality. The rules were fairly simple in the past. Charts did not get released or copied without a client's written consent or by subpoena. Health care practitioners and their staff were bound by law not to reveal any health information to anyone. Even with a subpoena many states specifically preclude the release of information relating to AIDS on a given client without the client's specific written permission. This did not pertain to other reportable public health information; it also did not apply to law enforcement agencies.

The situation was limited by technology in the past, but it has changed remarkably because of computers, e-mail, the Internet and electronic claims submission. People lost jobs, bank loans, life insurance policies and were otherwise compromised because their medical records (and other private information) were easily accessible on the Internet. In many cases the information was incorrect and the loss of livelihood and other important rights triggered a great deal of concern. While a few states had laws governing aspects of client privacy, there was no national system in place, especially with the advent of electronic information sharing.

The U.S. Congress passed the Medical Records Confidentiality Act of 1995 in an effort to establish uniform privacy protection for personally identifiable health information. On one hand, clients gained access to any health information about themselves and it gave people a chance to correct this information. In 1998, the Children's Online Privacy Protection Act was enacted to safeguard children online.

A far more comprehensive strategy was passed in 1996 known as the **Health Insurance Portability and Accountability Act**, or HIPAA. The final regulations were released by the Department of Health and Human Services effective February 26, 2001, and health care providers (and other agents) are mandated to have it in place by April 2003. The Federal Register describes HIPAA in approximately 700 pages. It can be downloaded off the Internet if you want to read it all. This section gives you the "bare bones" as it relates to your practice.

HIPAA has three major purposes: (1) to protect and enhance the rights of consumers by providing them access to their health information and controlling the inappropriate use of that information; (2) to improve the quality of health care in the United States by restoring trust in the health care system among consumers, health care professionals, and the multitude of organizations and individuals committed to the delivery of care; and (3) to improve the efficiency and effectiveness of heath care delivery by creating a national framework for health privacy protection that builds on efforts by states, health systems, individual organizations and individuals.

Who are the covered entities under HIPAA? Section 1172(a)(1) describes "health plans, health care clearinghouses and health care providers who transmit any health information in electronic form in connection with a transaction referred to in section 1173(a)(1) of the Act." **If you have read this far and are thinking that because you do not use electronic claims submission (ECS) you are exempt, think again.** If all your information is kept on paper, you do not have to comply on the surface; however, if you plan to fax, e-mail, or in any other way electronically send information, you are responsible. Nor are you exempt if you bill insurance and any of the other entities (e.g., a health care plan) electronically submits your typed claim form. In any event, plan on complying with HIPAA. As an ethical practitioner you have a duty to protect your clients' privacy.

The very first regulation deals with electronic transactions. The most common transaction of this type in most offices is ECS. Prior to ECS (and still used by many health care practitioners), health information was recorded and maintained on paper and stored in offices. Breaching confidentiality usually took a physical exchange of these papers or a verbal exchange of information. Today, most of this information is transmitted electronically, literally at the push of a button. In seconds a person's very private information can be shared with anyone who can access it.

The good news about electronic transmission is the increase in speed of delivery of effective care. In the practitioner's case it is not just about getting paid faster. The health information can be vital to that client's life. Obviously a balance must be maintained between safeguarding private information from abuse, fraud, prejudice and negligence and sharing the same information for the client's benefit.

Health information is often shared with consulting physicians. If a client is referred to you by a neurologist, that referral includes a diagnosis, possibly MRI results, other diagnostic tests and a telephone conversation between the referring doctor and you. The referral

http://cms.hhs.gov/hipaa
http://www.hhs.gov/ocr/hipaa
http://www.hipaa.org
http://www.hipaadvisory.com

information may also be disclosed to the health insurance company, managed care organization, or employer (if it is Workers' Compensation). How about getting a faxed MRI report or lab test? Although most of the time this is done without the client's knowledge, but is innocently directed toward the client's benefit. Will this information delivery method change under HIPAA? Yes.

The four parts to HIPAA's "Administrative Simplification" are:

- Electronic Health Transactions Standards
- Use standard code sets and ansi formats (except for claims and first injury reports).
- Unique Identifiers for Providers, Employers, Health Plans and Clients
- Each practitioner who transmits electronically is assigned a National Provider Identifier (NPI).
- Security of Health Information & Electronic Signature Standards
- Uniform levels of protection of all health information that is housed or transmitted electronically. An electronic signature is required for all hipaa transactions.
- Privacy and Confidentiality
- Limits the non-consensual use and release of private health information; gives clients new rights to access their medical records and to know who else has accessed them; restricts most disclosure of health information to the minimum needed for the intended purpose; institutes criminal and civil sanctions for improper use or disclosure; and establishes new requirements for access to records by researchers and others.

Failure to heed the HIPAA regulations will result in civil and criminal penalties, starting at $100 per person per violation and not exceeding $25,000 per year per person. The penalties get worse for knowingly violating HIPAA, especially if the offense is "under false pretenses" where there is a potential fine of up to $100,000 and/or imprisonment up to five years. If the offense is with intent to sell a client's information the penalty is up to $250,000 and 10 years imprisonment.

Complying with HIPAA

Here are some simple steps to take regarding HIPAA compliance:

1. Take client privacy and confidentiality very seriously. The penalties for violation are steep and there are felony charges that could potentially cause the loss of your license.
2. Designate someone in your office (or hire an outside party) to create a process to handle protected health information.
3. Train office staff on how to handle protected health information, including under what circumstances protected health information may be disclosed.
4. Use consent/authorization documents that the client signs.
5. Do not discuss **any** medical information with any third parties unless **written** consent/authorization has been obtained.
6. Be careful when discussing a client's protected health information with office staff; disseminate it on a need-to-know basis.
7. Assign User IDs and passwords to anyone with access to electronic information (e.g., computer billing software, voice dictation programs).
8. Contact your practice management software company and make sure the version you are using is HIPAA compliant.
9. Use passwords and security programs to protect and maintain computer files.

Get your assigned **National Provider Identifier:**
www.aspe.hhs.gov/admnsimp/faqnpi.htm

10. For e-mail obtain written consent from the client and use encryption software. Use electronic signatures to authenticate who sent the e-mail.

11. Use auditing software to monitor who sent what and when.

12. Create a policy for the destruction and retention of medical records that also includes e-mail communications.

13. Design a client information sheet that explains the following: how you use their information; the storage method for client files; the circumstances under which you may disclose client information; and the procedure for clients to see or obtain copies of their files.

8: Recourse Policy

What happens if the client is dissatisfied with the services provided or products purchased? Some practitioners refund some or all of a client's money if the client is not satisfied. Others give another session without charge. Discuss the concerns with your client regardless of your final action. Often the dissatisfaction results from a lack of ongoing communication. Keep in mind the power differential that exists in helping relationships may affect the client's ability to utilize a recourse policy. Because of this power differential, it is recommended that the policy statement include options involving a third party or mediator in the discussion. This kind of information serves to level the balance of power.

Working With Minors

Working with minors requires special consideration. While legal definitions of who is a minor differ from state to state, the purpose of all such definitions is protective. They establish a baseline for restrictions and safeguards that protect persons not yet recognized as adults.

Ethical standards also have a protective purpose yet published guidelines often do not specifically address work with minors. Due to the intimate nature of somatic therapy, it is especially important to discuss how working with children and teenagers differs from working with adults, and to consider how ethical standards are maintained.

> "
> The ultimate lesson all of us have to learn is unconditional love, which includes not only others but ourselves as well.
> "
>
> —Elisabeth Kubler-Ross

Special Considerations

While you should be even-handed about how you apply ethical standards to clients, you must certainly bring heightened awareness and sensitivity to ethical issues when working with children. One positive effect of laws regarding minors is to broaden the sense of responsibility toward youth so that all adults, not just their primary caretakers, share in this responsibility. In a session with a child the practitioner may feel a similar broadening of responsibility for the child's welfare. It is helpful, then, for the practitioner to consider what special factors may clarify ethical decision-making to support the child's best interests. The three questions that begin this exploration are: What is the child's stage of development? Who is part of the therapeutic constellation? What are the therapeutic goals?

The Child's Stage of Development

Physical growth is, of course, a consideration in a session but it is only one of multiple arenas where the child develops. Emotional, cognitive and social development also need to be taken into account. For example:

- Young people whose cognitive development is delayed may need the support of familiar people or places to receive the benefits of hands-on therapy.

- Girls who begin to menstruate at an early age may experience unresolved feelings about their bodies and generally do not develop a corresponding emotional maturity until years later.

- An infant who was separated from its parents immediately after birth for a prolonged period will likely have different needs and responses to touch therapy compared to an infant who achieved early bonding with parents.

By blending together, as much as possible, a complete picture of the child from these various aspects, a practitioner may design and implement a session that correctly meets the individual child's needs.

The Therapeutic Constellation

When a practitioner works with a minor, the therapeutic relationship expands beyond practitioner and client to include other caretakers. These may be one or both biological parents, adoptive parents, foster parents, social workers, or health care providers. Defining who is part of the therapeutic encounter is an important early step when working with children. The practitioner needs to know who is providing additional information about the child, who is helping to establish treatment goals and to whom the practitioner must communicate about the progress of therapy.

Many practitioners value the autonomy and independence of their role in the therapeutic relationship. When working with minors, this individualism may need to be tempered for the child's best interest. The expanded therapeutic relationship can benefit the child by bringing together multiple concerns and multiple skills for the overall purpose of enhancing the child's well-being.

Any wide therapeutic constellation can raise complex issues of authority, responsibility and decision-making. The practitioner determines how much to base the therapeutic encounter on what the child says and how much on what the adults say. In cases where the integrity of the caretakers comes into question, a practitioner may need to make the difficult decision to break therapeutic confidence. States require professionals who work with children to report cases of suspected child abuse and a practitioner must act ethically on behalf of the child even if doing so may compromise the expanded therapeutic relationship.

Therapeutic Goals

A practitioner must consider the therapeutic goals in light of the other two issues, i.e., the child's stage of development and the expectations of the care-taking adults. Elicit the child's input as much as possible in the process of choosing and evaluating goals. When children see their contributions as central to their own healing process, therapy often proceeds more smoothly and achieves greater success. Specific goals with clear check-points and end-points, clearly communicated among and agreed upon by all parties, go a long way toward ensuring that ethical standards are maintained in the work.

Infants and Children

A strong educational component underlies most work with infants and young children. Part or all of the session may be devoted to how the family can utilize touch in a healthy way at home. When a practitioner works with adult clients, she has their implicit permission to touch by their request for an appointment. When she works with children, she must explicitly ask even the youngest clients for their permission before touching them, and model both listening for the child's cues and responding appropriately to negative cues. The practitioner also teaches caretakers to do the same at home, thus allowing children to develop a sense of autonomy about who touches them.

Any practitioner who works with children should both like children and relate well to them. A sense of humor is a great ally: young children tell you immediately and honestly what they think about your work. Young children also tend to respond quickly to hands-on techniques. Practitioners need to keep their expectations, plans and timing flexible, since a session may complete sooner than planned. Put a pro-rated fee schedule in place and clearly communicate your payment policies to the child's caretakers.

In general a parent or other caretaker should always be present in the room when a practitioner works with an infant or young child. If the sessions become an established part of care, the caretaker may float in and out of the room while remaining nearby and accessible to the child. Occasionally, the practitioner may wish to interview the child alone and should ask both child and caretaker for permission.

Teenagers

Our culture does not offer many non-sexual ways for our young people to receive touch after the age of about 12. Manual therapies at this age can be a vital, positive part of a young person's changing body awareness and developing sense of self. They also provide our youth with a way to continue to receive the sustenance of nurturing touch, which feeds them physically, mentally, emotionally and spiritually.

Preteens begin to develop more autonomy from parents or other caretakers and come to rely more on peer relationships for social and interpersonal support. At this point young people may not wish for a caretaker to be present during their sessions and yet may not feel completely comfortable alone with the practitioner. An ethical way to approach such a situation is for the practitioner to ask the young client if she would like anyone else present in the room during the session. The presence of a friend or sibling can help the young client feel safer and more in control of the therapeutic encounter. If you are going to be alone with a minor, state very clearly to the minor and the parent together that you have no secrets in the treatment room concerning what you do, that the minor must feel free to tell the parent everything that happens because you do nothing in the parent's absence that you would not do with the parent present. Also urge the minor to tell you if anything is uncomfortable or does not seem acceptable.

During the teenage years rapid physical changes are matched by the youth's constant adoption of different personality traits, philosophies, ideals and values. A practitioner working with a teenager may feel that a different person is on the table at every session: this observation is close to the truth. Again, flexibility is key. Continue to ask permission to touch and offer options when there are choices that do not affect therapeutic outcome: "Do you want to leave some or all of your clothing on?" "Shall the work be done in a standing, sitting or lying position?"

In therapeutic situations the practitioner is in charge yet the client is in control. The practitioner must be in charge as the expert determining protocols and procedures. The client is in control because nothing may be done without the client's informed consent. The minor still certainly has the right to withhold consent but it should be clear what is being chosen. Obtain input and alignment by asking questions such as: "What is the goal for today's session and how does that relate to the overall goal of our work together?"

Somatic practitioners can serve as important role models for teenagers in many ways. The practitioner who models self-care teaches the youth about body awareness and taking care of one's self. A young man who hears from his practitioner that "no pain, no gain" is a lie may later stand up to the football coach who tells him to play to the point of injury. Ethical professionals who treat young clients with respect and dignity reinforce their image as persons worthy of respect.

Informed Consent

If you have ever felt the powerlessness of undergoing a medical procedure without fully understanding what to expect, you know the importance of *informed consent*. If you have ever felt the frustration of not having your hair cut the way you specifically requested, you know the importance of informed consent.

Informed consent, a concept that arose in the medical field in the early 1960s, served as the initial nudge of a major shift in consumer empowerment known today as "patients' (or clients') rights." Prior to the establishment of informed consent, the client was relatively powerless in relationship to a doctor's authority over medical and health care matters. Doctors and other medical professionals held a certain power over their clients simply because they had knowledge to which patients were not privy. Diagnoses, prognoses and procedures were secretive and mysterious; patients were the uninformed bystanders in their own health care.

Because of informed consent, clients have the right to know about and fully participate in their own care. The client, or his guardian, must now give full consent for most care except in emergencies where the client is incapacitated. The client also has the right to withhold or withdraw consent at any time. The consent given is not considered valid unless the client is informed about all procedures he is expected to undergo, the reason for it, the possible risks and benefits, and reasonable alternatives to the procedure. Most importantly, the client must understand the information given.

See Appendix A, pages 263-264, for sample **Informed Consent** forms.

It has become customary practice for the providers of many services outside the medical venue to practice the concept of informed consent. The consumer is now advised about what needs to be done or what is expected to happen before the service is rendered and the consumer must agree, either verbally or in writing, to the service. For example, when you take a vehicle to be serviced for an undiagnosed problem, the mechanic contacts you after the diagnosis is made and before the work is done, to tell you what is needed and the estimated cost. You can opt to say, "Go ahead and do the work," or "Don't do the work." If more complications arise during the repair process, you are notified, and you must give your consent again. Like clients' rights, consumers' rights are protected now more than ever.

In theory informed consent appears to adequately protect both the service provider and the consumer. At least legally when the provider imparts information, offers an explanation of what is to occur, and the consumer gives full consent after being informed, litigation is less likely to occur. In the professional relationship that occurs between a somatic practitioner and a client, viewing informed consent only from a legally debatable standpoint is inadequate. Informed consent between a practitioner and client provides the foundation and framework of an ethical and safe experience.

Informed consent also entails informing clients of what professional services you can legally and ethically provide as well as any limitations. Under the best of ethical conditions informed consent is a twofold agreement in which the client and practitioner share an objective for the treatment or procedure and its outcome. The objective is explained, discussed, fully understood and agreed upon by both the client and the practitioner before the treatment begins. Ethically speaking, the client needs to be *well-informed*, not *merely* informed. Most practitioners are very adept at offering information to their clients. The following ideas are presented for your consideration, and as reminders, of the many ways in which we can keep our clients well-informed:

- Introduce yourself when a new client arrives for her appointment with a firm and friendly handshake and let her know that you are the practitioner with whom she will be working.
- Use a client agreement form to eliminate any misunderstandings about what your services are and are not.
- Be aware of why the client is seeking your services. Ask this question during the initial contact or add the question to your medical history form, but be sure to ask, "Why are you seeking these services at this time?" Follow this up in subsequent visits by asking the client at each pre-treatment assessment what her goal is for the session. When possible, meet her expectations; if it is not feasible or possible, explain why.
- A client reports on the medical history form that he is seeking massage to lower his stress and relieve his low back and hip pain. During the pre-treatment assessment you ask the client his goal for today's treatment, which is his very first massage experience, and he says, "To help my back pain." Before beginning the massage you inform the client: "After assessing you, (your complaints of pain, postural and range of motion assessments and medical history), I would like to do a general relaxation massage treatment with some special focus to your low back and right hip area where you're experiencing pain. Since this is your first massage, I'll introduce your muscles to being massaged and use this first session to evaluate your response before I use deeper treatment methods. Does that sound like what you had in mind for today's treatment?"
- Do not assume that your client is familiar with your treatment process. Inform clients about what to expect by referring them to that section of your Policy Statement or offering them a "Welcome" form to read after they fill out their medical history.
- During the treatment, verbally inform the client when you are moving to more vulnerable areas, such as the anterior neck, medial thigh and abdomen.
- Verbally inform the client when you are about to lean your own body against the table, or climb onto the table to assist your body mechanics or to facilitate stretches.
- Inform the client when your work deepens and check if it is tolerable.
- Get permission from the client before varying from the agreed upon treatment plan or using a new modality.
- Several minutes before the treatment ends, inform the client that the session is nearing completion and ask if she would like you to focus on an area that may need more attention.
- If a client is in a semi-sleep state, gently get her attention and tell her if you are about to do something that could be considered jarring (e.g., performing tapotement, applying stimulation to acupuncture needles).
- Keep in mind that there should be no surprises for the client. Remember that information, knowledge and the right to refuse offer personal power to the client who is in a vulnerable or relaxed state.

- Inform the client about what to expect after the session. For example, when suitable, tell the client that he may experience soreness or tenderness the next day.
- Cover all bases so that neither you nor the client face a situation without some preparation about what to expect beforehand. Let the only surprise be how much the client enjoyed the experience and how impressed she was by the way she was considered and nurtured during the treatment.

Declining Potential New Clients

Is it ever ethical for you to refuse your services to a potential new client? Of course, the answer is "yes!" There are a number of situations where saying no to a new client may be the correct thing to do.

A Full Practice

Having enough clients to fill your appointment schedule well in advance is wonderful. Nevertheless, your refusal of new clients should be handled in such a way that the clients maintain a positive image of you and the profession. Remember your goal is to maintain a high quality of service for every client. Keep ready a list of the names and telephone numbers of other local practitioners whom you recommend. This list should be based on your direct knowledge of these practitioners, including the type and quality of work they do and that they are accepting new clients. Two examples of polite ways to tell someone that you are not taking new clients are: "I appreciate your call and I am unable to accept any new clients at this time. I know several local practitioners whom you can call...." "Currently all my appointment slots are filled with established clients. May I recommend some nearby practitioners whose work is similar to mine...?"

Inability to Help

There are times when you do not believe you can help a specific client. Sometimes a telephone or pre-treatment interview makes it clear the client needs a specialized type of treatment or wants to work with a practitioner who specializes in specific populations such as pregnant women, athletes or seniors. Also, the client may have a functional problem best addressed by a different type of somatic practitioner or the client may best be served by psychotherapy or life coaching. Unless you are trained in the specialty indicated, you are ethically obligated to refuse treatment and refer the client elsewhere. Again, be prepared either with the name and number of an alternate practitioner known to you, or with suggestions of health care facilities, web sites, or toll-free numbers where clients can find more information. Many practitioners do not charge a new client for a first session if they discover their skills do not match the client's needs. If this occurs, you can say something like, "From the information you have given me, I believe you will be better served by a specific modality I'm not trained in. You can find out more about this technique and obtain a list of local practitioners from...."

Countertransference

The most delicate reason of all to refuse treatment is when a practitioner experiences countertransference with the client. An ethical practitioner carefully examines such situations before making the decision to refuse. The countertransference may make itself known to you through the following ways: a feeling of great attraction or repulsion to the client; a sensation of intense dislike toward the client; a vague lack of affinity with the client. The fundamental question for practitioners to ask themselves is, "Can I give this client clear, caring, compassionate energy in the course of a treatment session?" If the honest answer is no, the client must be referred elsewhere.

See Ethical Principles, pages 19-20, for details on **countertransference**.

Personal issues can hinder practitioners from working compassionately with clients. Especially in the earlier stages of one's career, a practitioner may bring unresolved issues into relationships with clients. As he gains experience and maturity in dealing with people, he usually resolves many of these initially disturbing issues. A supervisor or peer group can offer tremendous support, perspective and wisdom. Usually the longer a practitioner stays in business, the broader spectrum of people he feels comfortable treating.

Consider, for example, a client who is obese, has a disability such as an amputation or has severe scarring from a burn. Ideally, these conditions would have no negative impact on a practitioner. If a practitioner knows he has difficulty maintaining a professional and caring attitude in this situation he is ethically bound to refer the client elsewhere. This practitioner should also consider discussing his difficulty with a supervisor to see whether the personal issues can be resolved.

To refuse to treat somebody based solely on their disability is not only unethical, it is often considered illegal.

Regardless of experience, a practitioner may find herself attracted or repelled by a potential new client. When she determines that her best course of action is to refuse to work with that client, she needs an ethical, neutral and non-hurtful way of expressing this refusal. The practitioner's statement should be less about her or the client and more about the appropriateness and quality of the service the client seeks. Following are examples where an inappropriate response is contrasted to a neutral, positive, ethical refusal.

INAPPROPRIATE: "I had a bad experience in my childhood with a relative who had a wartime amputation. I'm afraid I just wouldn't be comfortable working with you."

INSTEAD: "I don't believe my skills are developed enough to give you the standard of care you deserve. Let me offer you the names of practitioners with more experience in this area."

INAPPROPRIATE: "You really remind me of my former boyfriend. I'm working on my issues with him right now, so it's probably best if I refer you elsewhere."

INSTEAD: "I think my ability to help you is limited. I would like to refer you to a very skilled, experienced and compassionate practitioner who can give you better care."

Dismissing A Client

A practitioner may appropriately decide to stop seeing an established client for any number of reasons. Although ethical considerations differ from one situation to another, the practitioner should consider in each case how best to communicate the decision to the client and whether referral elsewhere is appropriate. In some circumstances "firing" a client from an established therapeutic routine may instead be a time to review treatment goals and possibly renegotiate a new contract based on new expectations.

If a practitioner is unable to treat a client for whatever reason, that practitioner should refer the client to another practitioner. It is not appropriate to simply deny treatment to a client. If a client's condition is out of your scope of practice or requires modalities you do not prefer to utilize, refer the client to an appropriate practitioner who can help. If you do not like the client or have serious concerns about countertransference, refer him out, do not simply dismiss him.

Discomfort

A practitioner should terminate work with a client who makes the practitioner feel unsafe or who makes continued sexual advances. Referring this client to another practitioner in the same field could pose ethical difficulties. More appropriate would be a referral to psychotherapy where issues of aggression or of infatuation with one's counselor frequently form a therapeutic fulcrum. In contrast the hands-on session is not a setting where such issues are dealt with and the practitioner can explain these facts to the client in a non-judgmental way when communicating the end of the professional relationship. For instance the practitioner might say the following:

> "I find that your [sexual comments] interfere with the effectiveness of our work together. Since our sessions aren't an appropriate place to resolve these issues, I've decided the best course is to stop our work together. Let me offer you the names of some excellent psychotherapists with whom you might look at these issues more closely."

If you are a primary care practitioner and a client does not pay his bill, you cannot refuse to treat him on this basis; you must refer him out. In some professions refusal to treat a client is called "abandonment" and it is illegal.

Transference and Countertransference

Situations can arise in therapeutic encounters where the intensity of transference/countertransference is beyond the ability of the practitioner to cope. For example:

- The client who becomes overly dependent or inappropriately demanding, and the practitioner is unable to set a workable boundary.
- The client suffers from some emotional disorder that threatens the practitioner.
- The client is a survivor of trauma, abuse or incest for whom the therapeutic session elicits hyperarousal.
- The client asks the practitioner for help outside his scope of practice: "Can you help me not feel depressed?" "I'm angry and fight with people all the time. Will this work help that?" "I need to eradicate this cellulite. Will these sessions help?"

See page 221 for more information on **hyperarousal**.

Discussions with a supervisor or peer group can help the practitioner determine when (and how) the practitioner could continue the therapeutic relationship by making appropriate changes, and when to let the client know their work together needs to end. Communicating this decision can be very difficult even when the decision to stop working with these clients is an ethical one. Affirm both the client and your work together while also expressing the limits of that work. In addition, the question of appropriate referral requires much thought. A same-field referral would be acceptable if you know the other practitioner has training and experience specific to the client's needs. For example, some practitioners hold concurrent licensure as psychotherapists or work closely with psychotherapists on certain issues. Otherwise, a psychotherapy referral as discussed in the last scenario may be most appropriate. The practitioner could say the following:

> "I've become aware that something you're asking for in your therapy with me (e.g., emotional support, memory processing) is outside my expertise. Although I feel our work together has gone well, I believe we've reached the limits of how much I can help you. I have enjoyed having you as a client and want the best for you as you continue your healing process; therefore, I'd like to offer the names of some excellent practitioners who offer a more suitable type of therapy."

Lack of Results

In a similar way, a practitioner may decide to end a therapeutic relationship because the client is not benefiting from the treatment being provided. In contrast to the above scenarios, however, in these cases the problem presented by the client is appropriate to the type of work being offered. A client who suffers from chronic headache or low back pain, for example, can reasonably expect a somatic practitioner to offer techniques that may help the problem. Nevertheless, not all techniques are effective with all problems, nor do all practitioners possess the same training or skill level. So that both client and practitioner can measure the effectiveness of the therapy, set parameters by keeping records of predetermined checkpoints (number of headache-free days, level of intensity of pain, distance walked without pain) or by predetermining a certain number of sessions after which progress is measured. If these parameters indicate the therapy is not working, it is appropriate for the therapist to terminate treatment and offer referral elsewhere.

> "We had the six sessions we agreed to when we started, and you've noticed very little change in your back pain. Clearly the type of work I am doing isn't effective for you. I would like to suggest a few other practitioners whose work differs from mine and wo might better help you."

Completion

There is the happy circumstance where you finish what you can do for your client; your work was effective and the therapeutic goals were reached. If clear parameters are set around the work, both practitioner and client recognize when this happens; nevertheless, it is the practitioner's responsibility to communicate this ending to the client. Here, ending does not necessarily mean completely stopping the therapeutic relationship, although the client should certainly be given that choice. The practitioner can ethically present other options to the client—for example, ongoing maintenance sessions, or a change to another form of somatic work in which the practitioner is trained. Acknowledge the successful completion of specific therapeutic goals and give the client information about what can come next.

> "The problem you came to me with has been resolved. Congratulations on seeing this process through to its successful completion! I have enjoyed having you as a client and if you wish to continue sessions with other goals in mind, I would be happy to work with you."

The Team Approach

Many somatic practitioners are joining forces with other health care providers and creating associations and partnerships. It is also becoming more commonplace to hire practitioners as employees in clinics. These alliances can be quite beneficial for the practitioners as well as for their clients. Unfortunately, too many people develop these alliances or take jobs in companies without creating a proper structure to clarify expectations and guide interactions, thus creating an environment where ethical dilemmas arise. The major areas for friction are: incompatible personalities; conflicting visions of the image of the business, the desired clientele and how the business should operate; marketing; client care; and finances. We explore the team approach from this vantage: the general concept of working in a group practice; issues specific to working in clinics, spas and salons; and case management.

Group Practice

Group practices can be formed as an association of individual practitioners, under one roof, who each have their own separate businesses. Often the individual practitioners contribute toward common expenses, such as rent, utilities, marketing and even the cost of hiring a receptionist. So long as the individual members only share common expenses and do not share revenues or profits, each separate business is separate for tax purposes as well.

If the association also shares revenues or profits, that association may be treated as a partnership, which requires different reporting for tax purposes. If revenues/profits are shared, the individuals should consider creating an entity, and reporting as an entity for tax purposes.

An association should also avoid holding itself out as an entity or joint venture. If enough facts are cited by a complaining party, each member of the association could be liable for obligations of the other members. Filing partnership papers, or creating a written partnership agreement, is not required to be legally considered as a partnership: the key to determining partnership status is the "appearance" that the business is indeed operating as a partnership, or holding itself out as a partnership. Thus if someone were to file a lawsuit against an associate of yours, you could be held jointly and severally responsible.

Group practices can also be formed within one legal entity. In this case, all expenses, profits and liabilities are incurred by that entity, and allocated among the owners (although not necessarily on an equal basis). The entity may be a partnership, corporation or limited liability company, depending on the goals of the individuals involved and various tax considerations. Each entity requires careful thought as to legal, tax and practical considerations of the owners.

Pitfalls in a group practice can be circumvented by delineating in writing the rights and obligation of each individual. List all of the particulars that are important to each person in running the business. An agreement between members of an association should include the following: the purpose and major goals of the association; expectations and duties of each practitioner; how common expenses are allocated to the members, objective consequences for failure to fulfill obligations; procedures for handling problems (conflict resolution); and a dissolution (or buy-out) agreement. In the case of a group practice operating in an entity, the agreement should also include specific terms of allocating collection of revenue, as well as allocation of expenses. Note that the allocation of income should focus on actual collections, rather than what may be billed but not paid. Also develop a general business plan, an agreed-upon Standards of Practice and a Code of Ethics.[12]

> *The law of self-fulfilling prophecy says that you get what you expect. So why not create great expectations and the highest vision possible of yourself and your world?*
>
> —Mark Victor Hansen

Financial obligations can be a major source of entanglement in an association. In an association, often one individual is required to assume responsibility for each common expense (e.g., rent, utilities and telephone). If at all possible, include everyone's name on the lease and clarify the group's shared budget. In an entity, also prepare financial projections, have a written agreement of each person's financial obligations; determine how revenues and expenses are split, and designate who, in writing, is authorized to make minor decisions, major decisions, pay minor expenditures and incur major expenditures on behalf of the entity.

Many group practices incorporate product sales. Although product sales are a great diversification method, three significant challenges arise: choosing the product lines; determining who is responsible for overseeing sales; and disbursing the profits, particularly when a client sees more than one practitioner in the group setting. Note: if your business is a partnership, the funds can be commingled. Be sure to create an action plan for product sales including goals and budget.

Cooperative marketing is one of the strongest benefits to being in a group practice and it is often an area where conflicts arise. Determine what percentage of marketing is done jointly. Develop a marketing plan with goals, target dates and a budget. Before placing long-term advertising (e.g., a shared advertisement in the Yellow Pages), create a payment agreement to cover the possibility of an associate leaving.

In most group practices each individual is responsible for *booking* his own clients. This gets fuzzy when clients come in from shared marketing activities. Avoid misunderstandings, resentment and unethical behavior by creating a new client booking policy that evenly distributes new clients among the practitioners.

Clinic Issues

Many somatic practitioners are working in clinic environments. The concept of multi-discipline or multi-practitioner practices is fantastic for excellent client care. However, in reality there are two very different motivations for setting up multi-care practices. The first motivation is to provide an environment where each client has one chart for the office and may access all of the different specialty practitioners in the center. The designated case manager coordinates the client's care plan between the different practitioners and oversees the progress. Each case is discussed at group meetings so that all minds involved can arrive at the best treatment(s) and ongoing care.

The second motivation to set up this type of clinic is financial. Several practitioners of the same or different specialities join together to share overhead. They each maintain a separate practice with their own clients and really do not promote inter-office referrals. This lack of cross-referrals is often due to the fear of losing clients to another practitioner. This motivation is for the benefit of the practitioners, but certainly not for the benefit of the client.

Other major concerns about joining a clinic are: the possibility of needing to alter your style and scope of practice to suit the clinic's visions, policies and procedures; and the controversy of being hired as an independent contractor versus employee.

Be sure the clinic attracts the kind of clients with whom you want to work, provides opportunities for you to use your favorite modalities and allows you to work at the pace and in the style with which you are comfortable.[13] Before working in such a setting, determine if you can live with the clinic's policies for dress code, finances, logistics, practitioner/practitioner interactions, client/practitioner interactions and marketing.

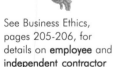

See Business Ethics, pages 205-206, for details on **employee** and **independent contractor** status.

Most practitioners discover they need to alter their treatments in a clinic setting. The time you spend with clients and the actual work you do may be determined by the lead primary care provider. You could be told what to do, how to do it, when to do it and the time allowed to work. You may even experience a sense of detachment from the client because someone else usually handles the greeting, scheduling, payment, paperwork and sometimes even the follow-up. On the positive side freedom from administrative tasks provides you with more hands-on time with your clients. In addition, your clients benefit from your association with the clinic because the setting provides access to managed care and possibly to state-of-the-art equipment that you otherwise might not afford.

Case Management

One of the prime advantages to working in a group practice or clinic environment is the opportunity to do case management. You better serve your clients when they have access to a variety of health care providers under one roof who actively work together for the optimum well-being of clients. For this to succeed what is required is communication, time, cooperation and shared values. Ethical case management is conforming to professional standards of conduct in coordinating client care.

The Case Management Society of America defines case management as a collaborative process that assesses, plans, implements, coordinates, monitors and evaluates options and services needed to meet a person's health needs.[14] In manual therapies, case management is the process of assessment of an individual case and facilitating the type of treatment and treatment schedule for the condition(s). The purpose of case management is to help clients more effectively reach positive health outcomes.

The key skills needed for case management are critical thinking, communication and collaboration.[15] *Critical thinking* is a scientifically based process used for gathering, synthesizing, prioritizing, analyzing and evaluating information. Critical thinking is essential for effective problem solving and decision-making. *Communication* is the ability to send and receive information. Practitioners must be proficient in effectively working with a broad range of people to carry out the case management plan and achieve the health outcomes desired. Obtaining accurate information from sources requires strong interpersonal skills and rapport with clients, families and providers. Another key role in case management is *collaboration*. The ideal environment is where all practitioners who work with a specific client communicate periodically about that client's treatment and progress. Throughout the case management process, practitioners also empower clients by educating them about their care and involving them in it.

In somatic practices the case management process consists of five steps: assessment; planning; implementation; coordination; and evaluation.

- **ASSESSMENT** is the process of collecting pertinent information about a person's situation to identify needs and develop a plan. When a client initially comes into your office, a health history is taken. After the intake is completed, an examination is performed, and the phase of the condition (acute, subacute, or chronic) is determined. Information about general physical health, functional capacity and age is also gathered. From the combined information from the history and examination, an *assessment* follows. After the assessment has been determined a treatment plan is formulated.
- **PLANNING** is the process of setting up specific objectives, goals and actions to meet identified needs. Individual treatment goals differ among clients with the same condition. Both practitioner and client must communicate to ensure they are working

Being challenged in life is inevitable, being defeated is optional.

—Roger Crawford

toward the same treatment goal. Without good communication the two perceptions may differ dramatically, thus leading to unnecessary treatment or poor case management.

- **IMPLEMENTATION** of the plan begins once the treatment plan has been formulated.
- **COORDINATION** of services is required if other providers are involved in the treatment plan.
- **EVALUATION** measures the quality and outcomes of services and is done to determine if the plan is producing the desired results. At this time any necessary modifications in the treatment plan are made. The intervals for further re-evaluations are determined by the speed and amount of progress, the frequency of reports from other sources and the timing of key decisions. If a case is progressing smoothly, maintenance monitoring occurs infrequently. The client should be treated until the symptoms are completely resolved or until they reach maximum improvement. As the client recovers, she should be educated on the importance of home care. Home care is the continuance of the treatment in the home environment (shifting from office treatment to more self-care). Case management continues along a continuum of care; as the client moves along the continuum, the case management process follows.

Tips For Effective Case Management

CLINIC INTERACTIONS

Agree on the definition of case management and what it entails, including the degree of interaction between the practitioners. Secure an Independent Practitioner's Agreement, Employee Agreement, Partnership Agreement, or Associates Agreement that includes such issues as "inter-office referrals." If the agreement states that cross-referrals inside the office are to take place and they do not, the owner of the practice is in breach of contract. Invest the money for an attorney to draw up the agreement and be professional enough to hold the owner of the practice to the spirit of that agreement. If the owner does not, this is not the best environment in which to stay. (Keep in mind that it is not wise to totally rely on referrals to fill one's practice.)

MULTI-DISCIPLINED PRACTICE WITH PRIMARY AND NON-PRIMARY CARE PRACTITIONERS

Multi-disciplined practices draw a variety of cases. If all the practitioners network, clients enter the clinic looking for different levels of expertise and modalities. Consider the following:

> A client comes to the clinic and initially sees a massage therapist. After treating the client for a short time, the therapist realizes that the problem is not progressing as it should and refers the client in-house to the chiropractor. The ethical question is, who is the primary care provider in this case now? The massage therapist was first to treat the client, but the chiropractor is of higher licensure and has a larger scope of practice.
>
> The practitioner of higher licensure and scope must take over as case manager and in this example the massage therapist must yield to the chiropractor's expertise. This is not only ethical, it is the best scenario for the client. The massage therapist may continue to treat and to provide supportive input into the client's care plan.

MULTI-PRACTITIONER CLINIC WITH LIKE PRACTITIONERS ONLY

There are groups of like-specialty practitioners who join for their financial benefit as well as the benefit of the clients. Each practitioner has her own clients and all practitioners share responsibility for all cases. They cover time slots for each other and vacation time.

Ideally, they practice in similar manners and are willing to exchange clients readily with continuity of care. This is usually a one-chart office where support staff coordinates the clients' care as the clients see multiple practitioners throughout their case. This type of clinic works only if the entire office functions well as a team.

LEAD PROVIDER OR CASE MANAGER DESIGNATION

A lead primary care provider (or designated case manager) determines the type and frequency of treatments and coordinates the collaboration of the health care team. The other practitioners are obligated to comply with a prescription for the treatment types and frequency.

PRESCRIPTION RENEWALS

If a client needs his prescription renewed to continue treatment and you are not the lead provider, you must manage the case as you have been instructed and consult with the lead primary care provider. If a client wishes to continue working with you and the renewal is not granted, the client must first be released before he can see you on a private basis.

SWITCHING PRACTITIONERS

What happens if a client is unhappy with her treatment from one practitioner and wants to change to another one within the practice? Both practitioners involved should be professional about the switch and make it easy for the client. Each client has individual needs. Just because one practitioner cannot meet those needs, it does not reflect on his abilities. The request for change simply means that the initial practitioner was not the right one for the client. If this scenario causes bad feelings, the practice suffers, and the clinic dynamics will jeopardize the care of other clients.

WALK-IN AND NO APPOINTMENT CLIENTS

Clients who enter a multi-practitioner practice should be signed in and taken in the order of arrival. If both scheduled and non-scheduled clients are seen on the same days, the scheduled clients should be seen on time for their appointments with the non-scheduled taken between in order of arrival. One practitioner should be designated in the practice to take walk-ins, or a rotation agreement should be designated for the day. Clients understand that they are usually unable to choose whom they see if they do not have an appointment.

CASE MANAGEMENT COORDINATION

Communication and coordination are the foundation of ethical case management. Ideally, arrange weekly meetings to discuss case management goals. Review the next week's client load prior to the weekly meetings. Update your treatment plans and be prepared to discuss them. Make sure that you are educated in the proper terminology to readily communicate with the other health professionals in their language regarding client care. Present your treatment plans concisely and with supporting information to gain cooperation. Be willing to compromise for the client's best interest, setting aside self-interest. Unfortunately weekly meetings may be unrealistic, particularly in clinics that see hundreds of clients each day. Most likely in these environments the client case coordination happens sporadically.

Ethical
Practice
Management

Spa and Salon Issues

Many spas and salons are expanding their scope from simply furnishing beauty services to offering health care services. It is commonplace to find a variety of providers such as massage therapists, acupuncturists, physical therapists, estheticians, energy workers and nutritionists employed at these facilities. Many practitioners work part time at a spa or salon part time to augment their private practices. This can be boring, frustrating and financially disadvantageous unless you work where the schedule is fairly full or you receive a base pay when no clients book sessions. Working in these businesses also requires conforming to a set image and structuring your treatments to align with the company's schedule, policies and philosophy.[16]

Spas range in image from holistic wellness centers to posh pampering resorts. Salons range from crowded bustling turnstiles to lush elegant day spas. The requirements in terms of attire, interactions and skills vary with the environment. Some spas ask practitioners to expand their skills to perform other services (e.g., hydrotherapy, wraps and paraffin treatments) when not doing their primary service. The expectations surrounding what you do when not working with a client depend upon the company philosophy and your employment status. Some facilities expect practitioners to assist wherever they are needed—from greeting clients to cleaning. Oddly enough, these expectations may be present even when practitioners are not paid for non-client interactions.

Major concerns of working in a spa/salon are similar to those in a clinic. Before hiring on in this environment, determine if it attracts the type of clients you want and allows you to work at a comfortable pace and style. Consider the people who frequent these establishments, the kinds of services they require and the manner in which they expect to be treated.

Marketing is another area that is often a source of conflict. In a spa you do not have to do marketing or schedule clients, but there is no guarantee that your work hours are filled. Many practitioners discover to their dismay that to increase the client flow they need to market their services. For instance, massage and other health treatments are of primary concern to spa visitors, but they are the least utilized services in salons.

Create an environment that encourages cooperation and ethical behavior by doing the following: review policy and procedure manuals (discuss areas of concern and clarify ambiguous policies); determine logistical requirements such as who prepares the room for a session; set explicit duties and responsibilities; create clear financial contracts; specify your role in the marketing plan; and clarify the expected types and levels of communication between practitioners as well as practitioner/client interactions.

> *There is nothing permanent except change.*
>
> —Heraclitus

In Conclusion...

Ethical practice management calls for high standards and personal integrity on the part of every somatic practitioner. Respecting the responsibilities of belonging to a profession, the practitioner can feel confident in interactions with governing bodies, colleagues and clients. In addition to the practitioner enjoying a sense of pride from maintaining an ethical practice, clients will receive the best possible treatment and the whole field is enhanced.

Chapter Highlights

- A professional is a person who conforms to the standards of a profession; has or shows great skill; engages in a given activity as a source of livelihood; follows a learned profession.
- Professionalism stems from your attitudes and is manifested through your technical competency, your communication skills, your ability to manage boundaries, your respect for yourself and clients, and your business practices.
- Ethical violations are unprofessional. However, not all unprofessional behavior is an ethical violation.
- The basis for true professionalism lies in integrity.
- People who possess integrity behave ethically, honor confidences and keep their word.
- Scope of Practice (SCOPE) regulations define, clarify and regulate what professionals do.
- The four key factors that influence SCOPE are: the law; educational training; competency; and self-accountability.
- The three regulatory methods affecting SCOPE are: licensure; certification; and registration.
- Licensure requires practitioners to obtain a license to perform their services.
- Certification is a voluntary option which may offer the use of vocational titles that would help distinguish professional services from adult entertainment.
- Registration is the means by which a government agency keeps track of practitioners by informational record keeping.
- Assessment skills are a systematic method for gathering information to make informed decisions about if and how treatments should proceed.
- Diagnosis is the assignment of a name or a label to a certain group of signs or symptoms.
- While local licensing laws govern your SCOPE and determine what you can and can't do, educational training individualizes SCOPE.
- Ethical practitioners must be mindful about the limitations of their training, regardless of what they are lawfully permitted to do.
- A good motto is, "When in doubt, refer out."
- Self-accountability is the cornerstone of ethics because ethics is much more than what you claim to be: it's about who you are and what you do when no one's watching you.
- Standards of Practice describe the underlying principles of a given field, the expectations of professional conduct and the quality of care provided to clients.
- A policy statement is a useful vehicle for creating boundaries that encourage trust, safety and comfort. It explicitly defines the expectations for both clients and practitioners.
- The eight major areas to cover in your policies are: type of service; training and experience; appointment policies; finances; client/practitioner expectations; personal relationships; confidentiality; and recourse policy.
- Confidentiality is defined as the client's guarantee that what occurs in the therapeutic setting remains private and protected.
- While you should be even-handed about how you apply ethical standards to clients, you must certainly bring heightened awareness and sensitivity to ethical issues when you work with children.
- The three major factors that impact ethical decision-making while working with minors are the child's stage of development, the therapeutic constellation and the specific therapeutic goals.
- In general, a parent or other caretaker should always be present in the room when a practitioner works with an infant or young child.

- Informed consent between a practitioner and client provides the foundation and framework of an ethical and safe experience.
- In therapeutic situations the practitioner is in charge, yet the client is in control.
- Informed Consent is a twofold agreement in which the client and practitioner share an objective for the treatment or procedure and its outcome. The consent given is not considered to be valid unless the client is informed about all procedures he is expected to undergo, the reason for it, the possible risks and benefits, and reasonable alternatives to the procedure.
- The client has the right to withhold or withdraw consent at any time.
- Informed Consent also entails informing clients of what professional services you can legally and ethically provide as well as any limitations.
- Sometimes declining or dismissing a client is the ethical choice.
- The major areas for friction when working in a group environment are: incompatible personalities; conflicting visions of the image of the business; the desired clientele and how the business should operate; marketing; client care; and finances.
- If you're in a group practice, strive to include everyone's name on the lease; clarify the group's shared budget and do financial projections (with a caveat against jointly making major purchases unless you're indeed partners); draw up contracts outlining each person's financial obligations; and determine how profits are split and designate who is authorized to make minor decisions, major decisions, pay minor expenditures and incur major expenditures on behalf of the entity.
- Most practitioners discover that they need to alter their treatments in a clinic setting. The time you spend with clients and the actual work you do may be determined by the lead primary care provider.
- Case management is a collaborative process that assesses, plans, implements, coordinates, monitors and evaluates options and services needed to meet a person's health needs.
- Ethical case management is defined as conforming to professional standards of conduct in coordinating client care.
- The key skills needed for effective case management are critical thinking, communication and collaboration.
- Spas/Salons often advocate practitioners expand their skills to perform other services (e.g., hydrotherapy, wraps and paraffin treatments) when not doing their primary service.
- Some facilities expect practitioners to assist wherever they're needed—from greeting clients to cleaning—even when practitioners don't get paid for non-client interactions.

Discussion Questions and Activities

- Think about someone you regard as being very professional. Identify the ways that person manifests professionalism. Describe how you feel when you are with this person.
- Describe yourself in terms of professionalism.
- Describe how you imagine others see you in terms of professionalism.
- List the changes you would like to make in terms of demonstrating professionalism.
- Discuss the advantages and disadvantages of licensure, certification and registration.
- Review your state's (or city's) laws and regulations. Identify any items of concern.
- Describe the characteristics that determine competency and list ways to objectively identify competency.
- Describe the activities and modalities that are within your Scope.
- Identify areas and activities that technically fall within your Scope but might be questionable for you to do.
- Determine the areas or circumstances that are high risk and might tempt you to go beyond your qualifications.
- Identify past actions or circumstances that you would prefer no one knew.
- List factors that could contribute to different Scopes for colleagues in the same field.
- Describe the ways in which your Scope might be different than your colleagues' Scopes.
- Review your profession's Standards of Practice and identify the following: items that you highly value; statements that are vague; standards that you do not agree with; additions you would like to include.
- Create/refine your Policy Statement.
- Identify the policies you might feel uncomfortable enforcing.
- Clarify how you handle the "bending" of policies (e.g., a client forgets her checkbook, a client who thought you were going to bill the insurance company).
- Describe situations where it could be easy to inadvertently break confidentiality.
- Identify circumstances when it is okay or even necessary to break confidentiality.
- Specify actions to minimize confidentiality problems.
- Describe situations where there might be a conflict between the desires of a parent and a minor.
- Design an Informed Consent form.
- Identify reasons why you might refuse to work with a particular client.
- Describe potentially uncomfortable situations in which you would need to terminate working with a client. Role-play these encounters and list actions you can take to overcome the discomfort.
- Create an "ideal" partnership/associate agreement.
- Design a "New Client Booking Policy" that evenly distributes new clients among all of the practitioners.
- Describe your ideal picture of working in a group environment where case management is part of the protocol.
- List reasons why you would be reluctant to refer clients to an associate.
- Identify reasons why an associate would be reluctant to refer clients to you. Designate options to counter this reluctance.
- Brainstorm ways to overcome reluctance for associates in a group practice to incorporate case management.

7

Business Ethics

- Attitudes About Money
- Fee Structures
- Tips
- Barter
- Gift Certificates
- Taxes
- Product Sales
- Referrals
- Marketing Materials
- Legal Issues
- Insurance Issues
- In Conclusion...
- Chapter Highlights
- Discussion Questions and Activities

Running an ethical business challenges the practitioner to maintain healthy boundaries and to operate from deeply held values. Ethical conflicts can arise when practitioners feel oppressed by laws and regulations, particularly those that are archaic or put unreasonable burdens on practitioners. Sometimes a practitioner may feel confusion about what is legal and what seems the right thing to do. Practitioners may feel forced to find legal loopholes to justify their choices. These dilemmas require thoughtful choices. Truly ethical businesses require a commitment from the practitioner. The business reflects the person who runs it. *The Power of Ethical Management*[1] relates ethical behavior to self-esteem: people who feel good about themselves withstand outside pressure, and do what is right rather than what is expedient, popular or lucrative.

Business ethics covers the major ethical issues that relate to managing a successful business: general finances; setting fees; tips; barter; gift certificates; taxes; product sales; referrals; marketing materials; complying with local, state and federal laws; regulating bodies; insurance coverage; slander/libel; contracts; civil lawsuits; employees; client custody; and insurance reimbursement.

As with all ethical issues, running a business presents many choices, dilemmas and challenges. In this chapter we review the concepts, beliefs and information that affect a practitioner's ability to build and maintain an ethical, professional and solid business or business relationship.

Attitudes About Money

Running a business that is both ethical and financially successful can be challenging since many people do not have a healthy relationship with money. We may wish it were not the case, but money plays an important role in our lives. Some people innately handle money well while others find it difficult to balance their checkbooks. Few people are taught how to manage money. The only formal training people receive happens if they take economics, finance or accounting courses. Ironically, most people taking those courses are the ones who are comfortable with the concept of money in the first place.

Consider the inaccurately cited biblical quote,[2] "Money is the root of all evil." The original quote is, "For the *love of money* is the root of all evil." Money is simply a method of exchange for goods and services. Originally people traded one thing for another. Money evolved as a method to simplify that exchange. Money is not a mysterious entity. Unfortunately, we imbue it with emotional significance and other qualities because most of us do not understand how to relate to the concept of money or how to manage money in a rational way—and that is where trouble brews.

In her article on money operating systems Lu Bauer wrote, "Yet, we all grow up dealing with money daily in a myriad of ways. We have had to develop our own guidelines and do our own learning, primarily by watching how money was handled in our families of origin. Unfortunately, this is often a case of 'the blind leading the blind.' Parents are not even aware they are teaching those watching children. People also learn about money from comic books, stories, teachers, church, friends and their parents, family legends, radio and television shows, and advertising. If your family was struggling financially, you may have been led to believe that strong values and love were missing in those rich families on the other side of town. Also, you were probably told that it is not okay to ask or talk about money. If your family was better off than others were, you learned not to show

See Ethical Principles,
pages 7-8, for details on
values.

it. Most people grew up with an array of mixed messages such as: a purpose in life is to acquire as much money as possible, so you can attain a higher status and respect in society, yet you wouldn't want anyone to know what you had or to be seen as a 'show-off.' You may have been further confused by parents who demonstrated differing money styles; one might have been thrifty, even a hoarder, while the other might have been happily spending and acquiring. Such families have a lot of tension around money issues."[3]

Many people in the helping professions proudly wear the "poor but pure" badge. Besides contributing to financial insecurity, this attitude often leads to questionable business practices. Many practitioners experience difficulty in charging appropriate fees for their services and many are uncomfortable charging anything at all. Income is often in direct proportion to one's self-esteem — especially for those of us in the health care field. It is imperative to recognize the difference between service and sacrifice.

> When a massage therapist first opened her practice, her fees were dictated by every hard luck story she heard. Her altruistic approach bankrupted her emotionally and drained her financial resources. What finally tipped the scales? She finally realized she was allowing her clients' money issues to be more important than her time. Several people had made comments such as, "I just can't afford to come here," and her heart strings were pulled and she scrambled to find a way to "help" them. Those same people would reveal during sessions that they recently went on a shopping trip, complain about how much it costs having their hair or nails done every week, grouse about how frantic having the new addition to their home has made them, mention an upcoming vacation, or leave and climb into a new car. It wasn't until she really began to listen and observe that she was able to assume the responsibility of her own life. Up to that point she had been robbing her clients of the opportunity to acknowledge the value of taking care of their health.

When it comes to money, everything is relative. An interesting shift occurred with the above scenario: when the massage therapist put a value on her services, so did her clients. Now she rarely receives complaints about her fees.

In his zeal to be "of service" a somatic practitioner felt it was his responsibility to provide his services to everyone who needed it. He worked 6-7 days a week, often charging at a sliding scale or *pro bono*. He had a substantial practice with very few clients paying his full fee. After years of dedicated work, he was still renting an apartment, driving the first car he bought, couldn't afford to take a vacation to care for himself and had little savings for retirement. He felt good about helping so many people and realized he hadn't cared for himself. In so doing he was now burnt out, worried about his future and unable to focus as clearly on his clients' needs.

The key to service, as well as life, is balance. Oftentimes those in the wellness field care for others instead of caring for themselves. While it is noble to care for others, it is necessary to care for oneself in all aspects. This is a lesson that must be learned; otherwise, ultimately you will not help either yourself or others.

Suze Orman, author of *The 9 Steps to Financial Freedom* states, "Before we can get control of our finances, we must get control of our attitudes about money, feelings that were shaped by our earliest experiences with it. Opening ourselves to abundance — not only of the pocketbook but also of the heart is what's necessary for true balance and freedom."[4]

Fee Structures

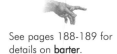

See pages 188-189 for details on **barter**.

The exchange of currency or barter is an integral aspect of the therapeutic relationship and helps establish boundaries. Many practitioners charge family members and friends a different rate than "regular" clients. While this practice is generally legal, it may pose ethical dilemmas. In addition some practitioners charge different rates for cash paying clients versus those who pay with a credit card or bill their insurance company. Consistency of rates charged is the key. Unfortunately, even acts of kindness can lead to questions of financial impropriety.

> A naturopath in a small city noticed that over the past year the other naturopaths had raised their rates. The dissenting practitioner decided that since he was making ends meet he didn't want to burden his clients with an increase. Six months later he noticed that he wasn't increasing his client base even though he was charging a lesser amount than his competitors. He was also not making ends meet any longer. He then decided to raise his rates in hopes that his current clients would understand. He received several comments from clients who felt his work was well worth the price. Interestingly, he also gained more calls from people inquiring about his services.

A delicate balance exists between charging too much for the services you offer or too little. Either way your practice suffers. By charging too little people will wonder whether there is something wrong with your skills or perhaps think that you are a novice trying to get started. Charge too much, and they might think that you are arrogant and they are not getting their money's worth.

It is essential to approach the following financial activities with thoughtful consideration: different rates for different clients; price reductions; sliding scales; package deals; and credit.

> *Money motivates neither the best people, nor the best in people. It can rent the body and influence the mind, but it cannot touch the heart or move the spirit; that is reserved for belief, principle, and ethics.*
>
> —Dee Hock

> An acupuncture client obtained insurance coverage for 10 sessions. At the end of the 10 sessions the client had received relief but wanted to continue with maintenance treatments. The client asked for a reduced rate for the sessions. He told the practitioner that rate reductions are a common practice amongst health care professionals when a client pays in cash—after all, the acupuncturist wouldn't need to wait for payment and nobody else would know anyway. The practitioner stated that she bills all her sessions (cash, credit card or insurance) at the same rate. It was unfair to expect a rate that was less than she charged her current cash-paying clients particularly since she would be putting in the same amount of effort and skill that had brought the client to this point. The client left without booking a session stating that he'd think about it. The practitioner decided not to contact the client about whether he would continue as she didn't want to compromise the value of her work or the relationship with other clients should they somehow find out.

In the Ethical Principles and Ethical Practice Management chapters we discussed self-accountability. The following scenario exemplifies the way in which the capacity for self-accountability determines financial ethics.

A physical therapist in private practice for eight years decided to raise her fees. While she enforced the increase with most of her clients, she decided not to inform several clients who had been with her for many years, allowing them to continue to pay the former fee. During the next two years she considered bringing those few clients up to the same rate as the rest of her clients but for various reasons decided not to raise their rates. Recently, one of the clients who wasn't affected by the increase had an appointment. At the end of the session, the client handed the practitioner cash to pay for her session, and while the client was in the restroom, the practitioner went to put the money away. As she did, she noticed that the client had given her twenty dollars too much. It appeared that the bills were new and had probably stuck together. "Hmm," thought the practitioner, "Perhaps I'll keep it. I certainly deserve this extra 20 dollars since she saved a lot more than this amount in not being affected by my increased rates over the past two years. So, this isn't stealing. If I didn't count it and just put it away, I wouldn't even have known she gave me extra. She'll probably never realize that she gave me more than required...I deserve to keep it,...it's her mistake."

The practitioner continued to ponder what to do. As she let herself explore the issue in her mind, she found her thoughts shifting to, "It is clear to me that if my business partner or another client were there observing me when I discovered the extra money, there would be no indecision; I would inform the client and give it back to her. Yet, here I am, with only myself to answer to with this ethical decision, and the answer isn't so clear as to what I should do. If I keep it, how will I feel about this tomorrow, or the next time I see her? Probably guilty and remorseful. How would I feel if she did this to me? Probably betrayed, and I would think she was dishonest and unethical. What would I do if a colleague brought this problem to me? I would tell her to return the client's money. How could I face this client again, knowing I didn't tell her about the money? What if she gets in her car and goes to get that $20 bill and she realizes she gave it to me? I'd have to lie and say I didn't notice. Now I'm stealing *and* lying." When the client returned from the restroom, the practitioner informed her about the extra money and returned her $20. When the client left, the practitioner felt good about her decision, realizing full well how both ethics and accountability take on new meaning when the only one to answer to is herself.

Offering different rates for different clients can lead to other ethical dilemmas. If you offer a rate to a client that makes you feel resentful, you may begin to justify lapses in your own standards. Thoughtful decisions about what you charge and why, along with self-accountability, lead to consistent ethical choices. You must be very clear about the nature of the price reduction (e.g., celebration, anniversary, thank-you for referrals, promotion) and follow the same policies for everyone.

A chiropractic client recommended the chiropractor to a friend. The friend had several sessions with the chiropractor. The two friends were having lunch one day and during their chat, the one friend thanked the other for the recommendation as the chiropractor had greatly helped her. She mentioned that paying $35 a visit was really worth the relief she had gotten. Her friend was taken aback, as she was paying $45 per visit, but said nothing. Her chiropractic visit was the next day. She felt a little resentful and wondered why she paid more than her friend. She spent the evening debating with herself whether it would be appropriate to mention it to the chiropractor. When she arrived at the office, she was uncomfortable and couldn't relax during the session. The chiropractor sensed something was different but hesitated to say anything. The therapeutic relationship has been compromised.

In the previous example the chiropractor might have been offering an introductory special or some other type of discount program. While this is not unethical, the first client now questions the chiropractor's motives and behaviors—which damages the therapeutic relationship.

Sliding Fee Scales

When a client cannot afford your fee, sometimes you need to let the client go. Another option is to reduce the per-session cost by offering clients a prepaid package plan. Or, if the client truly has financial difficulties, you could consider working with a sliding fee scale.

Sliding fee scales provide an objective method for allowing certain people to pay a reduced fee for your services. Sliding fee scales can be awkward. It is tough to set one up in advance of the first session unless a client has said something to you while booking the appointment. In general, most practitioners do not advertise a sliding fee scale unless they work with a target market that needs it (e.g., people on meager fixed incomes).[5]

Usually what works best is to give parameters. A frequently used model that seems least offensive and fair is determining fees based on income level. For example, your sliding scale statement might look like this:

My standard rate is $75 per session. If this presents a hardship for you, then I will accept a sliding scale fee based on your combined family annual income level. If the total amount earned is less than $15,000 annually the fee per session is $30, $15,000-20,000 = $45, $20,000-25,000 = $60, $25,000+ = $75

Be cautious when offering any type of discounted fee or doing *pro bono* work. Keep clear boundaries. Make certain that you have lucid policies so that the therapeutic relationship does not get damaged, you do not feel used and the client retains a sense of dignity.

Prepaid Package Plans

Prepaid package plans encourage people to book sessions more frequently, infuse extra income into your bank account and save clients money. Examples of prepaid incentives are: purchase three sessions and receive a $5 savings per session; purchase seven treatments and qualify for a 20 percent discount; and purchase five sessions and receive the sixth one free. The most important thing is to keep it simple. Do not overwhelm yourself and your clients with a plethora of options.[6] The main caution here is to limit the number of sessions in a package (a rule of thumb is three months or 10 sessions). You can always sell another package once the first one is completed. Consider the following scenario.

A practitioner wanted to take a training course that cost $3,000. One of her regular clients knew about it and told her that she would be willing to cover the training cost for weekly treatments for one year. The practitioner was ecstatic! Everything proceeded fine until about the eighth month. The client missed one of her appointments. The practitioner called the client to find out if anything was wrong, reminded her of the 24-hour cancellation policy and told her that she would waive it this time, but any future cancellation without notice would be a forfeit of that week's treatment. The following month the client missed several appointments—again without notice. When she finally showed up for an appointment, the practitioner initiated a conversation about the behavior. The client made several excuses. Then she said that she felt the practitioner hadn't been giving her usual energy into the sessions and the client wasn't sure she wanted to continue. The practitioner considered the situation and offered the client to transfer the balance of the sessions to someone else. Unfortunately, the client felt the practitioner should've refunded the balance, was angry about the proposed solution and never gave those sessions to anyone. In retrospect, the practitioner said if she had to do it over again she would've refunded the balance of the sessions. More importantly, she would never agree to such a long-term contract again.

Credit

Allowing a client to receive treatments on credit is rare in service professions. The three most common reasons for extending credit are: the fee has to be billed to a third party such as an insurance agency, attorney or a client's employer; a client forgets his checkbook; or a client has cash flow difficulties.

When billing a third party, make the client sign a statement saying that if a bill is not paid within a specified time (e.g., 60 days) the client is responsible for payment. Create a formal IOU with a payment schedule for clients experiencing cash flow difficulties.

Tips

The topic of accepting gratuities is complex. Some professions would never consider it because of the problems inherent with transference: since there is no guarantee that a client is feeling equal in power in the relationship, it is unwise and often unethical to take extra money. This includes extravagant gifts such as the use of a vacation home. The gray area concerns gifts that are more symbolic such as garden produce or homemade cookies. Graciousness is a delightful skill. It recognizes and affirms positive intentions. The acceptance of a flower can be a healing moment. However, if a client were to always bring something extra for you or offer you an expensive gift, it would be prudent to state that you are well compensated for your time and nothing else is needed.

Most people feel awkward about tipping. They are not certain when it is appropriate or how much to give. Are you supposed to tip mail carriers, hair stylists, pet groomers, auto mechanics, estheticians, gardeners and physicians? Do you tip them if they work for someone else, but not if they are the owners of the business?

Unfortunately, practitioners who work in settings such as spas usually receive minimal remuneration and rely on their tips. To complicate matters, many spas are expanding their services and employ a wide variety of practitioners including acupuncturists, nutritionists, massage therapists, movement specialists and physical therapists. This puts clients in a quandary about tipping protocol. Of course, if the practitioners were receiving appropriate fees for their work in these settings, tips would not be an issue. Clients, however, are not usually aware of the arrangements between the spa and the practitioner.

Many spas provide envelopes printed with the word "gratuity" for clients to leave tips. The manner in which this is handled makes all the difference. It is one thing to tastefully display the envelopes at the front counter; it is another to post a sign by the envelopes that says "I've helped make your day, now help make mine (hint, hint)."

Another downside to accepting tips is that it creates expectations: you do not want clients worrying about whether to give you a tip. Even worse is the anxiety clients might experience if they give you a tip one time and not the next. Will you think they did not like the session as much? Will they receive the same level of service next time? This tension defeats the therapeutic value of the work.

If you decide that in your setting, you elect a professional standard that does not accept tips, you can make a clear choice. If someone asks you about tipping, you can say something like, "I appreciate the acknowledgment and a tip is not expected in a therapeutic relationship." You can also give the client options such as donating the tip to your favorite charity or starting a scholarship fund for people who normally could not afford your services. Another idea is to thank the client and ask her instead to tell her friends about your services. Remind the client that gift certificates are a wonderful way to introduce individuals to your services.

Gratuities can make you feel appreciated, yet money is not the only way to express appreciation. Given that many people have money issues, it is not necessarily the best form of gratitude. Encourage people to simply say, "Thank you!" and have that mean something.

Barter

Barter is the exchange of goods and services. This cashless transaction method is not confined to traditional native cultures. For some, it is the preferred method of managing finances. Others use barter only occasionally to control their cash flow.[7] Bartering is not a casual activity. According to the International Reciprocal Trade Association (the governing body in the barter industry), approximately 500,000 companies in North America (mainly small businesses) transacted more than $4 billion in barter sales in 2001. Worldwide, approximately $8 billion was traded through barter companies, up 12 percent from the previous year. Barter affords a simple, legal method to conserve cash outlays. If you trade for something you need, then you can use your cash for other purposes. Also, bartering is an excellent method for expanding your client base.

Direct Barter

Many health care providers already barter on a direct basis. They identify services and products they want and then approach appropriate business owners with a trade proposal. Quite often, a client initiates a barter transaction. These direct trades work best if the items or services are of equal value. You can use gift certificates for trades and get gift certificates or vouchers from the person with whom you are trading. For instance, if you are bartering chiropractic services with a printer, ask the printer to give you a voucher for the amount you normally charge for an office visit. Then when you are ready to do a printing job, you redeem your vouchers. Here is another example: Let's say a restaurant owner wants to trade you meals for massage. You charge $60 for your massage. One method is for the restaurateur to provide you with a $60 voucher for each massage. Another idea is to transact a trade for a set amount, such as five massage certificates for $300 worth of restaurant vouchers (in varying denominations). The beauty of the latter idea is that the certificates and vouchers can be redeemed by anyone. If you do not want to eat $300 worth of food at that restaurant, give the vouchers as gifts or use them for trading with someone else. Your client does the same with the massage certificates, ultimately bringing you additional cash-paying clients.

Two major problems with direct barter arise from inequitable trades and trading for goods or services you do not really need. The following scenario demonstrates the first concern of inequitable trades:

> You want to hire someone to clean your office. You do not really have the cash to pay for that service, so you consider approaching someone to barter. Although you may find an office cleaner, it may not work if the person becomes resentful when five hours of labor (at $15 per hour) equals one hour of your service.

The second problem of trading for items and services you do not really need relates to setting good boundaries. It might be tempting to accept a barter offer from a potential client particularly if you feel that the only way the person will utilize your services is if you agree to trade. If this occurs, remind yourself that your time is valuable. If the trade is not for something you want for yourself or for a gift, then you are essentially giving away your session.

A successful barter arrangement requires that all parties feel good about the trade. This may be difficult to achieve if the client feels in a position of less power than the practitioner or if the client has difficulty speaking up for herself. In these cases it is important for the practitioner to encourage the client to be totally honest about her sense of fairness in the arrangement. This is particularly important if the value of the services exchanged is subjective, such as the value of a painting for a struggling artist who has difficulty putting a price on her work. Sometimes a barter may be based on time rather than money. For instance, one practitioner may be trading with another who charges twice his fee but they are giving each other equal time. What the arrangement actually ends up being does not matter as much as having both parties feel good about the exchange they have agreed upon. Both of these problems can be eliminated by membership in a barter network. Contact The National Association of Trade Exchanges or The International Reciprocal Trade Association for listings of barter organizations in your city.

Financial Considerations

Treat barter as cash; after all, it is taxable income. The trade dollars you spend on business expenses are deductible; the personal expenditures are usually considered draw/profit and are not deductible. The barter exchange organizations report each member's income to the IRS via the 1099-B form.

Do not pay more for an item through barter than you would pay in cash. Before making a purchase, check prices with other vendors. Most barter members are ethical but some charge higher prices to trade customers than to cash customers. Also, do not accept bartering transactions that you cannot fulfill. For example, a barter member wants you to provide ongoing wellness care to 50 employees. At first, this seems great until you realize that this would take between 16-20 hours per week of your time. This would not allow you much time for cash clients. This transaction becomes more feasible if you know another practitioner who could work with you.

The National Association of Trade Exchanges
440-205-5378
www.nate.org

The International Reciprocal Trade Association
585-424-2940
www.irta.com

Gift Certificates

Gift certificates infuse income into your practice and provide an easy way for clients to share your services with their family, friends and colleagues. They are also a valuable marketing tool to generate new clients. They serve as a goodwill promotion when you give them as presents or donate them to charities.[8]

Some people advocate increasing your revenue stream by aggressively selling gift certificates with a short expiration term. This way the majority of certificates expire before being redeemed and you receive the income without having to perform any services. While this might appear tempting, carefully consider the long-term consequences of the bad will this generates. When you sell a gift certificate, you are exchanging one form of currency for another, albeit not as universal as government scrip. A gift certificate sale is essentially a contract you have made with the purchaser to provide said value. Confiscating that monetary value simply by creating a short-term expiration date demonstrates a lack of integrity. Indeed, doing so in a way to make redemption difficult or unlikely is fraud.

> A somatic practitioner gained four new clients because another practitioner refused to honor gift certificates after the expiration date—and this refusal was to someone who had spent $1,000 on Christmas gift certificates for two family members. The gift giver and the recipients felt extremely "ripped off" by the previous practitioner. Even though the new therapist uses an expiration date on her certificates, she calls the purchasers one month prior to the expiration date and suggests they contact the recipients. If someone waits until the last day to call for an appointment, she extends the expiration date for one month. If the recipient still doesn't redeem the certificate, it reverts back to the purchaser. She tells clients her procedure when they purchase gift certificates because she doesn't want their money to be wasted.

In some states it is illegal to put an expiration date on paid gift certificates (after all, the person gave you money in good faith). Also, in many of those same states gift certificate income must be put into a trust fund.[9] Keep in mind that these rules do not apply to gift certificates or discount coupons you give away as part of your marketing strategy. These rules apply only when an exchange of money takes place.

The Downside of Gift Certificates

Some practitioners are concerned that gift certificates increase in value if not redeemed quickly (particularly if prices go up in the time between when the certificate was purchased and then redeemed), and thus they "lose" money. If you feel this way, consider putting the money into an interest-bearing account to make up for any fee increases. Another option is to put a dollar value on the certificate instead of a certain number of treatments. Many practitioners (reluctantly) admit that they do not always give their best service when a client pays for a session with a gift certificate (particularly when cash flow is tight). This is another example of where self-accountability comes into play for the ethical practitioner. An idea for circumventing the potential for a lack of enthusiasm on your part is to put at least half of all gift certificate revenue into a savings account and transfer the funds into your checking account when the certificate is redeemed. Otherwise, if you sell a lot of gift certificates, you could find yourself in the position of working for an extended period of time without receiving "new" income.

Taxes

Your financial belief system is the context for all your financial dealings. Taxation is a topic fraught with emotional charge. Many people resent the amount of money they pay in taxes (or how that money is spent) and use this anger to justify shady business practices. The two most common practices are concealing income (mainly cash payments and barter) and exaggerating expenses.

Charting makes it more difficult to hide income although we have all heard stories and seen movies where businesses keep duplicate sets of books. Beyond the simple fact that this is illegal, it makes record keeping a nightmare! Most practitioners would not consider such an extreme action as keeping duplicate books or falsifying records. The more common occurrence is pocketing cash payments—particularly when it is unlikely that the client will return or if you do not chart and your clients do not ask for receipts.

Business deductions are not always obvious and the thousands of pages of tax codes make this subject impenetrable for most people. The two areas most prone to entice people to be less than honest are purchases made by the business that are mainly used personally, and extravagant (or unnecessary) travel expenses. Keep accurate records and work with an accountant to find legitimate ways to reduce your tax liability.

A taxation area that many practitioners choose to ignore is state sales tax. Unless you live in a state that does not levy sales tax, you are required to collect (and remit) sales tax on product sales—regardless of the volume. Contact your State Department of Revenue to apply for a Transaction Privilege Tax License. Most states charge a one-time fee of less than $20. The frequency of how often you must submit reports and the collected sales tax varies. Usually you are required to fill out a form on a monthly basis for the first year, then if the volume is low, the state might reduce it to quarterly or even annually.

Discuss tax collection requirements with the state as well as the company from which you buy products for resale (e.g., certain food-based products are not taxed). Also, if you purchase products to resell you do not need to pay sales tax to the company that sells you the product. Unless you purchase products from out-of-state vendors, the companies often ask for your Resale Number (which is on the Transaction Privilege Tax License).

An ethical practitioner keeps precise records, declares all income received, refrains from inflating expenses and accurately files governmental reports.

> "
> Laws control the lesser man. Right conduct controls the greater one.
> "
> —Chinese Proverb

Product Sales

Product sales can be a lucrative adjunct to a practice, yet some disciplines discourage (or even prohibit) their members from selling products. This censure stems from a concern about the power differential that exists between practitioners and clients. Clients assume that you are an authority and may feel influenced to purchase products to please you or because they think you know everything. Even if you take great care not to exploit this power differential, you must nevertheless be careful not to manipulate or coerce your clients.[10]

Ethical sales are based upon educating your clients on the benefits of certain products and then allowing them the opportunity to purchase them from you.

The major issue here is: are you influenced in some way by the money that product sales generate, or are you selling products to clients simply because they need or want them? Exercise caution and check your motives to make certain that you are not "pushing" a little harder because your income is down or because the multilevel marketing program you are involved with requires you to meet a targeted sales volume.

Only sell products that you know are reliable, are suitable for use by your clients and are a natural extension of your business. For instance, if local statutes permit, it is totally appropriate for a somatic practitioner to sell health care products that are designed to assist in the relief of pain and promote well-being. Examples of these items are hot and cold packs, ice pillows, relaxation tools, support pillows and similar ergonomic devices, essences (such as aromatherapy), specialty lotions, self-health books and videos.

Ethical products sales is not about hype or "hard-sell" tactics. The point is providing your clients with easy access to high quality products that help enrich their well-being. As a health care provider, your clients depend on you to give them accurate information. You must know every one of your products well and convey that information to your clients. If your client really enjoyed the cervical hot pack you used during the session and wants to purchase one, you would educate the client how to use the pack and under what circumstances not to use it.

Your clients lose faith in you (and no longer stay as your clients, not to mention the loss of goodwill) if you fail to adequately inform them about the appropriate use, benefits, limitations and possible side effects or contraindications of the products you sell.

Ultimately, selling products is no different than "selling" your services—simply share your enthusiasm about them. If you make your products visible, accessible, attractive and affordable, your clients will buy them when it is appropriate.

Nutritional Supplements

In the quest to diversify their practices many practitioners sell nutritional supplements. The major concern is that practitioners may be working beyond their scope of practice unless they are a nutritionist, herbologist, or extremely well-versed in this subject.[11]

The use of herbs and vitamins has expanded so much that a new industry term, "nutriceuticals," has been coined and the government has its eye on regulation. In the 1970s the Food and Drug Administration (FDA) attempted to reclassify chamomile as a narcotic—and almost succeeded. Comfrey became a target and more recently herbs such as ephedra are under scrutiny. The FDA on more than one occasion has said that certain supplements are not safe. What qualifies a somatic practitioner to say that they *are* safe? Recently legislation was pending in the United States to require a physician's prescription for these types of supplements. The bill did not pass, but it serves as a warning. Clearly, most consumers do not want the government to take away their freedom to choose and purchase supplements from wherever or whomever they desire. Unfortunately, the more that people irresponsibly sell products without proper education, the more likely the government will intercede.

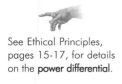

See Ethical Principles, pages 15-17, for details on the **power differential**.

Some practitioners' waiting rooms look like small health food stores. It is highly unlikely that those practitioners know much about all the products they carry. Perhaps clerks in health food stores do not know that information either, so what is the problem? Essentially, the ethical and legal responsibilities significantly differ in a client/practitioner relationship versus a customer/retailer relationship.

If there is a product(s) that you really believe in and want to make available to your clients, educate yourself on the product: the contents, suggested applications, possible adverse reactions and contraindications. Keep in mind that just because something works for you, does not mean it is beneficial to the next person. Also, "works" is a tricky word. Beware of anecdotal evidence. Results are not always proven or reliable. The possibility exists that the product could ever be harmful to someone else. When discussing nutritional supplements with clients, you need to discuss the potential side effects (such as a "healing crisis") in addition to explaining the benefits.

The more informed you are about the products you carry, the less risk is involved for yourself and your clients. If you are interested in herbs and vitamins, consider taking courses on the subject—or even pursue a degree in nutrition or herbology. Another option to ensure that you are providing your clients with information and products that are in their best interest is to team up with a nutritionist or herbologist. The marketplace is flooded with nutritional supplements and the general public is looking for direction. As health care providers, your clients naturally rely upon you to provide them with information, products and services to enhance their well-being. Proceed cautiously when incorporating nutritional supplements into your practice.

Referrals

Thanking people for referrals seems straightforward, yet such a simple gesture can be easily misconstrued. The key is the nature of the business relationship. Consider situations where current clients refer new clients to you. Whether you give them a free session, a discount off a future session, a plant, a fruit basket or even money, it still can be viewed as a kickback (although most of us hold it as a thank-you). Again, there is very little problem with these types of rewards because the client talking to a friend is usually on an equal power level.

It becomes an ethical issue when a person in a power differential relationship makes a recommendation to a client and the practitioner receives financial remuneration for the referral. Might the concept of a referral fee come to outweigh the client's need for the best possible objective referral? The bottom line is that a kickback is a kickback. Health care providers are responsible for serving the client to the best of their abilities. Accepting payment for referrals clouds that ability and puts their ethics in a compromising position. In all cases this creates a conflict of interest. In many professions it is illegal; this practice of accepting payment for referrals, or referring to clinics or laboratories in which the provider has a financial interest, is known as rebating. Severe penalties can be levied on practitioners who violate laws of this nature. It is appropriate to refer within a health system network or preferred provider list. It is not appropriate if the referral is based on the prospect of financial gain.

The gray area involves the little thank-yous. Be cautious so that there is no hint of impropriety. How much can you do as a thank-you without it appearing like a bribe?

A holistic practitioner who is also a nurse states, "As nursing employees, we were also prohibited from accepting personal gifts of any kind, even food, from the patients, from the medical staff, or from ancillary businesses such as pharmacies and home health agencies. These items had to be offered as 'gifts at large' to the unit, or it was considered something like a tip, or even worse, a bribe. When asked for recommendations [referrals], the staff had to offer a list of all the agencies/professionals available in the area and decline to offer personal recommendations in their role as employees of a facility, since their referrals might be subjective, and reflect, for good or ill, on their employer."

Marketing Materials

Marketing materials are often essential to a successful practice. Done with good taste, accurate information and honest intentions, these materials serve to enhance individual practice and the overall field. The major concerns about marketing materials are making exaggerated claims, utilizing misleading ploys, displaying inappropriate images, not following regulations and misrepresenting credentials.

Exaggerated Claims

Be certain that you can back your claims, including the verbal ones. It is impossible to know with absolute certainty that a given person will respond in a specific manner. Some clients present with symptoms that appear easy to manage but are not. In addition, everyone has their own pace of letting go and healing. Avoid statements that promise results in a specific time frame such as, "You'll be better in just five sessions." Assuming that your techniques help with everything is not wise, so do not say things like, "Oh, that isn't a problem, we can easily get rid of that." You might say, "In the past I've helped several people with this problem. This type of treatment may be very helpful for you, too, but it also may not work for you. It is difficult to predict a guaranteed positive outcome. I will do my best to help you and if it doesn't seem to be working in a [month, six weeks], I'll refer you to someone else."

Promising cures seems obvious to avoid, yet many practitioners approach or even cross that line. Check out brochures and advertisements by professionals in your field. The telephone Yellow Pages supplied these examples of statements that convey intent to help while avoiding blatant promises to cure:

- We Can Help You With....
- We Can Help Give Back Your Quality of Life
- Offering Options, Quality & Sensitivity
- Feel Better Than You Thought You Could
- Get The Relief You Deserve
- Relaxation to Rehabilitation
- Why Live With Pain?
- Specializing in....

Guarantees

Guaranteeing satisfaction is different from promising a cure. A clearly defined guarantee reflects confidence. A massage therapist in Wisconsin found an effective way of guaranteeing satisfaction by posting the following statement in her treatment rooms:

> ### Essential Massage Center Guarantee
> If you do not notice a reduction in pain or feel more relaxed after receiving a massage from one of our highly trained therapists, we happily refund the price of the session.
>
> Minor soreness, while not to be expected, does occasionally occur following a massage session. We fully expect that you will feel better within 36 hours.
>
> If after 36 hours you continue to feel that the massage has had no positive effect, your session fee is refunded.
>
> This policy applies equally to gift certificate clients.

Misleading Ploys

Sometimes words are misleading, so choose them carefully. We have all seen headlines that convey multiple, unintended meanings. Ask several people to read your promotional copy and tell you how they interpret your presentation. Clearly state the parameters if an offer has limits (e.g. "Good through March 15, 2010." or "Free to the first 10 new clients.") Avoid the "bait-and-switch" routine: do not offer a reduced price and then claim that you have sold out or the offer expired; do not offer something for free and then require the client pay something to receive the "free" service or product. Not only are these ploys unethical, they create ill will and alienate clients.

Inappropriate Images

Marketing materials should be dignified and convey professionalism. Consider the following suggestions for any visual promotional product (e.g., business cards, fliers, brochures, display advertisements in telephone books and magazines, billboards and television commercials):

- Hire a professional photographer to take pictures of you or your clients.
- Use high quality artwork. Be sure it is royalty-free or get reprint permission.
- Avoid sensationalism.
- Be sure your photos and artwork are not provocative: view pictures from all angles because sometimes images look fine from one direction, but suggestive from others. Refrain from using "glamour" shots.
- Make certain that photos do not portray results that you cannot guarantee, such as showing someone in a wheelchair in one panel and running a marathon in the next.

Follow Business Regulations

Check your city, county and state rules and regulations regarding marketing. For instance, some places have marketing regulations such as: your license number must be listed on all promotional materials; you cannot use certain media such as billboards; or you are limited in the depiction of benefits.

Misrepresenting Credentials

Honestly and accurately represent professional qualifications, competence, education, training, experience and affiliations. If you list a specialty, be certain you back this up with appropriate credentials: training and time invested in integrating the modality. Oftentimes practitioners cite numerous adjunct modalities in their promotional materials. A brochure that lists a variety of treatment modalities you practice is quite different than calling yourself a specialist or master in something—particularly after taking a weekend course.

Hold yourself responsible for a higher standard than anybody else expects of you.

—Henry Ward Beecher

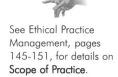

See Ethical Practice Management, pages 145-151, for details on **Scope of Practice**.

Legal Issues

Legal issues vary by profession and locale. A professional practitioner who intends to do business for the long run wants to comply with all legal requirements. Attending to the legal aspects of a practice shows respect for the community, the field, the client's welfare and the practitioner's own values. The principal aspects are: complying with local, state and federal laws; maintaining appropriate insurance coverage; slander/libel; negotiating and complying with contracts; civil lawsuits; employees; and client custody.

Comply with Local, State and Federal Laws

The two words "laws" and "regulations" make most people cringe at least a little bit. Few practitioners enjoy dealing with bureaucracy even though the results are often beneficial. Complying with laws is usually straightforward—of course, this means being cognizant of the laws in the first place. Ignorance of the law is not a good defense; in fact it is *no* defense. The difficulty arises when your values or morals conflict with one of those laws.

> *Average people look for ways of getting away with it; successful people look for ways of getting on with it.*
>
> —Jim Rohn

A reflexologist moved to a new city and was looking for a home/office. She found a house with a "mother-in-law" space that included a bathroom, small kitchen and a separate entrance that provided privacy. This space was connected to the family quarters by a breezeway. The home was purchased prior to checking the city zoning codes. Surprisingly, she was restricted from using the space as the zoning board considered her profession was a "medical" practice which required her to have office space in a professional building. Her home office granted privacy and separate restroom facilities. She believed she was providing what was necessary for her clients. In her opinion the regulation was unjustly classifying her as a "medical" practice. Her choices were to ignore the regulation and quietly build her practice, go before the zoning board and request a variance, or succumb to the regulations and allow her mother-in-law to move in.

The two major options when encountering restrictive or archaic laws and regulations are to ignore them or change them. Changing the regulations is the best long-term option although many people do not have the time (or possibly money) to invest in such a pursuit. The bottom line is that when you choose to disregard laws and regulations, you are acting unethically. At the very least, most professional Codes of Ethics state that you must abide by national, state and local laws. Some people feel their actions are justified; nevertheless, the result is still a chink in their ethics. The other consideration is the extent to which you are in violation. The penalty for disregarding a regulation or breaking the law can be as slight as a modest fine or as severe as loss of licensure or even imprisonment. If you make a choice that technically violates a law, you must be prepared to pay the consequences. Investigate potential consequences before deciding what to do.

Insurance Coverage

Maintaining adequate business and malpractice insurance coverage is crucial and some localities require specific coverage. Accidents happen, and nature has been known to strike devastating blows; without proper coverage you could be out a considerable amount of money. The United States is a highly litigious society, and no one is shielded from the possibility of a lawsuit even if his behavior is above reproach. A practitioner might win the case, but without insurance most practitioners would be hard-pressed to afford the astronomical costs of litigation. Be sure to carefully read your policy. For instance, some policies do not cover sexual misconduct while others cover the litigation costs but not the damages awarded if you are found liable. Also, some insurance companies will nullify a policy if the practitioner does not uphold all local, state and federal legal requirements.

Slander and Libel

The two major forms of defamation are slander (verbal) and libel (written). Telling everyone about a bad experience you have had with another health care practitioner or denigrating a modality that you feel is not beneficial is tempting. Most practitioners have overheard uncomplimentary conversations about providers and read similar postings on Internet news groups. Be careful of what you say so that you do not malign a colleague or are not sued for defamation.

Make sure that you state your concerns about another professional or organization as your opinion. It is fine to be emphatic and say, "I won't do business with this person!" Always stick to the facts. The minute you start embellishing the truth you could find yourself in trouble. For instance, saying someone is a crook could be actionable, but stating that you never received payment or you found the treatment to be ineffective is acceptable from a legal standpoint. Keep in mind that just because you do not work well with a particular practitioner, or certain modalities are not effective for you or are contrary to your belief system, does not preclude others from receiving benefits. Determine your intent before saying anything that may be construed as "bad-mouthing" or gossip. These types of actions often reflect more poorly on you than the practitioner or modality in question.

Action can be brought against you if you try to interfere with someone's right to contract. The term for this is Tortious Interference with Contractual Relations. The measure is if you stated something that is not true and contacted someone who is doing business with that person. For instance, you could be held liable if you know a clinic has hired a practitioner and you contact that clinic and bad-mouth the practitioner, causing the practitioner to be fired. Although a seeming paradox, this does align with the many professional Codes of Ethics that require members to report alleged violations by other members. Again, you can state facts, but be cautious about the wording. Gary Wolf, attorney at law in Tucson, Arizona, says, "Truth is the best defense for a defamation claim."[12]

Copyrighted Materials

Many practitioners copy materials to aid in client education without realizing that they are violating copyright law. If it looks copyrighted, assume it is. This applies to pictures and cartoons as well. The "fair use" doctrine allows limited reproduction of copyrighted works for educational and research purposes. The relevant portion of the copyright statute provides that the "fair use" of a copyrighted work, including reproduction "for purposes such as criticism, news reporting, teaching, scholarship or research" is not an infringement of copyright.[13]

Unfortunately, many practitioners and teachers take this to mean they can copy short sections of books or magazine articles to give to clients or use as handouts in workshops, classes or free presentations. This is usually not the case.

The two main objectives of copyright are to protect an author's right to obtain commercial benefit from valuable work, and to preserve the author's right to control how a work is used. Copyright law is mostly civil law. Unlike criminal law, you are not "innocent until proven guilty." Also, be aware that new laws are being enacted to move some forms of copyright violation into the criminal realm.

Fair Use Factors

The law evaluates the following factors to determine if a particular use of a copyrighted work is a permitted "fair use," or a copyright infringement:

- The purpose and character of the use. This includes whether such use is of a commercial nature or non-profit educational purposes.
- The nature of the copyrighted work.
- The amount and substantiality of the copied portion in relation to the copyrighted work as a whole.
- The effect of the use upon the potential market for, or value of, the copyrighted work.

Although all of these factors are considered, the last factor is the most important in determining whether a particular use is "fair." Where a work is available for purchase or license from the copyright owner in the medium or format desired, copying all or a significant portion of the work instead of purchasing or licensing a sufficient number of "authorized" copies is unfair.

Almost all materials are copyrighted the moment they are written—a formal copyright notice is not required. Copyright law makes it technically illegal to reproduce almost any new creative work (other than under fair use) without permission and copyright is still violated whether you charge money or not. Facts and ideas cannot be copyrighted, but their expression and format can. Ask yourself why you are reprinting (or taping) those materials and why you could not have paid for copies. Obtain permission to use the work from the copyright owner and always give proper credit.

Photocopy Request Information

Most authors/publishers gladly give permission to copy or excerpt material as long as it is not part of a money-making venture. It is customary to send a request to copy a copyrighted work to the permission department of the publisher of the work. Companies such as Copyright Clearance Center, Inc. will obtain permission for you (for a fee of course). Permission requests should contain the following:

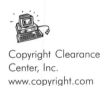

Copyright Clearance
Center, Inc.
www.copyright.com

> " Conscience: self-esteem with a halo. "
> —Irving Layton

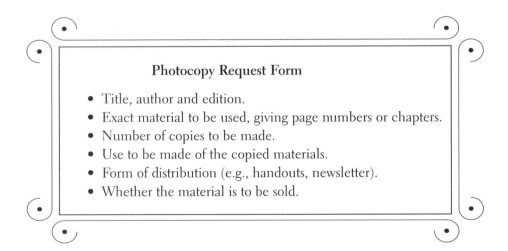

Photocopy Request Form

- Title, author and edition.
- Exact material to be used, giving page numbers or chapters.
- Number of copies to be made.
- Use to be made of the copied materials.
- Form of distribution (e.g., handouts, newsletter).
- Whether the material is to be sold.

Contracts

Legal forms and agreements are an integral part of any business relationship, yet people often avoid written contracts. Whether you are interested in a one-time only interaction or a long-term affiliation, delineate in writing your roles and expectations. Clear written agreements serve several purposes: they help avoid problems; they provide a predetermined method for resolving conflicts; and they keep you focused on your goals.[14]

A binding contract does not need to be written on a piece of paper with the word "Contract" emblazoned across the top. In business arrangements all that is usually required is some written form (letter, memo, or a full-blown contract) that describes what is to be contracted, the terms of the exchange, parties' signatures and dates. Keep in mind that once you agree to the terms of a contract, you are bound by it. Unfairness is rarely a legal ground for nullifying a contract unless it is outright fraud. Also, most states uphold verbal contracts as legal and binding.

The dullest ink is stronger than the sharpest memory.

—John Rickenbacker

Ideally, you would come to the negotiating process with a sample of your own contract and a checklist of key elements you want addressed, review the other party's contract and create a specific contract that is mutually agreeable to both of you. If the other party insists on only using her contract, make sure to obtain responses (preferably in writing) to all the items in your checklist. Verify that all parties initial each change whenever items to the contract are deleted or added. Rewrite the contract if it contains a significant number of changes.

You may be tempted to not write a "formal" contract for presumably simple transactions, particularly if it is just a "one-time" event, such as a cooperative marketing project or a short-term equipment rental. Yet it is usually those seemingly negligible occurrences that cause regrets. Invest the time in clarifying what is truly important to you in a business relationship. Even if you are currently involved in a business relationship and do not have a contract, you can always design one now. Each situation is unique and one contract will not suit all situations. Once you have the basics done, you will find it much simpler to alter any contract.

Questionable behavior is rare when everything is working smoothly. The problems arise when one party is not happy about something or when it is time to end the relationship. Some people let the "little things" accumulate until they explode. Contracts assist all parties in clarifying and maintaining ethical behavior.

Business relationships end for many reasons: one party wants to move in another direction; the association has run its course; the project is complete; the parties do not want to work together any longer. Most people do not know how to cleanly end relationships. You significantly reduce stress in ending a business relationship if your contract includes a dissolution clause that clearly describes how to terminate the association and what to do if there is an impasse.

Dispute Resolution

The options for resolving a dispute with a business associate, a client, or a landlord include: ignore it; attempt to resolve it yourself; submit to arbitration; engage in mediation; take it to court. Stewart Levine details the following seven steps to conflict resolution in his book, *Getting to Resolution: Turning Conflict into Collaboration*[15]: Adopt an attitude of resolution; listen carefully to each party's stories; allow a preliminary vision to arise with all parties, allow people to express their disappointment and then bring everyone into the current moment; agree (at least in principle) to create a new vision; design the new agreement; acknowledge resolution.

Many people are moving away from expensive, stressful and time-consuming ways of resolving disputes. They are also reluctant to engage in the traditional "positional" dispute resolution where each person takes a position and then uses a win-lose approach to getting what she wants. People are recognizing the many benefits in using interest-based bargaining, where parties engage in collaborative problem-solving that is based on the needs, desires and concerns of each party. In that way each person fulfills his goals. Mediation is an extension of this idea and can be the best choice when those involved cannot resolve a conflict by themselves: it provides the disputants with an opportunity to communicate and understand each other's points of view, create options and control solutions.

Attorney Joan C. Calcagno states, "When disputants participate in problem solving and decision-making, they are more likely to follow through with the agreement made to resolve the dispute. An enhanced working relationship is one of the many satisfactions that can result from a mediated solution to a dispute. Mediation is, at the least, less costly and time consuming over the long term and can be the way to finding innovative, mutually beneficial solutions and preserving important relationships. Faced with a dispute, consider proposing mediation to the others involved."[16]

Civil Lawsuits

Many lawsuits levied against practitioners by their clients could be avoided by keeping clear boundaries and using effective and compassionate communication skills. Luckily the number of lawsuits filed against complementary health care providers is fairly low. This is reflected in the reasonable malpractice insurance rates. For instance, massage insurance policies can be purchased for approximately $100 per year; acupuncturists pay from $500-$1,200 per year; and chiropractic policies start at about $2,000 (depending on the state and inclusions).

When, after weighing the advantages and disadvantages, a client chooses to bring a civil lawsuit, time limitations may foreclose that action. These limitations, enacted at both the state and federal level, are referred to as "statutes of limitation" since they contain a specified time limit after which a suit may not be filed, regardless of the merits of the claim. For malpractice lawsuits statutes of limitation vary from state to state but generally range from two to three years. Special limitation periods are often written into statutes that are tailored to specific legal avenues or causes of action.

Fairness underlies the rationale behind statutes of limitation. The enacting body or reviewing court attempts to balance the right of defendants to timely notice and settlement of claims with the right of plaintiffs to judicial resolution for civil damages. This balancing of interests can result in exceptions to the applicable statutes of limitations. The most commonly used exception in boundary violation cases is the discovery rule which suspends the running of the statute of limitations until the victim discovers or should have discovered the injury and its cause. The discovery rule benefits victims of boundary violations who may not connect the harm suffered to the offending practitioner until long after the damaging acts occurred.

If a client decides to pursue litigation, the process usually begins with filing a complaint in court. This document spells out the basic theories of legal duty and allegations of the practitioner's liability and damage to the client. In response to the complaint, the practitioner, usually through counsel, files an answer in which the practitioner responds to the allegations and asserts defenses. A prolonged period known as discovery follows the initial interchange between the parties to a lawsuit. During this period both sides endeavor to gather (or discover) as much information as possible about the proof of the claim or the practitioner's denial/defense of the claim. Although state and federal rules govern the extent of discovery, the scope is very broad. Friends and family of the victim usually become involved in the process and may be required to testify or provide other information to the practitioner's counsel.

Discovery

The discovery period encompasses mechanisms discussed below. The stress of these intrusions into the victim's (and the accused perpetrator's) private life can be extreme and debilitating. Conduct this type of action ethically, focusing on your integrity and honesty.

INTERROGATORIES are written questions asked of either party and must be answered under oath. In most instances the party answering the interrogatories provides a draft of the answers along with any corroborating documents to his attorney. The attorney then formalizes the answers which the responding party reads and signs, if correct. The attorney's duty is to present the information accurately and in the best possible light for the client. It is the client's responsibility to make sure that in doing so, the information is truthful.

DEPOSITIONS involve the oral examination of a witness during which an attorney asks questions that the witness answers under oath. Any person, including the parties to the lawsuit and others having information relevant to the lawsuit, may be summoned to a deposition. Typically, a deposition takes place in an attorney's office in the presence of the attorneys for both sides and a court stenographer.

REQUESTS FOR PRODUCTION OF DOCUMENTS are written requests by the attorney for either party addressed to the other party and seeking the identification of documents that are relevant to the case. When a party responds to a request for production of documents, copies of the documents described are usually provided to the requesting party. In a malpractice case a common document request would include the records of the health care provider and medical records of any prior or subsequent treating practitioner or physician of the client. The client's journals or other personal papers could be examined under a request for production. Keep in mind that you are legally obligated to provide the information even if the information may be damaging. The temptation may be great to alter or destroy documents; however, the risk, worry and liability of being discovered is not worth it.

REQUESTS FOR MEDICAL OR PSYCHIATRIC EXAMINATIONS are common. These involve examination of the client by a neutral physician or psychiatric practitioner if the client claims in the lawsuit that she suffered medical or psychiatric injuries. The examination provides an ostensibly unbiased opinion concerning the client's present condition, past history and prognosis.

Malpractice Actions

The legal theory underlying most civil lawsuits filed by clients against exploitative health care practitioners is negligence. The most commonly invoked form of negligence action is the suit for malpractice. To prove a claim for malpractice the client must establish four elements by a preponderance of evidence. This means that the client must prove that her version of events is more likely than not to be true. The quality, rather than quantity, of evidence determines whether the client has proven her case. The jury must determine whether one party's evidence is more believable, more trustworthy or more accurate than the other's, regardless of the number of witnesses testifying.[7] This represents a much easier burden for the client to satisfy than in a criminal case which requires proof beyond a reasonable doubt of all of the elements of a crime.

The elements in a malpractice case that a client must prove by a preponderance of the evidence are (1) a duty of care owed by the practitioner to the client; (2) a breach of that duty; (3) a causal relationship between the breach; and (4) damage to the client. In malpractice actions the breach of the practitioner's duty is determined by measuring the actions of the offending practitioner against what is expected from others practicing the same profession. Thus, the standard for judging health care practitioners is that they be "held to the standard of care and skill of the average member of the profession."[18] This measuring stick is called "the standard of care."

A client goes to a practitioner for a wellness treatment and when the treatment ends has difficulty getting off the table due to severe back pain that wasn't present before the session. This pain continues for several weeks and the client is unable to work. The client files a malpractice suit for pain, suffering and lost wages. Through the discovery process the lawyers learn that 10 years ago the client suffered debilitating back pain for a period of three months and couldn't work during that time.

Regardless, the practitioner was still held liable. In this instance had the practitioner done a thorough intake interview, it might have alerted him to this prior condition resulting in the exercise of greater caution.

A person is involved in a car accident, goes to the emergency room and is diagnosed as suffering from a mild whiplash injury. Her major symptoms are general achiness and a mild headache. She makes an appointment with a practitioner in hopes of alleviating the discomfort. She experiences a moderate improvement after the first two sessions but after the third one she experiences an increase in neck pain. When she arises the morning following the treatment, she has severe neck and head pain and is unable to rotate her head more than a few degrees in either direction. She files a malpractice suit against the practitioner.

The practitioner demonstrates that whiplash injuries often have a delayed onset of symptoms up to 2-3 weeks. The practitioner's notes clearly documented objective and subjective progress after the first two treatments. According to the treatment notes the same procedure was followed in each session. The case was resolved without any judgment against the practitioner; mainly due to the evidence presented which included treatment notes and the testimony of an expert witness who confirmed the common occurrence of delayed pain onset in whiplash cases.

A practitioner breaches the duty owed to the client if the treatment rendered falls below the applicable standard of care. In the first scenario the preponderance of evidence indicated that the standard of care was low, while in the second scenario it could not be shown that a causal relationship existed between the treatment and the damage to the client.

Employers' Liability

The employers of health care practitioners who commit boundary violations can also be held accountable for the actions of their employees under two distinct theories of liability: vicarious and direct. Vicarious liability, also known as the doctrine of *respondeat superior*, holds an employer liable for the acts of an employee. It is usually a prerequisite that when the wrongful acts were committed, the employee was acting within the scope of his employment. The theory holds the employer vicariously liable for someone else's behavior even though the employer did not commit the act. Instead, the employer is deemed to have control over the employee when the employee is at work, even if the employee is working away from the place of employment or the employer is not physically present at the time the wrongful act occurs.

By contrast, direct liability involves the employer's own negligence in hiring, retaining or supervising employees. Consider this flagrant example of negligent hiring:

> A security company hires a person with a long record of violent crime as a
> security guard in an apartment complex and provides that person with a gun.
> The person hired uses a master key to enter an apartment with the intention
> of robbery and shoots the startled inhabitant.

Clearly the employer has a duty to investigate the background of persons to whom weapons or access to property is given. Other potential areas of concern are not necessarily obvious. A possibility that could easily occur is that of a health care practitioner who moves after losing his license for sexual misconduct and applies for a job at a clinic in another state. That new employer might be found directly liable for subsequent sexual misconduct by the practitioner if no inquiry were made into his background or if an inquiry was made yet no action taken. In many states colleagues, supervisors and referring professionals risk liability for victims' injuries when they knew or should have known of the misconduct and failed to take appropriate steps to stop it or warn the victim.

State Licensing Boards and Professional Organizations

Some victims of boundary violations by health care practitioners choose to file a complaint with the state licensing board (that regulates the profession) or with the professional organization of which the perpetrator is a member. These actions can be taken alone or in conjunction with the civil or criminal actions. One potential result of a licensing board complaint is the offending practitioner's loss of a license to practice. This loss serves two purposes for the victim—to deprive the practitioner of a livelihood and to prevent the victimization of others by the same practitioner. These results, however, are not guaranteed. Often, state licensing boards do not possess the necessary resources to pursue all cases through adjudication. Secondly, a practitioner may forego her license but continue to practice. In many cases the offending practitioner agrees to settle a civil case out of court for a sum of money as long as the victim agrees to refrain from reporting the practitioner to the licensing board.

A successful complaint to a professional organization might also result in revocation of the perpetrator's membership in the organization or some other sanction. As with license revocation, though, this event does not preclude the practitioner from continuing to practice. Although a potential benefit of an ethical or licensing board complaint may be confidentiality of the proceedings and findings, confidentiality requirements vary among states and professional boards. In those states that do maintain the victim's confidentiality, the victim may pursue these avenues without fear of public exposure. In addition, both of these options can be more "victim friendly" since the victim is not cast in the adversarial role inherent in a civil lawsuit. A licensing board prosecutor typically presents a victim's case to a state board. The inquiry is more concerned with fact finding and determining whether the practitioner meets the criteria for licensing than with assessing the victim's emotional and monetary damages.

Who Pays?

One result of civil litigation is the award of monetary damages. In cases involving abuse by health care practitioners, the funds awarded help ensure that the victim of the abuse is able to afford treatment for the psychological or physical damages suffered. For a variety of reasons the most likely source of the funds used to compensate the victim is insurance, either of the offending practitioner or the practitioner's employer. Few practitioners can financially afford to pay a large monetary award. Furthermore, few people would risk the possibility of being held personally responsible for such payments. Most practitioners, therefore, obtain malpractice insurance if it is available to them. In most malpractice lawsuits the insurer pays any judgment amount and provides the insured with defense counsel.

Even with insurance coverage, however, a practitioner may be responsible for some of the damages awarded the victim. If the practitioner refuses to settle out of court for a sum agreed upon by the insurer and the victim's jury award turns out to be higher than the settlement offer, the practitioner may be liable for the difference. The defense attorney assigned to the practitioner also represents the insurance company; therefore the insurer controls the case. If the practitioner wants personal representation, he can hire an attorney at a substantial cost.

Many malpractice insurance policies specifically exclude intentional acts from coverage. They also write exceptions into policies for sexual misconduct or set a dollar limit on any payments for sexual misconduct. Some require a separate rider for sexual misconduct coverage. Other policies pay for the costs of a lawsuit yet do not cover monetary damages if the practitioner is found liable for sexual misconduct. The insurer may also refuse to renew a policy once a sexual misconduct claim is filed.

These are important considerations both for the practitioner and the client. If the practitioner is denied insurance coverage, the expense incurred in defending against the claim and the potential that a large verdict is returned can lead to financial destruction and bankruptcy. For the victim the lack of a reliable source of payment of damages can mean that he cannot afford the treatment needed to recover from the injuries suffered at the hands of the exploiting practitioner. Thus, in an effort to avoid denial of insurance coverage, a victim's attorney focuses on boundary violations other than sexual contact to establish the practitioner's negligence. A knowledgeable attorney also seeks to avoid insurance exclusions or liability caps by raising other legal and public policy arguments.

Several other avenues for compensation may be available to victims. In some jurisdictions the licensing board can order the practitioner to compensate the victim for treatment costs. In a criminal prosecution the court may order restitution for the victim, or the victim may access funds from crime-victim assistance centers.

Employees and Independent Contractors

It is common for practitioners to be hired as independent contractors and not as employees. This is usually done because the clinic/spa owner wants to avoid the costs associated with being an employer. With employees, in addition to the responsibility of having enough money for their paychecks, the following needs to be done: match their FICA (Social Security and Medicare) deductions; pay FUTA (Federal Unemployment Taxes) which is calculated at a percentage of the employee's first $7,000 of wages annually; pay state unemployment taxes; provide workers' compensation; withhold state and federal taxes; deposit withheld taxes (the requirement varies from weekly to monthly to quarterly, depending on the amount); file regular returns; send W-2 forms to employees annually; and in most instances offer benefits such as health insurance, paid vacations, sick leave and retirement plans.[19]

The main advantage to those who hire independent contractors is not having to withhold income tax or social security tax from independent contractors. But if you pay an independent contractor $600 or more during the year in the course of your business, you must file a form 1099-MISC at the end of the year. In most instances it is much easier and less risky to terminate a contracted practitioner than to fire an employee. Also, your liability is reduced in terms of malpractice if you have hired an independent contractor who is required to carry his own insurance.

The potential pitfalls of working with non-employees include paying a higher price for their services and not having control over their work in terms of timeliness and quality. Many clinic owners lament that the level of professionalism and camaraderie is not the same among independent contractors as with employees. Plus, an independent contractor (by nature of the classification) is less likely to actively build your business—after all, she has her own business to pursue.

The Internal Revenue Service (IRS) guidelines for determining employment status are fairly clear when it comes to clerical staff: in most instances an office-person is an employee. A gray area exists in hiring health care practitioners. In researching numerous spas, clinics and group practices, we discovered many of them walk a very thin legal line. A significant number of the so-called independent contractors that work for them would most likely be classified as employees under the IRS guidelines. Calling someone an independent contractor does not make it so.

Under common-law rules, anyone who performs services subject to the will and control of an employer, as to both **what** must be done and **how** it must be done, is an employee. It does not matter that the employer allows the employee discretion and freedom of action, so long as the employer has the **legal right** to control both the method and result of the services.

Two usual characteristics of an employer-employee relationship are that the employer has the right to discharge the employee and the employer supplies the employee with tools and a place to work. (Do not assume that you can get around this by having your "employee" provide his own specific supplies. "Tools" is a broad term that can include the equipment required in running a practice such as telephones and copiers).

If you have an employer-employee relationship, it makes no difference how it is described. It does not matter if the employee is called an employee, associate, partner or independent contractor. It also does not matter how the payments are measured, made or what they are called. Nor does it matter whether the individual is employed full time or part time.

The IRS has developed a list of 20 factors[20] that it uses to determine the status of employee or independent contractor. A practitioner can still qualify as an independent contractor even if some of these factors are present in the working relationship. The key elements to differentiating between employee status and independent contractor status in the health care industry involve the following: who regulates the type of work done and how it is performed; where and when the sessions occur; who determines the fee structure; who receives the money from the clients; who provides the equipment and supplies; who pays for client-related expenses; and who generates the clientele.

As an employer, you take a considerable risk by deeming a worker an independent contractor. If the IRS determines that your independent contractors are (or were) indeed employees, you may be required to pay fines (of up to 100 percent of the tax) in addition to the back income taxes and social security taxes. This can easily add up to a sizable amount. In the eyes of the IRS, it makes no difference if you signed an agreement that states you are contracting with an independent contractor—although a written agreement is advisable.

Minimize the risks of your independent contractors being reclassified as employees by taking the following steps: make certain independent contractors possess multiple sources of income; sign "independent contractor" contracts which clearly state the requirements of all parties while making it clear the contractors can pursue other clients; require contractors to provide their own tables, linens, products, music and other supplies; allow contractors to set their own schedules (make certain they work less than full time); have clients pay contractors directly; request copies of the contractors' tax returns; and require contractors to provide their own insurance and workers' compensation coverage. Complying with these suggestions still does not guarantee independent contractor status. If in doubt, you can request that the IRS determine whether a worker is an employee by filing Form SS-8.

If you decide to hire other practitioners as independent contractors, be sure to create a thorough contract. Hire a lawyer to review the contract. The several hundred dollars it may cost you in attorney fees is minimal compared to the potential fees and penalties the IRS are wont to impose.

Client Custody

Who retains custody of the client when a practitioner leaves a clinic setting or wants to see some clients at another location? This question is one that often elicits emotional upheaval and unethical behavior. Many practitioners work in other practitioners' offices, health clubs, salons, spas and clinics in the hopes of building up their private clientele. Problems arise if the expectations and boundaries are not clear. Consider the following:

> You provide physical therapy services for a health club. Several of your clients decide they would prefer to receive their sessions at home. Your ability to ethically take them on as private clients depends upon your agreement with the club. The club owner might not care whatsoever, particularly if she mainly views your services as an added value for membership. But the owner might be upset if the health club regards you as a significant revenue-producing adjunct or spends a lot of money marketing your services.

Another common occurrence is changing locations. For whatever reason you may no longer want to work at the hiring party's location.

> A somatic practitioner was hired as an employee at a wellness center. After five years she decided to have a child and wanted to reduce her hours and see clients in her home. Since she was an employee, the center didn't have her sign a contract. She had been seeing some of her clients for years and established a deep rapport. She wanted to continue working with her current clients in her home so she notified the clients of her plans to leave and gave them her home telephone number. The center's owner was angry and felt cheated because he had spent a considerable amount of time and money building the practice (the practitioner did very little marketing) and providing continuing education opportunities for all the staff. Ultimately, they came to an agreement and the practitioner paid the center the following percentage split for each client that she saw in her home: 40 percent for the first five sessions; 20 percent for the subsequent five sessions.

Avoid hurt feelings, and possibly a lawsuit, by clearly defining how you will deal with the future allocation of clients. Some options include: the leaving practitioner pays a fee for the client files, either a flat fee or a percentage of a specified number of sessions that each client books; the practitioner who leaves agrees to not see the clients for a specified time (e.g., three or six months). If you are a licensed health care provider, this could be a moot point since most states uphold a client's right to access any provider.

Insurance Issues

Insurance coverage for complementary health care treatments is an evolving issue. Careful attention and record keeping can maximize the benefits for both clients and practitioners. This section presents several current ethical dilemmas for somatic practitioners in the areas of documentation, insurance billing and communication with the health care team.

Responsibility for Payment

When is treatment finished? When does maintenance or wellness care begin? There is a fine line between the two especially if the condition is chronic. By identifying guidelines for delineating treatment versus wellness care, you can ethically apply those standards to the insurance issue: who pays for care?

The insurance issue is often clouded by people's beliefs and bad experiences. For instance, many people feel that insurance policies or case managers limit access to manual therapy and prevent clients from receiving the number of treatments necessary to recover from their injuries. Therefore, in the seemingly few situations where authorized treatment exceeds the number of sessions necessary for healing, practitioners often feel justified in continuing to provide care. Certainly, the clients are willing to continue: manual therapy feels good and is effective. And it makes sense to continue; after all, an ounce of prevention is worth a pound of cure!

According to standard insurance definitions, treatment is warranted until the condition is corrected or maximum improvement is made. These definitions also state that treatment must provide the client with appropriate instruction for follow-up, self-care and prevention of future occurrences. All maintenance and wellness care are the financial responsibility of the client unless otherwise specified by the insurance plan.

Sometimes it is obvious when the client has reached maximum healing: the client is pain free and fully functional. Other times, as with chronic pain, it is not so clear. In such cases, wellness is determined by the client's ability to manage pain and successfully modify activities. The focus is not on living pain free, but on quality of life: the client's ability to participate in everyday activities. Use these guidelines to determine when treatments are no longer necessary for resolving the client's condition:

- The client can function normally, or functional progress has plateaued.
- The client has no significant symptomology, or clinical progress has plateaued.
- The client demonstrates self-awareness by identifying situations (e.g., activities, emotions) that exacerbate his condition.
- The client applies self-care techniques to limit exacerbations and to remedy exacerbations when they do occur.

Test your findings by discontinuing care for a predetermined length of time. For example, if after four weeks without treatment a client is sufficiently symptom-free and active, care can be reduced to a monthly or maintenance level of care. Ongoing treatment is warranted if that client experiences an exacerbation or acceleration of the condition in spite of performing his self-care routines.

Most clients who reach maximum improvement for their conditions would benefit from wellness care. Encourage the client to return monthly for wellness care (for a predetermined number of weeks or months) after terminating treatment. During that time, provide care as needed and fine-tune the client's self-care instructions. If the client's health deteriorates without regular care, you have a case to reinstate insurance coverage. If the client administers appropriate self-care and maintains his health status, celebrate his accomplishments and invite him to continue monthly or quarterly wellness sessions, or refer him to someone who specializes in wellness care.

Preferred Provider Status

Insurance carriers contract with health care providers in an attempt to limit who provides health care services and how much the carrier pays for those services. Insureds enjoy discounts such as reduced co-pays or deductibles that may be waived for receiving health care services from preferred providers. Often insurance networks and insurance carriers can only support a limited number of providers. Set numbers of providers are credentialed for a given area based on the number of insureds that reside in that area. Once the quota is met, the network is closed to new providers.

Only credentialed practitioners are permitted to bill under the preferred provider contract. It is unethical and often illegal for non-credentialed practitioners to bill for services under the license of the credentialed provider.

Fee Schedules

Ethical billing practices include charging reasonable and consistent fees for services provided. It is tempting to charge higher fees to insurance companies because of the time and paperwork required for billing. However, it is unethical and in some cases illegal to charge insurance companies higher rates than clients who do not utilize insurance coverage for your services. This is commonly referred to as payer discrimination.

Unethical billing practices also arise when services are chosen because they cost more than other equally appropriate services, or when a practitioner bills for services that pay higher rates than the services actually performed. This course of action is tempting when insurance fee schedules delineate different fees for different manual techniques, as though one technique is better than another.

Healthy-We-Be publishes a fee schedule that charges $12 per 15-minute unit for therapeutic massage, $15 per 15-minute unit for manual therapy and $18 per 15-minute unit for energetic therapeutic touch. It is unethical to bill for four units of energetic therapeutic touch if other techniques were performed. It is also unethical to use only energetic techniques if other techniques would be equally or more effective.

The key to an ethical fee schedule is in its application. Be consistent and do not discriminate. Apply the same fee for the same service to everyone, regardless of the type of payer (this does not mean that you cannot offer a sliding scale). Provide the service that is most appropriate to the client, despite the reimbursement rate for the service.

Timely Documentation

Unethical charting practices occur when weeks, months or years later the chart is filled in because of a request for charts or because payment has been denied and rebilling requires copies of all treatment notes. Charting should be done in a timely fashion. It is difficult to remember a particular session after several other sessions have blurred the details.

The best time to chart is during or immediately after the session. Everyone has days, however, when the charts pile up and the practitioner does not get to them until the next morning. It is stressful but possible to recreate the session 24 hours later. However, few can record a session accurately weeks, months or years later.

Communication with Referring PHCP

As health care is currently structured a physician or doctor, and possibly a nurse, naturopath, acupuncturist or chiropractor (depending on the insurance policy and the state regulations), is considered *a primary health care provider* (PHCP). The PHCP is responsible to diagnose the client's problem, orchestrate treatment and refer to adjunctive therapists.

Communication skills are essential particularly when you are not the PHCP yet are working under the referring PHCP's direction, but not her supervision. Provide the referring PHCP with clear, complete information so that she can give the client the best possible treatment.

Occasionally you may find yourself disagreeing with the referring PHCP about a client's condition or treatment. Do not express this disagreement to the client. Instead, state your views to the referring PHCP calmly, professionally, tactfully, with the supporting evidence you have assembled. If your input is not considered or if you find that you cannot endorse the prescribed treatment, your best choice may be to withdraw from the case. However you choose to handle the situation, remember that the referring PHCP is the final authority and that it is unethical to undermine the relationship between the referring PHCP and the client. If the client approaches you with complaints about the referring PHCP's approach to the treatment plan, support the client in addressing the issues directly with the referring PHCP.

Permission to Consult with the Health Care Team

Request permission from the client to exchange information with the other members of the client's health care team. In many states practitioners do not need the client's consent to speak with referring providers. Nevertheless, it is a good idea to inform the client with whom information will be shared. When providing information to other practitioners, respect the client's confidentiality and limit those conversations to information pertinent to the client's condition. Omit your personal opinions about the client and any gossip or details that do not bear on the case. Refrain from discussing client cases in public where others who are not bound by confidentiality might overhear sensitive information.

In Conclusion...

Most health care providers care deeply for clients and strive to nurture and heal their bodies and souls. In an effort to be successful they are influenced by fears, needs, desires and spiritual longings. Ethical dilemmas are unavoidable. It is critical that practitioners take steps to encourage personal and professional growth and protect those they intend to serve by setting standards and reviewing their business practices regularly, and educating themselves on the laws that govern their profession.

Chapter Highlights

- Running an ethical business challenges the practitioner to maintain healthy boundaries and to operate from deeply held values.
- Money is simply a method of exchange for goods and services.
- Carefully consider offering certain clients different rates, price reductions, sliding scales and package deals and credit.
- Your financial belief systems are the context for all financial dealings.
- Be consistent in your fee structure.
- Be cautious about accepting gifts or tips.
- Treat barter transactions as you would any other method of payment.
- Honor all gift certificate sales, they are essentially a contract between the purchaser and the service provider.
- Set up a savings account for gift certificate income.
- Keep accurate records and work with an accountant to find legitimate ways to reduce your tax liability.
- You must collect and remit sales tax on products unless you live in a state that doesn't levy sales tax.
- Ethical product sales are based on your knowledge of the product, educating clients on the benefits and allowing purchases without manipulation or coercion.
- Accepting referral payments can cloud and compromise ethical standards and in some cases is illegal.
- Marketing materials should refrain from making exaggerated claims, using misleading ploys, displaying inappropriate images, or misrepresenting credentials.
- Marketing materials should be dignified and convey professionalism.
- The principal legal aspects of running an ethical business are: complying with local, state and federal laws; maintaining appropriate and adequate insurance coverage; slander/libel; honoring copyright laws; negotiating and complying with contracts; civil lawsuits; employees; and client custody.
- Maintaining adequate business and malpractice insurance coverage is crucial and some localities require specific coverage.
- To avoid problems with slander and libel, give your opinion, don't embellish on the facts and state the truth.
- Copyright law makes it technically illegal to reproduce almost any new creative work (other than under fair use) without permission and copyright is still violated regardless of whether you charge money.
- Create contracts and agreements to circumvent problems, provide a method for conflict resolution and keep goals in focus.
- Minimize the likelihood of costly civil lawsuits by keeping good boundaries and communicating effectively.
- In malpractice actions the practitioner is held to the standard of care and skill of the average member of the profession.
- Employers can be held responsible for the actions of their employees.
- You may be responsible for some of the damages awarded in a malpractice suit even with liability insurance.
- Know the IRS regulations and create independent contractor agreements to minimize the risk of having independent contractors reclassified as employees.

- Many practitioners work in other practitioners' offices, health clubs, salons, spas and clinics in the hopes of building up their private clientele. Problems arise if the expectations and boundaries are not clear.
- At the beginning of a business relationships, establish how clients will be allocated when a practitioner leaves a business.
- Ethical dilemmas are unavoidable but can be mitigated by setting standards, reviewing business practices regularly and being educated about laws that govern your profession.
- Ethical insurance billing and payment depends upon knowing when treatment is finished and maintenance begins.
- It is unethical and often illegal for non-credentialed practitioners to bill for services under the license of credentialed providers.
- Ethical billing practices include charging reasonable and consistent fees for services and providing the most appropriate service regardless of the reimbursement rate.
- Charting should be done in a timely manner.
- Effective communication is essential between the somatic practitioner and the referring primary health care provider.
- Refer client disputes over treatment plans back to the referring health care provider.
- Obtain permission from clients to exchange information with other health care providers.

Discussion Questions and Activities

- Describe your relationship to money.
- Recount your family history with money.
- What circumstances would prompt you to offer a sliding fee scale?
- What will you charge family members and friends for your services?
- If your family/friend rate is different than your standard rate, describe why.
- What types of package plans could you offer and what are the benefits and disadvantages?
- When is it appropriate to take a tip?
- What are your parameters for accepting tips or gifts?
- Describe instances when a barter exchange worked well for both parties.
- Describe instances when a barter exchange did not work well for both parties.
- How can you ensure that your barter transactions are handled ethically?
- List ways to ethically sell gift certificates and manage those sales.
- What products are appropriate to sell in your practice?
- What products are inappropriate to sell in your practice?
- What experiences have you had in purchasing products from a health care provider?
- Describe how you can sell products without using "hard-sell" tactics or taking advantage of the power differential.
- Describe examples of marketing materials that you feel are in questionable taste.
- Describe examples of marketing materials that you feel are blatant examples of unethical marketing.
- Peruse a local telephone Yellow Pages for health care advertisements. Find examples that are ethical as well as ads that are questionable or that exaggerate claims.
- You took a weekend touch therapy course that is part one of a multiple series. It meets the CEU requirements for renewing your license. Do you advertise this modality and list it on your business cards and brochures?
- What are your guidelines for listing a specialty in your repertoire of services?
- The zoning ordinances in your area states that you cannot treat clients in your home. You are in a tight financial situation. You want to turn one room in your two-bedroom domicile into a treatment room. What do you do?
- You read a flier that states: "Workshop to Help You Pass the Massage Licensing Examination." The charge is $35 for two hours of lecture and practice test questions. You know the presenters of this workshop. They were students with you at school and both did poorly in anatomy class, yet somehow managed to do well on their examinations. You suspected they had cheated in school. You heard that they were gathering test questions from the licensing exam by therapists who could remember the questions. What do you do?
- What would you do if you are changing the name of your business and discover that someone else in a neighboring city has an already established business with the same name? What if that person never registered the business name?
- What do you do if your client tells you that she is considering working with a practitioner that you do not feel is ethical?
- What do you do if a colleague tells you that he is considering working with a practitioner that you do not feel is ethical?
- Discuss the types of business arrangements where a contract would be beneficial.

8

Special Considerations

In Cases of Trauma

- Understanding Trauma and Abuse
- The Core of Trauma and Abuse
- The Benefits of Touch Therapy
- Prerequisites for Working with Survivors
- Body Memories and Flashbacks
- In Conclusion...
- Chapter Highlights
- Discussion Questions and Activities

O n the average, one of every five clients a practitioner sees has a history of some kind of trauma or abuse. Whether or not you are aware of it, in a large percentage of your sessions the client in your treatment room may be a survivor. Even the client might not know it. To avoid ethical complications every practitioner who uses touch needs basic knowledge about trauma and abuse survivors and a clear protocol for working with these particular clients.

This chapter offers practitioners ethical guidelines and techniques for working with clients who are survivors of physical, emotional or sexual trauma. The technical and emotional skills needed to work effectively with this population are learned over time with ongoing training, supervision and increased self-knowledge. Please note that the written information in this chapter is not a replacement for in-class, hands-on training in working with this population. We strongly believe that any practitioner who chooses to treat survivors of abuse and trauma is ethically bound to seek continuing education and ongoing supervision.

If you choose to specialize in working with survivors of trauma and abuse, you will find great rewards. But even if you do not choose this focus, we believe you will find the following information is of fundamental importance to practicing ethically.

"
If you can learn from hard knocks, you can also learn from soft touches.

"

—Carolyn Gilmore

Understanding Trauma and Abuse

Touch therapy can provide a valuable healing environment for the abuse survivor. Practitioners minimize the risks of retraumatization by being sensitive to the experience of the survivor and its effect on their work together. Psychologist Melissa Soalt eloquently describes the dilemma faced by the survivor as he enters therapy: "Being present in one's body is a double-edged sword for survivors: on the one hand working through the body can stimulate the trauma and evoke confusing or frightening feelings; on the other hand, it is this very ability to be present and in one's body that ultimately allows one to feel more grounded and thus safer and more in control."[1]

Many responsibilities fall upon the practitioner. When a practitioner begins work with an abuse survivor, she may be the first person to touch the client's body since the abuse. The practitioner minimizes potential errors and creates a safe environment for the treatment process when she has awareness and understanding of the factors surrounding abuse and recovery.

Sometimes, the client who is a survivor of abuse exhibits physical symptoms which indicate the presence of unresolved trauma. Examples of such symptoms include chronic fatigue, insomnia, chronic joint and muscle pain throughout the body and a weak immune system.[2] Other reactions to the abuse experience are flashbacks and intense memories. It is useful for practitioners to understand the origins of these reactions, know how to recognize them and appreciate the contribution of the touch treatment to their resolution.

The TARA Approach for the Resolution of Shock & Trauma:
303-499-9990
www.Tara-Approach.org

The Potential for Harm From Reckless Treatment

Chris Smith, the founder of Trauma Touch Therapy and a survivor of abuse as a child, had some early experiences with types of bodywork that encouraged cathartic emotional releases. Although such releases may feel beneficial at first, Smith now believes that they ultimately increase rather than decrease the traumatization.[3] Smith is one of a large number of professionals who believe that bodywork undertaken in isolation from other therapies, or in a context that does not allow the client to integrate the experience, has more potential to harm than to heal. Below are several examples of the negative effects of touch therapy when done without appropriate knowledge and training.

A practitioner was approached by a client who wasn't in psychotherapy and wanted to address her abuse issues through bodywork. The practitioner had very limited training in working with survivors but wanted to assist the client in her healing process. In the course of their work together the client began to have flashbacks during the treatments. The practitioner felt she should let the client fully experience these memory experiences and would process what happened afterward. After several weeks of treatment the client began to experience more uncontrollable, intense and disabling flashbacks on buses, in the supermarket and frequently upon entering the practitioner's office. The practitioner's lack of training in this area resulted in a damaging situation for the client and a lawsuit against the practitioner. In this case the practitioner did not understand the significance of the flashbacks and how to deal with them. She did not realize the client needed psychotherapy and other support systems in place; she herself lacked outside supervision to guide her work when questions or difficulties arose.

This harmful situation occurred because the practitioner did not understand that recovery from abuse proceeds in stages, and that her client was in a very early stage of this process. Therefore, the practitioner did not know what the client needed to proceed safely with her recovery. This client was not psychologically ready to delve into her past.[4] The boundaries and support systems necessary for effective treatment were not adequately in place.

Another practitioner performed deep and somewhat painful bodywork on a woman who was an abuse survivor. Only months later into the process did he discover that often, after sessions, she collapsed in bed for two or three days to recover from nightmares, light sensitivity, emotional pain and turmoil.

Clients with a history of abuse often lack the ability to adequately protect themselves when a practitioner errs. Treatment mistakes occur when a practitioner works too deeply or inadvertently violates a boundary. Because survivors often have trouble recognizing their boundaries, they may ask for treatment that is inappropriate, or they may be unable to let the practitioner know if they are feeling violated. Practitioners must understand abuse issues to structure the treatment session at a level appropriate for the survivor's needs. This determines how a practitioner approaches a session. Consider the following story.

A woman came into a massage therapist's office and immediately began removing all of her clothing. The therapist quickly covered her with a blanket and gently asked her to dress again since they were going to start with an interview. During the interview and history the woman reported that she was an abuse survivor and only felt comfortable removing her socks and shoes.

The practitioner who works with survivors must possess a gentle and enduring patience, for the pace of the treatment may be very slow. For instance, a practitioner could literally work on a survivor's hands or feet for two or three months. Many clients report taking up to a year before they can have their backs and legs touched when they are unclothed. Patience can nurture healing, and well-informed care can minimize the potential for harm in the treatment process.

The Core of Trauma and Abuse

Trauma Touch Therapy Training: Contact the Colorado School of Healing Arts
303-986-2320

Before discussing how to work with clients who have been abused, it is important to understand what constitutes abuse and the complexity of its effects. Janet Yassen,[5] Coordinator of Crisis Services at the Victims of Violence Program at Cambridge Hospital and co-founder of the Boston Rape Crisis Center, defines sexual abuse as "unwanted or inappropriate sexual contact, either verbal or physical, between two or more people, that is intended as an act of control, power, rage, violence and intimidation with sex as a weapon." Physical abuse is defined as the use of force or violence to cause pain or bodily harm which is used as an instrument of intimidation, coercion or control. Emotional abuse is the infliction of emotional harm by verbal intimidation or neglectful behavior to intimidate, demean or hurt another person. Mind control abuse can be defined as the act of undermining a person's free will through the control of behavior, information, thoughts and emotions.

The trauma experience has a physiological effect even if the trauma is not physical in nature. The diaphragm and muscles of the chest contract restricting breathing; muscles at the base of the occiput and pelvis often contract; energy frequently withdraws to the center of the body leaving the extremities cold; and there is an overall shrinking and contraction of the physical organization of the entire body.[6] Severe trauma may cause loss of muscle tone.[7] Symptoms of the breach in psychic integrity from abuse include depression and anxiety.[8] At its core, the intent of all abuse, whether sexual, emotional or physical, is the same: to dominate, humiliate and gain control of another person. It is a traumatic event, perpetrated by another person, that violates the basic bodily and psychic integrity of the victim.

The Types of Sexual Abuse

Sexual abuse ranges from inappropriate seductive behavior and sexual touching to sexual intercourse. Sexual abuse includes rape, gang rape, date rape, partner or spouse rape and incest.

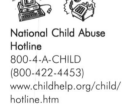

National Child Abuse Hotline
800-4-A-CHILD
(800-422-4453)
www.childhelp.org/child/hotline.htm

Incest defines a specific kind of abuse which has particularly devastating effects. In the narrow, legal definition, incest is the sexual abuse of a person by a family member who is related by blood or marriage, such as a father, mother, uncle, aunt, sister or brother. Within the psychological community incest is more broadly defined to include sexual violations by trusted individuals with regular access to a child or care giving responsibilities, such as family friends, child care providers or clergy.

Sexual abuse rarely occurs as an isolated event. Violations are often accompanied by other types of mental, physical and emotional torment. Emotional abuse such as put-downs, insults, demeaning comments and sudden irrational acts intended to instill fear are common. In the case of incest, this may also include the withdrawal of love and affection or threats to hurt other family members as a weapon of control.

Sexual abuse can also involve more than one perpetrator or more than one victim. Examples of this include some religious cults and secret societies, or organized criminal activities such as pornography rings. These are systematic forms of violation in which the victims are subjected to sadistic torture and may be drugged to become compliant.

The Prevalence of Sexual Abuse

The statistics on sexual abuse are staggering and difficult for most people to fathom. The National Violence against Women Survey found that in the United States, one of six women and one of 33 men has experienced an attempted or completed rape as a child or an adult; specifically 18 percent of surveyed women and three percent of surveyed men said they experienced a completed or attempted rape at some time in their life.[9] Other research has found that approximately one in every five women and one in seven men have been sexually abused by the time they are 18 years old.[10]

Tip: Keep a telephone list of the safehouse hotlines in your area.

To look at this another way 18 to 20 percent of the U.S. population or approximately 50 million people have been sexually abused. The 1984 Royal Commission on Sexual Offences Against Children and Youth reported that in Canada 22 percent of women and 10 percent of men experienced some type of sexual abuse before the age of 18.[11] Some professionals believe that these numbers are an exaggeration while others think they are low due to under-reporting. If these numbers are hard to believe, reduce the total by a factor of half, or even two-thirds, and the tally is still a frightening number. It is difficult to determine whether sexual abuse has always been this prevalent and is only now being more accurately reported, or whether it has increased due to the dissolution of the family and other social factors.

There have been several periods over the last hundred years during which sexual abuse has been exposed, discussed and acknowledged but it has only been since the mid-1970s that the social and political context has provided an ongoing, welcoming atmosphere for research and wide acceptance. According to Herman,[12] the women's movement provided the political environment to support the ongoing research and recognition of the extensive existence of sexual abuse.

State by State Abuse Hotline and Organization Directory: www.brokenspirits.com/directory/states

Although more girls than boys are sexually abused, one research study finds that the number of boys who have been sexually abused is greater than previously thought.[13] Most of the abuse is perpetrated by men, although women do abuse both male and female children. Thus, a practitioner could generally expect that approximately one in five clients is likely to be a survivor of sexual abuse, and many others were victims of other types of physical or psychological trauma.

Types of Physical Abuse

Physical abuse of children is more common than imagined and shows itself in obvious forms such as violent beatings, corporal punishment, food deprivation or aggressive tickling that does not stop. Other types of physical abuse includes spousal battery, the threat of violence as a means of control, and the use of physical torture as discipline of spouses and children. More women are injured by battering than are injured in car accidents and it is estimated that each year millions of children directly witness acts of domestic abuse.[14] Physical assaults and muggings are commonplace as well.

All forms of physical abuse leave scars that close people off to themselves. Various forms of emotional and body oriented therapies can help these individuals reclaim themselves and their bodies.

Types of Emotional Abuse

Emotional trauma is experienced by everyone to one degree or another: a loved one dies; a love relationship ends badly; an accident occurs which severely curtails our activities. Most individuals experience these traumas and then move on. However, when emotional abuse occurs, the extent of the trauma may go beyond the individual's ability to effectively cope. Whereas physical abuse inflicts harm directly to the body, emotional abuse inflicts harm to the psychological well-being of another.

We define emotional abuse as the infliction of emotional harm by verbal intimidation or neglectful behavior. Direct verbal threats or attacks and taunting or belittling language used to intimidate, demean or hurt another are examples of emotional abuse. Emotional abuse occurs when a person, whether young or old, is regularly taunted, put down, shamed, berated, ostracized or humiliated.

Emotional withholding and emotional neglect also constitute abuse. In children dependent on adults for their care, abuse may take the form of consistent lack of response to a child's emotional needs, the inability of the adult to express appropriate emotion to the child, or neglect. Other forms of emotional abuse include when children are severely punished, dominated or forced to perform acts which go against their humanity.

Usually victims experience strong feelings of fear, shame, rage or despair. If the feelings are overwhelming, victims may enter a depressed or dissociative state in which they are cut off from some or all of their emotions. Emotional abuse is a means to overpower someone; it is always destructive and inevitably results in emotional scarring and long lasting self-esteem issues.

Cult Mind Control Abuse

Cult mind control abuse occurs when people are subjected to an extreme form of abuse that involves creating an alternate identity which is programmed to depend on a person or totalistic system. This creates a dissociative disorder leading to a number of other trauma-related symptoms. Members are deceptively recruited into a destructive cult (religious, political, "therapeutic" or business). Some people are born into such cults and never get the opportunity to develop their own identity until they break away.

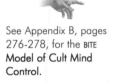

See Appendix B, pages 276-278, for the BITE **Model of Cult Mind Control.**

Mind control abuse includes the control of: behavior, information, thoughts and emotions to undermine a person's free will. Without specialized therapy, mind control victims can exhibit a host of psychosomatic complaints as well as the following: identity confusion; black and white, simplistic thinking; difficulty with decision-making; fear and panic disorders; sexual problems; sleeping and eating difficulties. Cult members are often encouraged to cut off from family and friends, and abandon education and career choices. They tend to speak with cult jargon and are either extremely aggressive in converting others, or are very secretive, deceptive and evasive when asked direct questions.[15]

The Effects of Trauma

Traumas come with life. They create stresses which often encourage us to engage in self-exploration. Most people quickly overcome mini-traumas; other events take years to undo. Additionally, there is a category of traumatic events that goes far beyond the norm. Individuals who have gone through severe or repeated trauma may be in a kind of shock for the rest of their lives while others work through the trauma by themselves or with help from others. Throughout the ages the brutality of rape and war have been consistently with us. Now the devastating aftermath these traumas create is beginning to be acknowledged.

Post Traumatic Stress Disorder

Sexual, emotional or physical abuse/trauma leaves profound and lasting effects on a person's psychological, cognitive and emotional functioning. The impact and symptoms of trauma are known as "post traumatic stress disorder," or PTSD.[16] According to dedicated researchers, including psychiatrist Judith Herman, who explored the effects of trauma in her groundbreaking book, *Trauma and Recovery*,[17] similar effects of trauma are experienced by survivors of sexual abuse, political prisoners, kidnap victims, concentration camp survivors, victims of terrorism and many soldiers who experienced combat in war. Other experts also include survivors of major accidents, childhood torture and medical abuse.[18] In her book, Herman summarizes three major symptoms of post-traumatic stress disorder: hyperarousal, intrusion and constriction.

National Center for PTSD
www.ncptsd.org/
facts/treatment/
fs_seeking_help.html

HYPERAROUSAL is a state of constant alertness to danger experienced by the survivor of trauma. The survivor's senses and body are poised to respond to the slightest movements, noises or provocations. A survivor may react with extreme irritation or alarm to situations that impart little effect on others. Often, she sleeps poorly. To the person in this state, all situations carry potential re-enactment of past traumas.

INTRUSION is experienced when past traumatic events recur as vivid memories interrupting the course of life in the present. "The traumatic moment becomes encoded in an abnormal form of memory, which breaks spontaneously into consciousness, both as flashbacks during waking states and as traumatic nightmares during sleep," writes Herman.[19]

CONSTRICTION occurs when the intensity and pain of an event is so severe that the survivor becomes numb and psychologically removed from the pain. The survivor registers the event in her awareness but in an altered state where she does not experience pain, attachment or emotion. The person may describe it as going numb, going deaf, or leaving the body. Also referred to as dissociation, in this state the trauma victim survives unbearable conditions from which there was no actual escape. One incest survivor described her experience of dissociation this way.[20]

PTSD Hotline
800-784-2433

> After I knew what he was doing, I used to separate from him. I used to feel that if I could just get close enough to the wall, that he couldn't touch me (yet I knew he could), but I used to go inside the wall and it was like he was touching someone else. I would just turn off and get cold."

Constriction can also be experienced as hypervigilance, an overfocused narrowing of attention onto one idea, one part of the body, or a particular sensation or feeling. Constriction carries over to the experiences of the present, affecting the ability of the survivor to feel both positive and negative emotions, physical sensations, or attachments to others.

Complex Post Traumatic Stress Disorder

People experiencing post-traumatic stress disorder alternate between the opposing psychological states of hyper-awareness and numbness in an effort to gain balance. Until significant aspects of the traumatic memories are explored and integrated, the survivor is caught between complete forgetting and the constant fear of reliving the traumatic experience.

Herman has proposed a new term, complex post-traumatic stress disorder (CPTSD)[21] for those subjected to prolonged, repeated trauma. Repeated traumatic abuse shatters a person's sense of self and relation to others. In an even more intense way, human contact, especially intimate contact, becomes associated with feelings of intimidation, pain, violence, rage, humiliation, disgust, shame and betrayal.[22] Further, a person who has experienced prolonged abuse during childhood has no guideposts for judging who is worthy of trust or which situations are truly safe. As a result of the violation of physical, sexual and emotional boundaries, a survivor of sexual abuse often has difficulty defining her personal boundaries with people in the present and is therefore at risk for further abuse.

The Three Stages of Recovery

Clinicians identified three distinct stages of recovery, from establishing safety, to remembrance and mourning, to reconnection. Others believe that the healing process stages are less clearly defined and more fluid. Most likely a continuum of the healing process exists. The three stages described by Judith Herman give practitioners a clear way to think about using touch while working with survivors in recovery. Throughout the therapy process the survivor could move back and forth between stages two and three, or experience two stages simultaneously.

1. SAFETY

The goal of the first stage of recovery is to establish physical and psychological safety.[23] The survivor learns to control his body and attend to his basic physical needs, (i.e., eating well, sleeping, getting regular exercise, having a safe place to live). As the client develops this immediate sense of safety, he can begin to exercise initiative and take charge of his recovery. It may take the client as little as a few sessions or as long as a few decades before she truly feels safe experiencing somatic treatments.

2. REMEMBRANCE AND MOURNING

The second stage of recovery involves remembrance and mourning. In the presence of safety, formerly unconscious, often fragmented, disguised and deeply buried memories arise. Forgotten and painful memories heal by being reconstructed and transformed into an integral part of a life story. This stage of recovery can be profoundly painful and prolonged as the person relives the pains and horror of the trauma, and experiences the accompanying grief and loss. "The telling of the trauma story inevitably plunges the survivor into profound grief," observes Herman. "The second stage of recovery has a timeless quality that is frightening. The descent into mourning feels like a surrender to tears that are endless. But it is by the remembering, telling of their story and grieving that the survivor can move toward integration of their trauma and eventually reconnect with ordinary life."[24]

3. RECONNECTION

In the third stage of recovery the survivor begins to look to the future and imagine a whole, intact self. The survivor recognizes her trauma but is not possessed by it. She feels more confidence in her ability to connect with the outside world and her capacity to appropriately give and withhold trust. A survivor in this stage often turns her experience into social action, having transforming effects on self and society.[25]

Anxiety Disorder Support, including PTSD:
Anxiety Disorders Association of America (ADAA)
11900 Parklawn Dr.
Rockville, MD 20852
301-231-9350
email: AnxDis@aol.com
www.hipusa.com/mental health/anxiety.html

Hotline listings:
www.find-a-therapist.com/ hotline.htm

Recovery Criteria

How does a therapist know when the survivor has achieved recovery from trauma? The following seven criteria identified by Lebowitz, Harvey and Herman,[26] help practitioners define in precise terms recovery from both chronic and acute trauma. Clients in psychotherapy may recover these seven fundamentals sequentially, but more often the progression is not so orderly. Progress in different areas varies. The criteria are as follows:

Memory

In recovery the individual develops the authority to control the remembering process. He chooses whether to recall traumatic events that previously intruded unbidden into awareness. Critical memory gaps are filled in and the survivor has available a meaningful, coherent narrative of his life that can be integrated with his ongoing life story.

Emotional Range and Tolerance

Many survivors live life in the affective extremes (numb, overwhelmed or flooded). Affective recovery is achieved when: emotional life is no longer experienced in the extremes; emotions can be felt, named and endured; and the full complement of feelings in a range of intensities is accessible to the survivor.

Memory and Emotion Links

Coping with trauma frequently necessitates unlinking the phenomenological experience. In recovery, feelings and memories are rejoined. Memories are recalled with affect that's appropriate in content and intensity. The survivor experiences feelings in the here and now about what happened in the past and can access or imagine what she felt at the time of the trauma.

Symptom Mastery

Symptoms associated with chronic and acute PTSD, including psychophysiologic ones, have receded or become manageable.

Self-Esteem

During the course of recovery, feelings of self-hate, badness and shame are replaced by a more positive and realistic view of self. Responsibility for the abuse is shifted from the victim to the perpetrator, adaptations needed for survival are acknowledged without undue shame and self-caring routines replace self-injurious ones.

Attachment

In recovery, disruptions in the survivor's ability to negotiate psychologically safe relationships are developed or repaired. Feelings of isolation are replaced by an increased capacity to feel connected to others, and previously polarized and distorted perceptions of other people become more realistic.

Meaning

Through the recovery process, the survivor assigns a realistic meaning to the trauma and to the self as a survivor. Views of self, world and others emerge that are complex and the survivor can incorporate the contradictory and ambiguous nature of reality. The survivor feels a realistic sense of hope and optimism about the future.[27]

> *Healing may not be so much about getting better, as about letting go of everything that isn't you—all of the expectations, all of the beliefs—and becoming who you are.*
>
> —Rachel Naomi Remen

The Benefits of Touch Therapy

As awareness of the prevalence of abuse has grown, an increasing number of survivors sought various touch therapies to help them reconnect with and reclaim their bodies. Psychiatrists, psychologists, social workers and counselors are referring an increasing number of their clients for touch therapy. The practitioner who understands abuse and the healing process is prepared to respond in a helpful and knowledgeable way.

Melissa Soalt, a psychotherapist and the founder of Model Mugging of Boston (a self-defense training program), has worked with many survivors and observes the following:[28]

- For survivors of abuse bodywork can be a very powerful adjunct to psychotherapy. The trauma from abuse typically results in dissociative numbing or repressive mechanisms that leave survivors feeling "empty" or vacant on the inside. With reconnection and integration (or a move toward wholeness) as primary therapeutic goals, working through the body can be a valuable tool toward this end. Because the body is such a direct medium, bodywork facilitates this process of re-entry and one's ability to feel more present.
- Bodywork can help survivors develop a friendly and compassionate relationship with their bodies. Sexual or physical abuse often leaves survivors feeling disgusted, shameful or even violent toward their body, as though their body betrayed or turned against them.
- Bodywork helps survivors experience their bodies as a source of groundedness and eventually as a source of strength and even pleasure.
- Working with a compassionate and skilled bodyworker helps rebuild survivors' sense of trust and reconnects them with the possibility of other genuine caring relationships.

When performed responsibly at the appropriate stage of the client's healing and with care and sensitivity, body therapy can be an important healing force in a client's life. Bodywork offers survivors a new and non-abusive way of being in touch with their bodies, to discover how their bodies feel and to discern their general level of health.

Establishing a Place of Safety

When the survivor of abuse enters psychotherapy, establishing personal and psychological safety with the psychotherapist is a crucial first step in the healing process. A touch therapy relationship builds on this experience. A healthy bodywork environment creates another opportunity for the survivor to establish an environment where she feels safe with emotions and the physical self. Somatic work offers safe touch with dignity and respect in a non-judgmental, non-sexual environment.

Regaining Body Control and Rebuilding Boundaries

Somatic therapies can be helpful in rebuilding personal boundaries damaged by trauma and abuse. During this time the client reacquaints himself with his body through sensual awareness of how the body is organized and what sensations trigger trauma response. The process of learning about these boundaries and managing the bodywork session helps to integrate the sense of body control.[29] Eventually the client stays grounded in his body while talking about the experience, bringing a new level of healing through reorganizing negative body response to positive somatic memory.[30] The client has the opportunity to construct new boundaries as the treatment progresses. For example, the client sets important boundaries by simply telling the practitioner where to touch and where not to touch. By being in charge of the session, the survivor gains another piece of control of his life associated with the body. Each experience of inviting, choosing and denying touch empowers the survivor.

A client described her experience of bodywork, expressing both the benefits and cautions needed to guide therapy in relation to boundaries:

> My 'talk' therapist person suggested to me that I might want to start to draw some boundaries around places in my body where I just didn't feel that I wanted to be touched. That was the beginning of the physical healing part, to say, 'No, I don't want you to massage below my waist and above my knees.' I felt like such a baby having to draw those lines, but it was such an important part of my recovery. The more I was empowered, the more I was able to say 'Stop' and 'No.' To rebuild those boundaries was incredibly important to me. But there are still times when I roll over, if I feel like my genitals aren't covered up properly, it's like an alarm goes off somewhere in my head and I still have a lot of shame about saying what's going on for me in the moment."[31]

Experiencing the Pleasure of Non-Sexual Touch

Touch that is neutral or pleasurable provides building blocks for a changed experience of the body. After safety has been established through repeated positive physical contact, the survivor usually begins to perceive the practitioner's touch as neutral and over time experiences touch without dissociation. Later on, pleasurable sensation which is not sexual is usually experienced by the client. This capacity to experience pleasure in a relaxed parasympathetic state while receiving tactile stimulation brings an expanded sense of self and a trust in life experiences.[32]

Another client described her experience this way:[33]

> Bodywork helped me learn how to be touched again—to relearn how to be touched. All the touch I had gotten was always abusive; sexually or physically abusive. I never knew that touch could be otherwise. Having a massage therapist helped me to trust again and eventually to relax. It was a wonderful way to learn how to go on to a normal life afterwards."

Reintegrating Body Memories

In conjunction with psychotherapy touch therapy assists the survivor in reaching hidden memories and integrating them into his present experience. Abusive traumas from the past cause the survivor to dissociate from the body and this experience often recurs when the body is touched. Renegotiating somatic memory by replacing a negative physical response with a positive memory reintegrates the experience so that the client achieves a more balanced and positive state of body awareness. Therapeutic touch may trigger the recall of memories to be processed in psychotherapy.

As clients connect with their bodies in a more positive way, they experience improved body image and feel less shame. Practitioners may find that these clients take better care of their bodies as treatments continue

Special Considerations in Cases of Trauma

Enhancing Psychotherapy Collaboration

Psychotherapists who recommend touch therapies for their clients see the bodywork practitioners as collaborators in the healing process. Many see touch as a valuable adjunct for some of their clients to reduce stress while others see it as a vital part of the task of reintegrating the body into the survivor's life.

In their collaborative book, *Embodying Healing*,[34] Robert Timms, PH.D., and Patrick Connors, C.M.T., write, "Working with the body is a powerful means of sidestepping the conscious mind and gathering information directly from the unconscious fund of knowledge." In their "psychophysical model" each professional brings separate skills and roles to the healing process. The psychotherapist helps the client integrate her emotional and cognitive insights, while the bodyworker helps the client increase her self-awareness and gain access to emotions and less conscious memories through direct touch.

Timms, a psychotherapist, describes the benefits of his frequent collaboration with Connors, a massage therapist, in the following way: "Often I find clients are better able to make cognitive connections in psychotherapy sessions that follow bodywork sessions. In most cases, the client's characteristic resistances are lowered and she or he is more available for therapeutic insight."[35]

Melissa Soalt writes, "In psychotherapy the therapist is often the one who holds the client's feelings until the client is more able or ready to have and own them. In this light, bodywork can both elicit feelings/memories and help survivors contain (i.e., stay with but not become overwhelmed by) these feelings, thus aiding in the psychotherapeutic process."[36]

Psychotherapists and bodyworkers collaborate in different ways. A sequential mode is when the client has a bodywork session in the first hour and a psychotherapy session in the next hour. A combined mode entails the psychotherapist and the practitioner working simultaneously with a client in one room, as described by Timms. (The combined mode, where psychotherapist and somatic practitioner work simultaneously, may present complex challenges, both rich in opportunity and possible difficulties.) Others work concurrently at separate locations, seeing a client weekly at their offices and communicating by phone as needed. Psychotherapists who regularly call upon touch therapists to support their treatment plan usually interview the therapists before they refer their clients to them.

Chris Smith's Trauma Touch Therapy method utilizes simultaneous but separate bodywork and counseling sessions. While the bodywork session may release memory and emotion, the counselor's role is to help the client integrate the experience in a meaningful way. In this manner, the practitioners in the two fields remain within their respective scopes of practice and avoid confusion of roles.

Prerequisites for Working with Survivors

The undertaking of a course of any type of touch therapy is a journey of courage for both the survivor and the practitioner. It places many demands on both the client's and the practitioner's resources. Certain prerequisites are essential and others very helpful in preparing the practitioner and the client for their work together.

Practitioner Prerequisites

The treatment of survivors requires a refined degree of self-awareness. Education to prepare for this type of work should include training in psychology, communication, sexuality, ethics, trauma and counseling, as well as actual hands-on techniques. The practitioner

> "The best time to plant a tree was 20 years ago. The second best time is now.
>
> —Chinese proverb

also benefits greatly from support networks that include peer counseling and supervision. Practitioners who lack information and formal training in this field risk harming their clients and themselves. Untrained and unaware practitioners are likely to: impose their own assumptions, needs and conflicts on their clients; retraumatize their clients during the bodywork session; and suffer what is known as secondary or vicarious trauma themselves.[37] The boundaries between practitioner and client can become blurred and the boundary of scope of practice can be unclear. In the book, *Victims of Cruelty: Somatic Psychotherapy in the Treatment of Posttraumatic Stress Disorder*, Maryanna Eckberg states that an experienced psychotherapist/bodyworker does not do bodywork on a client if the risks for transference, regression, or for eliciting sexual impulses are too great. She further adds that, "touch must contribute to the treatment process."[38] The untrained practitioner may casually give advice to a client whose real need is to receive a referral to another type of therapy.

See pages 228-229 for more information on **secondary traumatization.**

Psychological Understanding

A baseline knowledge of human psychology and specialized knowledge of issues related to abuse are essential to practitioners who wish to work with survivors. Fundamental psychological concepts relevant to the healing process include transference, countertransference, power differential, dual relationships and boundary issues. Practitioners must learn how to deal with flashbacks, body memories and psychological symptoms such as hyperarousal, intrusion and dissociation. The experiences of abuse survivors intensifies all these psychological aspects of the therapeutic relationship, and often has unexpected effects.

Practitioners must understand the mechanism of countertransference. The untrained practitioner may project her own feelings about the client's history onto the client and assume that the client's responses are the same as the practitioner's. In doing so the practitioner further disempowers the client and unwittingly adds to the client's sense of helplessness and hopelessness. Instead, the ethical practitioner learns to play a supportive role, helping the client find her own answers.[39] Practitioners who understand these concepts work safely and effectively and identify ways to avoid re-enacting the very traumas for which the client has come to receive treatments.

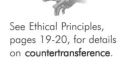

See Ethical Principles, pages 19-20, for details on **countertransference.**

Practitioners who work with self-disclosed abuse survivors respond to clients' needs in a helpful and appropriate manner. The actual hands-on techniques for working with survivors are no more physically demanding or difficult than with any other client. But these clients are mentally and emotionally challenging because more focus and attention is required.

Practitioners need to be sensitive to the messages a client sends (often without words) and create an empowering, non-hierarchical collaboration. The manner in which practitioners handle giving feedback and support to the client, and how the practitioners receive feedback from the client, is crucial in establishing and maintaining trust. The practitioners' reactions to a client's memories, inadvertent boundary crossings and anger at treatment errors makes or breaks the relationship. Making mistakes is not the problem because every practitioner makes mistakes. What is important is how the mistakes are handled. How the practitioner deals with his own feelings will be keenly perceived by the client's radar and strongly affect the therapeutic relationship.

Issues and Motivations

Ethical practitioners strive to understand their own issues and motivations. Taking a closer look at why one chooses to become a touch practitioner is an important step. We all choose careers for different reasons. Awareness of conscious, as well as unconscious, motives helps the practitioner focus on what needs to be addressed to work effectively with a vulnerable clientele. Making friends with many clients, or talking about oneself and one's life with clients, or having difficulty telling a client that the practitioner cannot help, may all indicate a practitioner's unresolved or neglected issues that will interfere with the effectiveness of the work.

> A practitioner decided to work with the body because his family never touched him after he was 12 years old, except when he was punished. And as an adult he was only touched sexually. He wanted to learn about touching that wasn't punitive or sexual.

> A practitioner spoke of how she was never verbally intimate or physically close with anyone in her family and that her work satisfied her need for non-sexual intimacy. She also realized that she was using her work as a way to avoid developing intimate friendships.

> A practitioner realized she needed to re-enter therapy after learning she was overstepping her clients' boundaries by asking invasive questions. Her questions related to her own intense curiosity and weren't really relevant or useful to the therapy. In other words, her interventions with the client served her needs and not those of the client.

Clarity about where and how the practitioner gets her personal needs met for touch, intimacy and sexuality is an important aspect of preparing to work with survivors. Undergoing personal psychotherapy is an excellent way for the practitioner to explore her level of awareness about these issues as well as the ability to communicate effectively. Psychotherapy is a good place to investigate and understand one's own unmet needs before and during the work with survivors because of the many strong feelings that may arise during this process.

Ethical Dimensions

The ethical dimensions inherent in bodywork are intensified in working with survivors. Having a clear ethical code that is thought through and adhered to is an important part of a practitioner's commitment to the survivor and the survivor's healing. Practitioners keep the treatment client-centered by paying careful attention to ethical boundaries including: relationships with clients outside the treatment context; respect for the client's confidentiality; precision with financial dealings; willingness to admit mistakes; and honesty if the situation goes beyond the practitioner's expertise.

Secondary (aka: Vicarious) Traumatization

Psychotherapists sometimes experience secondary traumatization when they work with survivors of abuse or psychological terror.[40] This is sometimes true of children of survivors as well.[41] They may even take on some of the symptoms of post traumatic stress disorder (PTSD). A somatic practitioner may also experience the fear, outrage and despair of the survivor client—particularly if her practice includes a large percentage of trauma victims. She may feel suddenly helpless in the face of the client's pain and emotions, emotionally vulnerable and unable to protect herself well.

During a session, if a survivor chooses to tell the practitioner about abuse experiences, the sharing may stimulate uncomfortable feelings in the practitioner, memories from the past and a stronger countertransference. The practitioner should process these feelings, memories or countertransference in a supervision session with a supervisor, in psychotherapy, or with a colleague called on for peer supervision or support. Sharing these kinds of feelings and thoughts with the client is inappropriate.

If a practitioner feels overwhelmed by something a client says, a countertransference is probably occurring. One practitioner might contain the feeling, finish the session and seek supervision afterwards. Another practitioner might say, "I'm feeling strong empathy with what you've just said. Would it be all right if I took a break for a moment to gather my thoughts?" Practitioners need a process to work through the feelings stimulated by their clients' stories of abuse, or their unresolved feelings will impair their effectiveness.

Supervision and Support

Setting up solid support systems for oneself before working with survivors is essential. Many issues and difficulties occur for the experienced practitioner as well as for the novice: transference and countertransference; feelings of vicarious traumatization of the practitioner; and tricky situations may arise in which the client unconsciously tries to re-enact the abuse. Arrange for regular supervision with a psychotherapist who is an experienced supervisor and who has worked with abuse survivors. Ideally this person has some familiarity with somatic therapies as well, but this is not essential.

Refer to the Supervision chapter, starting on page 241.

Client Prerequisites

Clients need to be in a place in their therapeutic process where they will gain benefit from bodywork. They should be in therapy and at an appropriate stage in their recovery. Clients must be ready and strong enough to deal with the increased intensity of the psychotherapy process that touch therapy often elicits.

Engaged in Psychotherapy

Before beginning treatment with an abuse survivor, it is important to confirm that the person is working with a psychotherapist and that the therapist has agreed that it is a good idea for the survivor to receive your type of treatment. Psychotherapy is the primary therapeutic relationship for working through survivor issues. (Survivor groups are also an essential part of the recovery and therapeutic process.)

Appropriate Stage of Recovery

Bodywork is generally most helpful as part of the third stage of recovery (reconnection), when the client is integrating her trauma experience and when she is building connections with the outside world.[42] Bodywork is sometimes helpful during the second stage of recovery (remembrance and mourning) as a means of making contact with the body, learning to like the body and in some cases to help recover memories.[43] The psychotherapist and client decide together if the time is right for a collaboration.

When treatment is undertaken too soon, it may trigger memories that the client is not prepared to handle. In these cases the client often experiences the hands-on work as recreating the trauma experience. There may be episodes of escalating intrusive symptoms, crying, sleep disturbance and increased flashbacks.[44] Bodywork is generally inappropriate during the first stage of recovery (establishing safety), which requires very careful building of trust and safety between the client and psychotherapist.

Consent to Communicate

Ongoing contact between the client's psychotherapist and touch practitioner should occur during the body therapy process. This may happen only at important junctures or once each month if the client is securely into the third stage of recovery. In other instances, weekly contact is required. When a client experiences a flashback or a very strong memory during a treatment, it is often useful for the practitioner as well as the client to communicate this to the psychotherapist. The psychotherapist may also make helpful suggestions as to where the bodywork might be concentrated at different points in the therapy. The client must be willing to give consent for this communication. This permission should be given in writing at the beginning of the first or second session and kept in the practitioner's files for his protection.

See Apeendix A, pages 263-264, for sample **Informed Consent** forms.

Before the work begins, the client must understand that sessions are confidential and only the psychotherapist, practitioner and supervisor involved discuss the client's sessions.

Special Boundary Issues

Certain boundaries are built into the practitioner/client relationship that are quite different from those between friends, colleagues or family members. How they are understood and applied has a profound effect on the quality of relationships with clients. This is particularly true for working with survivors of sexual abuse. Melissa Soalt describes her observations, "Because abuse disrespects and destroys one's boundaries, survivors typically have poorly developed boundaries. To feel 'safe,' many survivors resort to a familiar isolation and erect dense protective barriers. Conversely, survivors often describe feelings of defenselessness and vulnerability that are equated with having 'no skin' of one's own and therefore having no internal shock absorption. Everything feels 'jarring' and triggering and personal. Creating flexible and appropriate boundaries can be extremely challenging for survivors."[45] The boundaries of survivors have been crossed and broken repeatedly. Because of this past abuse, survivors are often unable to consciously recognize boundaries and protect themselves:

Refer to the Boundaries chapter, starting on page 25.

> I wasn't only molested by my father, but by my grandfather on my father's side. It was somehow accepted that my grandfather could put his arms around us, could pet our legs, could French kiss us when he greeted us, you know....
>
> This would be in public, and yet, there was my mom smiling, there was my dad, smiling and his French kissing me in private wasn't far from that. Where did I draw the line? I didn't know."[46]

Practitioners need to be very sensitive to the boundaries of touch both during and after treatments. For instance, when greeting or saying goodbye to a client do you shake hands, do you put your hand on the client's shoulder or back, or do you hug the client? These are all questions to think through and talk about when working with any client, and especially when working with a survivor. The boundaries of survivors have been so violated that they may be unaware of being violated, or are unable to protect themselves by saying no to unwanted touch even if they are aware of it. With survivors, the range of physical contact on and off the table must be handled very carefully.

Careful attention to boundaries help to empower the client and protect against excessive, unmanageable transference reactions. The practitioner who works with survivors must maintain clear, consistent boundaries to both provide and model a relationship with good boundaries. An important part of the touch therapy work is to help the client rebuild boundaries and thereby empower the survivor to protect himself or herself. The highest ethical standards on the practitioner's part are essential to the healing process.

Body Memories and Flashbacks

A memory is a remembered past experience that may or may not be painful. Memories appear along a continuum of consciousness, ranging from an integrated memory to a brief, faint recollection that is gone in an instant (unintegrated memory), to a flashback which is out of the person's control.

Integrated Memory   Unintegrated Memory   Flashback

An **INTEGRATED MEMORY** is a memory that may have been painful at one time but has been remembered, understood and accepted. The person may not like the memory but does not fight remembering it and copes with the details of the memory without being overwhelmed by it. An integrated memory has a tolerable emotional charge that does not consume the person.

An **UNINTEGRATED MEMORY** exists when a memory is so painful that parts of the memory are blocked and many of the details missing. If a memory is disturbing, it may appear and then be lost for periods of time. One person recalled having a clear memory that was painful, and then totally forgetting it within seconds—as if he were in a fog. Unintegrated memories stir up unresolved feelings and are usually quickly repressed.

Clients who feel indefinite, disturbing emotions when they are touched, are uncomfortable, but do not know why. This can be the result of a painful memory that is triggered, but is not yet able to emerge into consciousness.

A **FLASHBACK** is the experience of reliving or re-experiencing a traumatic event as if it is occurring or is imminent. When a flashback is triggered, concrete, distinct memories suddenly surface and intrude on the present. They can be triggered by touching any part of the body or by a particular feeling, sensation or experience. Sometimes the smell of an oil or the cologne the practitioner wears is associated with a past event. A flashback can be experienced as a momentary flash of memory or a movie that the client is in. When this transpires, "the individual is awake but appears to be in a state of altered consciousness and often has subsequent amnesia for what takes place. The experiences last from a few minutes to several hours...."[47]

The client may have intense emotional reactions such as fear, sobbing or feelings of rage with physical trembling. When the flashback is occurring the person is dissociated from the present. The client cannot tolerate the memory and splits off his consciousness and is no longer psychologically present. When a flashback occurs the task of the practitioner is to bring the client back to the present as quickly as possible.

Flashbacks differ from integrated memories. The body holds memories,[48] therefore when an emotionally charged area is touched, long repressed memories may be evoked.[49] Certain areas such as the mouth, throat, neck, chest, abdomen, buttock and inner thigh are more likely to hold memories of traumatic abuse than other areas. But this is not

See Appendix B, pages 268-275, for details on **treatment protocols** for working with self-disclosed survivors.

always the case. One survivor described feeling very upset when her partner put an arm around her shoulder. She recalled her abuser putting his hand gently around her shoulder when the ritual of her abuse was about to begin in childhood.[50]

Many variations exist along the continuum from integrated memory to flashback. For instance, one has a faint recall of an event triggered by a part of the body being touched or by a smell or a sound, but nothing of substance is recalled. A person can also have a very clear memory and find it so unacceptable that she re-represses it and cannot recall the memory later.

Here are some examples of how touch triggers different memory experiences:

- While her mouth and jaw were being massaged, one client described a memory of a very clear sexual encounter with her father. The client had no idea that she had been abused until that moment.
- Another client felt afraid whenever her left shoulder was touched. She only recalled the details of her abuse after years of psychotherapy.
- A third client had a momentary flashback triggered by a neck adjustment and went into a catatonic state for 20 minutes. This client was fully dissociated, not responding to verbal communication or touch.

When aware of the dynamics of body memory, the practitioner can help the client remember while remaining present and in her body. A skilled practitioner learns how to avoid inducing flashbacks and how to move the client back to the present if flashbacks occur.

Recognize Flashbacks

Recognizing when a client is experiencing a flashback is not always easy. On one end of the spectrum, the out-of-control flashback can be frightening to experience and easy to recognize. Other flashbacks are quieter and are over fairly quickly. Recognizing these subtle flashbacks requires a practiced eye.

One of the keys to identifying a flashback is to look at the client's eyes. The pupils are often dilated and the client has a faraway look as if she is "out of it," extremely tired, or using drugs. She has left her body or is out of touch with feelings, thoughts and sensations. She may stare into space, curl up in a ball on the table, refuse to respond when asked a question, experience a loss of sensation (especially in the legs), begin to cry, flutter her eyelids, or talk incoherently. Phrases such as, "No, no, what are you doing?" "Who are you?" or "Don't touch me, I'm scared!" may be spoken. The body may suddenly tighten, stiffen or shake uncontrollably.

Precautions

Physical touch to particular areas of the body is more likely to stimulate a flashback than others:

- In general, the "safest" areas to touch are the hands, feet, legs below the knee, arms, gently on the scalp and forehead, the middle and lower neck, shoulders, upper back area and the mid-back. The lower back in certain individuals holds a high emotional charge because the muscles there move the pelvis and inhibit movement during unwanted sexual contact. Feet and hands can also be trigger areas if the client's abuse involved being held down or bound.
- Proceed with caution when working with the following areas: the deep, sub-occipital muscles at the back of the head, the buttocks, the front and back thighs. Some clients never want these areas touched.

While *The Ethics of Touch* covers many aspects of working with survivors of trauma and abuse, nothing replaces in-person training including boundary setting and flashback role-plays with a skilled teacher or coach.

- Consider avoiding the following areas except in consultation with the client's psychotherapist: inside the mouth, the front of the neck, the throat, the abdomen and the upper portion of the inner thigh.
- Avoid working on a woman's chest, the breast tissue and the front of the pelvis (just above and to the side of the genitals). And of course, never work in or around the genitalia.

Still, no matter how careful you are, flashbacks sometimes occur. Certain hand techniques or past associations with specific types of touch, such as a gentle touch on the shoulder, may trigger a flashback. In working with a client over a period of time, the practitioner may help minimize the likelihood of flashbacks. Remember, when the client is reliving a flashback he may believe that abuse is about to occur or is occurring. The person may feel he is actually back in childhood re-experiencing the trauma. The practitioner, alert and conscious about his role in this situation, facilitates the client's awareness of the present and immediate surroundings. "Reliving" flashbacks does not offer the opportunity to learn from earlier experiences in a way that is useful.

Retrieve the Client From a Flashback

Follow these steps when you realize a flashback is occurring:

- Break contact with your hands and acknowledge that a flashback is happening before you do anything else. Say the client's name, e.g., "Rochelle, are you here with me?" and wait for a reply. If the client is in a flashback, there is usually no reply or a vague one that is uncharacteristic of the client's communication with you. Note: a flashback is not the same as an emotional release, where you would likely maintain physical contact with a client.
- Make voice contact. Using the client's name every time, say in a very calm voice, "Jane. This is Terry. We are here together." Or say, "Ralph, where are you right now? Are you here with me? This is Terry, I am here, with you. We are having a bodywork session." Ask questions such as, "Do you know where you are? Do you know who I am?" If the eyes are closed, say, "Ann, can you open your eyes and look at me?" or direct the client to look at an object in the room. "Let me know that you hear me," is another phrase to bring a client back.
- Eye contact is one of the best ways to stay in touch with a client especially when physical touch is often a triggering mechanism. Encourage the client to open both eyes and focus on you or an object. Eye contact is usually a very good way to bring a client back to the present.
- Cover the client with a blanket to create a safe, thick physical boundary around the body. Stand to the side of the table and make eye contact. The client's eyes are usually closed, or staring into space, not seeing you. The client may also cover her eyes with her hands.
- Follow any instructions that the client has given you about how to respond if she goes into a flashback.
- Encourage the client to sit up. This often helps to re-establish an adult reality. Ask if the client would like to sit up. If the client is not sure, encourage him to do so. If he says, "No," go with the client's preference. If you have the impulse to help the person sit up, first ask if it is okay. Do not touch a client in that state without permission. Instruct the client to sit on the table or move to a chair. Pull up a chair yourself and sit so you are neither above the client looking down, nor too close. Some clients are specific and ask the practitioner to sit off to the side, not directly in front.

See Dynamics of Effective Communication, pages 62-64, for details on **dealing with emotions**.

- Take time to talk about what happened, not probing for any details of the flashback. First, ask if the client feels able to talk about the process of what happened and what might be important from this experience to discuss with the psychotherapist. Then talk together about what you are going to do next, whether you are going to continue the hands-on session, or stop. If the occurrence is a first for the two of you, it is usually a good idea to stop the hands-on portion of the treatment.

Process Why the Flashback Occurred

Once the client has sufficiently recovered from the flashback, determine if you did anything to trigger the flashback. Was it something you said, a reaction to a specific part of the body you were touching, background music, or a scent wafting through the room? Gather as much information as you can in a gentle, noninvasive way. Ask if she felt or feels numbness in any part of her body, especially her legs. If numbing occurs, the effects of the flashback were very strong and are still occurring. This information influences your decision to continue or stop the hands-on part of your session.

If you choose to continue the session, check with the person frequently to see if she is present. Notice if the client becomes spacey and ask if she is beginning to feel numb physically, particularly in the legs.

If you choose to stop, leave the room and let the client dress before talking further. The routine of dressing and preparing to leave helps bring the person into the present. Call through the door once to make sure she is okay. Otherwise, you may return to the treatment room and discover that the client hasn't moved during your absence. When the client is finished dressing, sit down and have a more complete closure than usual.

Ask what was and wasn't helpful when you were assisting the client back to the present. Ask what you could've done differently, if anything, to be more supportive.

Plan for Client Safety

Ask if the client has plans after leaving your office. The client should be with people with whom he feels safe. If the client feels too disoriented or dizzy to drive or to travel alone, ensure his physical safety by arranging for a taxi or for someone to pick up the client. Most people recover within a half hour while others take longer. Help the client make emergency plans should another flashback occur. Talk about whom to call: a friend, partner, family member, psychotherapist, a hospital emergency room, or you.

Adjust Your Schedule

You may need to adjust your schedule and run overtime if a flashback occurs, particularly toward the end of the session. Extending a session should not become a habit. If another client is waiting, take the first opportunity which feels appropriate to tell your current client that you are leaving for just a moment to tell the next client that you are running a little late. This lets the current client know that you are conscious of the extra time needed and also want to show respect to the person who is waiting. It sets a professional tone and helps both clients feel comfortable at the same time.

Follow Up

Tell the client that you will talk to his psychotherapist about what happened during the session. Suggest that the client call and talk with the psychotherapist the same day as well. At the beginning of the next session again ask the client what was helpful and what wasn't. You may hear different information.

Checklist for Working with Trauma Survivors

The following checklist is adapted with permission from Stephanie Mines, PH.D.[51]

1. Spend time connecting with the client.
2. Consider using more subtle, gentle body therapy techniques that do not feel invasive.
3. Invest in education about trauma and shock and understanding their somatic impact. There are resource centers that offer such training.
4. Always remember to ask permission to touch. Be willing and ready to wait and not to touch.
5. Remember to establish a relational connection first. Never touch mechanically.
6. If a flashback occurs, bring the person back to the present immediately.
7. Keep in regular contact with the client's psychotherapist. Have clear, written permission from your client for these conversations.
8. Be gentle but clear about boundaries.
9. Behave as a team and set goals together.
10. Allow the client to control the pace of the treatment.
11. Have a time for closure at the end of each session.
12. Be present, inquire and never assume. Do not hesitate to check-in with your client, asking about her experience.
13. Develop a referral list of psychotherapists and counselors. Establish personal connections with these therapists before you refer clients to them.
14. Develop the skills that allow you to distinguish shock from trauma and to identify them when they are activated.
15. Receive bodywork or energy medicine treatment yourself to clear your own system of fatigue and repression, thereby preventing retraumatization and burnout.
16. Consider volunteering at a local safehouse for survivors of domestic violence or joining the bodywork team at an AIDS service agency. These organizations usually provide a volunteer training that is excellent education about the treatment of trauma.
17. Cultivate a supervisory relationship and bring issues to your supervisor or peer supervision group.

In Conclusion...

Touch therapy is a powerful adjunct in the recovery from abuse, and with this power comes the need for great responsibility on the part of the practitioner. The practitioner who provides ethical treatment for abuse survivors comes from a place of sensitivity, caring and the desire to help, as well as from one of detailed education, extensive training and ongoing supervision. Bodywork might be the first experience of pain relief or nurturing that survivors have on the physical level. It may be the path home.

See Appendix B, pages 268-275, for additional information and treatment techniques for working with self-disclosed survivors.

Chapter Highlights

- The ethical dimensions inherent in body therapy are intensified when working with survivors.
- Long-repressed pain may emerge as mental or emotional dis-ease or physical symptoms of musculoskeletal dysfunction and discomfort.
- Survivor symptoms and behaviors include hyperarousal, intrusion, constriction, dissociation and flashback.
- Chronic fatigue, insomnia, chronic joint and muscle pain and chronically weakened immune response may indicate unresolved trauma.
- Flashbacks, intense memories and unexpected reactions can result from abuse experiences.
- Cathartic emotional releases may increase rather than decrease traumatization.
- Body therapy isn't appropriate in the first stage of recovery where the client hasn't yet established safety.
- Treatment mistakes mainly occur when the practitioner inadvertently violates a boundary.
- Survivors often have difficulty recognizing where their boundaries are.
- Sexual abuse is defined as unwanted or inappropriate sexual contact, either verbal or physical, between two or more people, that is intended as an act of control, power, rage, violence and intimidation with sex as a weapon.
- Physical abuse is the use of force or violence to cause pain and/or bodily harm which is used as an instrument of intimidation, coercion or control.
- Emotional abuse is the infliction of emotional harm by verbal intimidation or behavior which intimidates, demeans or hurts another person.
- Mind control abuse is the act of undermining a person's free will through the control of behavior, information, thoughts and emotions.
- Sexual abuse ranges from inappropriate seductive behavior and sexual touching to sexual intercourse.
- Sexual abuse rarely occurs as an isolated event. It is usually accompanied by other types of mental, physical and emotional abuse.
- Mind control abuse involves creating an alternate identity in the person which is programmed to be dependent on a person or organization.
- Sexual, emotional or physical abuse is trauma that leaves profound and lasting effects on a person's psychological, cognitive and emotional functioning. This is often referred to as ptsd (post traumatic stress disorder).
- There are three major symptoms of ptsd: hyperarousal, intrusion and constriction.
- Hyperarousal is an exaggerated state of constant alertness to danger.
- Intrusion is when past traumatic events randomly recur as vivid memories in the person's present life.
- Constriction occurs when the pain of an event is so severe that the survivor becomes numb or psychologically removed.
- The three stages of recovery are: establishing safety; remembrance and mourning; and reconnection.
- Establishing safety refers to creating physical and psychological safety.
- Remembrance and mourning mean remembering traumatic events and experiencing the grief and loss that accompany the memories.
- Reconnection refers to the trauma survivor re-establishing trust and connection with the outside world.

- Body therapy is most useful when performed in the latter part of the second stage and the third stage of recovery.
- Skillful bodywork creates a safe place to help survivors reconnect with their bodies.
- The ethical touch therapy experience offers a safe place to be touched with dignity and respect in a non-judgmental, non-sexual environment.
- Somatic therapies help in the rebuilding of personal boundaries damaged by trauma and abuse.
- Touch that is neutral or pleasurable and non-sexual provides building blocks for a changed experience of the body.
- Trauma from the past can cause a person to dissociate from the body and this disassociation experience often recurs when the body is touched.
- Working closely with a psychotherapist, touch therapy can assist the survivor in reaching hidden memories and integrating them into the present experience.
- The psychotherapist helps the client integrate emotional and cognitive insights while the touch therapist helps the client increase self-awareness and gain access to emotions and less conscious memories.
- The treatment of survivors requires a fine degree of self-awareness along with training in psychology, communication, sexuality, ethics, trauma and counseling.
- A baseline knowledge of transference, countertransference, power differentials, dual relationships and boundaries is essential for the practitioner who wishes to work with trauma survivors.
- Practitioners who wish to work with trauma survivors need to understand their own issues, limitations and motivations.
- Practitioners who work with trauma victims are vulnerable to vicarious traumatization in which the therapist may experience fear, outrage and despair in identifying with the client.
- Practitioners need a place to work through feelings stimulated by their clients' stories of abuse or their unresolved feelings will get in the way of being effective.
- Set up a solid support system including an experienced supervisor before working with survivors.
- Trauma survivors need to be in the appropriate stage of recovery to best benefit from hands-on work.
- Undertaking treatment too soon may trigger memories that the client is not prepared to handle.
- In most cases the trauma survivor should be in psychotherapy at the same time he undergoes bodywork.
- Before beginning treatment, gain permission from the client to have ongoing contact with her psychotherapist.
- Because boundaries of survivors have been crossed and broken repeatedly, these clients are often unable to consciously recognize boundaries and protect themselves.
- Practitioners need to be sensitive to the boundaries of touch both on and off the treatment table.
- Careful attention to boundaries empowers the client and protects against excessive, unmanageable, transference reactions.
- Any part of the body can hold a memory. When an emotionally charged area is touched, repressed memories may be evoked.
- Memories appear along a continuum of consciousness ranging from an integrated memory to a faint recollection to a flashback which is out of the person's control.

- A flashback is the experience of reliving a traumatic event as if it's occurring in the present time.
- An integrated memory is a painful memory that has been remembered, understood and accepted.
- When a flashback occurs the person is dissociated from the present and the task of the practitioner is to bring the client back to the present as quickly as possible.
- A skilled practitioner learns how to avoid inducing flashbacks.
- Physical touch to particular areas is more likely to stimulate flashbacks.
- It is important that the client has a specific plan for the day after a flashback occurs.
- In the first session discuss your policies which should detail the boundaries of your professional relationship.
- Discuss the client's goals for somatic therapy.
- Invite the client to make suggestions; accentuate teamwork.
- Emphasize that the client is free to stop the session at any point.
- The client should be in control of where and how deeply the therapist works.
- A structured treatment creates safety.
- Move slowly from one part of the body to another, asking for the client's consent before proceeding.
- As the session proceeds, actively track the client for flashbacks or dissociation.
- The first few times you initiate a new movement, check in with the client to see if it's okay.
- Hold a closure discussion at the end of each session.

Discussion Questions and Activities

- Why is working with a trauma survivor not advisable in the first stage of recovery?
- Why does a survivor of trauma need to be careful about emotionally cathartic experiences?
- Relate the three stages of recovery to experiences in your own life.
- Discuss experiences you or others had with mind control abuse in which control of behavior, information, thoughts and emotions were involved.
- What are the physical effects and sensitivities of trauma on the body?
- Discuss and then have several people role-play the experiences of hyperarousal, intrusion and constriction.
- What are the elements of establishing safety in a somatic therapy practice?
- List examples of how a practitioner can help a survivor rebuild physical and emotional boundaries during a session?
- Explain the differences between a flashback, an unintegrated memory and an integrated memory.
- Discuss why a trauma survivor undergoing touch therapy should be in psychotherapy.
- What are the prerequisites for the practitioner working with trauma survivors? Discuss their importance.
- Why is it important for the therapist working with trauma survivors to understand transference and countertransference?
- Discuss helpful and unhelpful motives for working with trauma survivors.
- Describe situations in working with a trauma survivor where supervision would be useful and necessary.
- Discuss the prerequisites for the trauma survivor client interested in undergoing touch therapy to help deal with the traumatic experiences.
- What is the primary task of the practitioner when the client is experiencing a flashback, and why?
- What are the signs that a flashback is occurring?
- What is meant by secondary traumatization and how can it be minimized?
- List ways to lessen the power differential when working with a trauma survivor.
- Why is it unadvisable to engage in dual relationships with clients who are trauma survivors?
- Describe what "being present" actually means.
- Why is it important to maintain continuous communication when working with a trauma survivor? How might you maintain reasonably continuous communication without being intrusive?

9

Supervision

- ◆ The Role of Clinical Supervision
- ◆ Essential Elements of Helpful Supervision
- ◆ How to Find a Supervisor
- ◆ Peer Supervision
- ◆ In Conclusion...
- ◆ Chapter Highlights
- ◆ Discussion Questions and Activities

Overwhelming emotional and boundary dilemmas occur as a predictable aspect of the somatic practitioner's life. Practitioners need a shame-free, trusting relationship with peers or a supervisor to sort out such dilemmas. This relationship protects clients as well as the practitioner. Ethical clinical practice for all somatic practitioners includes self-awareness, self-monitoring and ongoing review of challenging or difficult cases with peers or a clinical supervisor.

Supervision creates a setting for self-care, support and nurturance. It is the right place for practitioners to receive appreciation for their good and useful work. Supervision assists practitioners in maintaining ethical practices and reduces burnout. The management of boundaries in professional relationships is complex. With increasing attention to boundaries, boundary violations and professional misconduct in the practice of all health care professionals and particularly in the touch professions, the fundamental importance of clinical supervision is clear.[1]

The crucial role of supervision in the training of all health care professionals has been widely acknowledged by practitioners and supported in the professional literature over the past 15 years.[2] Yet the core curricula in most training programs often neglect to teach practitioners how to deal with the intense feelings that arise in the therapeutic relationship. When the body is touched as a part of the therapeutic relationship, clients' feelings can become intensified. These feelings may be confusing and troubling, and at times diminish the practitioner's ability to deliver quality care.[3] Without solid models or communication tools, practitioners have to figure out by trial and error how to best manage the complex interpersonal dilemmas that arise when working with clients.[4]

The clients who come for care and treatment have wide-ranging vulnerabilities, multiple needs, past relationship troubles, unrealistic hopes and personal traumas. An important and integral aspect of being a health care professional includes tolerating and managing feelings that arise in our professional relationships with these clients.[5] This can be very stressful and difficult at times.

Practitioners need to be involved enough to feel for and care for clients, yet distant enough to decide objectively on and implement the best course of treatment.[6] Inevitably, feelings toward certain clients affect practitioners by bringing them closer, pushing them away, confusing or irritating them as professionals. Particular clients may challenge their capacity to manage their feelings, expose professional "blind spots," or touch on areas of personal vulnerability. This hampers practitioners' efforts to communicate directly and effectively which impacts their ability to deliver the best care. Discussing these issues in a supervision setting helps diffuse residual emotions and create balance.

The Role of Clinical Supervision

Clinical supervision has long been the "primary professional training model for mental health clinicians"[7] and more recently other somatic professionals have begun to recognize and use this forum to train students. Professionals who benefit from supervision include massage and bodywork therapists, acupuncturists, chiropractors, physical therapists, physical therapy assistants, occupational therapists, athletic trainers and other somatic practitioners. Clinical supervision is a valuable and necessary form of continuing education for all wellness professionals, and it is particularly important for practitioners who perform ongoing body therapy. Les Kertay, PH.D., states, "If you're interested in doing work that has emotional and spiritual impact on your clients, then the most powerful way of dealing

Like coals in a fireplace, we keep our sense of character warm by contact with each other. Set any one of us alone on the moral hearth, and we'll pretty quickly turn to a cold dark cinder.

—Rushworth M. Kidder

with the questions involved is to utilize ongoing professional supervision. Supervision is not about being told how to do your job, rather it's a place to process your clients' work and your experiences of being with them."[8]

Supervision can be done on a one-on-one basis or in a group. It is often useful to have supervision in a small group of practitioners who are doing the same kind of work. This broadens the base of learning and creates an additional support system for each member. If the practitioner is in a group situation where she can learn from others' experiences, it is possible to master the fundamentals of practice through witnessing other's learning and not relying exclusively upon her own professional trial and error. Hearing the fears and doubts of other practitioners who are feeling challenged by unusual client situations can help practitioners feel less isolated and alone.

In a group setting clinical supervision undertakes four functions: 1) addressing the relationship issues that arise between clients and practitioners; 2) functioning as a support group for the participants; 3) serving as a forum for didactic instruction on important psychological concepts (such as projection, transference, countertransference); and 4) training the participants in supervisory skills so that they feel confident continuing this helpful type of coaching by themselves at a later date without the supervisor. Clinical supervision provides an opportunity to discuss with a more experienced, psychologically savvy practitioner how to best help a client while promoting increased self-observation and awareness. In a group setting the supervisor will often invite other members to help guide a colleague toward the core issue underlying the problem. Practitioners can increase their tolerance and understanding and learn how to manage feelings in themselves and their clients through clinical supervision. Supervision is often a nourishing, protective, creative endeavor that greatly benefits the practitioner, client and the supervisor.

Identifying and understanding intense, sometimes objectionable, feelings in professional relationships is central to the management of professional boundaries. With inadequate preparation for managing intense, often startling feelings, practitioners run the risk of over-identification, engaging in destructive behavior, or developing restricted practice styles that do not benefit themselves or their clients.[9, 10] Supervisors are well suited to assist practitioners with identification and management of their feelings around these boundary dilemmas. Consultations may assist practitioners in sorting out clinical and interpersonal dilemmas, thereby protecting competent care of the client.

The clinical supervisor helps the practitioner define his problems and questions. This can be a surprisingly difficult job for both supervisor and practitioner. When a practitioner feels disturbed by *something*, the task becomes naming that something precisely and figuring out what kind of help is wanted. There is an important distinction between how the practitioner sees the problem and how the supervisor sees it. Rather than offering advice and telling the practitioner what to do, a good supervisor helps the practitioner explore what is happening internally, define where the appropriate boundary is for the practitioner and the client, and determine what action might correct the situation. In general these techniques—which draw on and validate the practitioner's problem-solving skills—lead to a more effective and empowering resolution.

Guidelines for Consultation

Ethical practitioners are committed to self-supervision concerning personal motives and ethical responsibilities. The following questions may facilitate self-supervision and assist practitioners in deciding when a consultation with a supervisor is indicated.

Sometimes our light goes out but is blown into flame by another human being. Each of us owes deepest thanks to those who have rekindled this light.

-Albert Schweitzer

There is only one corner of the universe you can be certain of improving, and that's your own self.

—Aldous Huxley

- Does the care of this client deviate from the usual professional standards of care for this client's problem? Were usual and customary professional boundaries stretched or violated? What is the clinical rationale for the unusual treatment approach?
- Are you aware of strong feelings about this client? Do you adapt your behavior according to your attitudes about this client? Do you feel intimidated, afraid, angry, powerless or especially close to this client? How do these feelings influence the care provided?
- Are you confused or conflicted about the relationship aspects of this client's care?
- Are you uncertain concerning the differentiation between professional and personal feelings and where to construct the professional boundary? Are you attracted to the client? Is the client attracted to you?

Scenarios

Consider the following scenarios illustrating boundary dilemmas practitioners have encountered and discussed in supervision. These scenarios depict the internal, interpersonal and clinical process of formulating the dilemma and constructing useful boundaries through supervision.

Scenario 1

In general practitioners are advised to listen to their own anxiety as a reliable signal that a problem or client relationship deserves further attention and work. When possible, it is useful to identify the source of the anxiety. When a client presents threatening behaviors, the practitioner needs to assess whether the client presents a real, physical threat and danger to the practitioner or the staff by evaluating the client's capacity for violence. Many somatic practitioners may not be competent or capable of assessing a client's dangerousness. A consultation with a supervisor or mental health professional may be necessary and indicated to assess a client under these circumstances, particularly if the client does not respond to verbal limits.

An acupuncturist found herself feeling frightened and disgusted by a client, a 40-year-old divorced man who was a recovering alcoholic with a history of impulsive, aggressive behavior. Although he had always been in control in her presence at the clinic, the acupuncturist overheard the client verbally abusing someone on the support staff. The acupuncturist wished to transfer the care of this client to an associate in the clinic to avoid her anxiety and sense of intimidation. She understood that this client had great difficulty with change and wondered if her wish to transfer his care was ethical and necessary. Did he present a danger to her and could she more effectively manage her anxiety and relationship with this client?

With clinical supervision the acupuncturist became aware of her nearly phobic dread of this client and explored what specifically frightened her about this man's behavior. Did this client remind her of someone in her life? Did she have difficulty being appropriately assertive? While she understood it was her responsibility to set limits, she confirmed she was uncomfortable with confrontation and had little experience as a professional exercising her authority when it involved conflict. She realized her conflict-avoidance stance was a lifelong pattern in personal relationships and this client might be triggering a personal set of experiences. The supervisor highlighted the practitioner's professional objective to become more comfortable with asserting herself in conflict situations, emphasizing the importance of these professional skills and responsibilities.

Through the process of supervision, the acupuncturist realized that several options were available to her. As a practitioner it was her responsibility to educate and protect clients and staff, and seek mental health consultations if necessary around safety issues. To ensure competent and safe care of her clients and support staff she needed to deal with her anxiety and difficulty with professional self-assertion through supervision. If she were unable to master her anxiety and assume professional authority with this man despite specialized assistance and ongoing supervision, she might not treat this client safely. If her sense of anxiety and terror with this man's anger continued to interfere with or compromised her clinical judgment, then she would have an ethical responsibility to refer his care to a colleague. This, of course, is the least desirable alternative, to be employed only after seeking assistance and trying to work with the client and the professional issues raised for the practitioner.

Through direct questioning, modeling and explanation, the supervisor demonstrated how professionals might assert themselves by setting clear boundaries and establishing a safe environment for both practitioner and client.[11,12] With technical and emotional support the acupuncturist decided she would try this approach and discussed with the client his inappropriate and scary behavior. While the client expressed his desire to air a grievance, he had little awareness of how frightening his behavior was to staff. He reassured her that despite his "loud bark" he wouldn't hurt anyone. Furthermore, he expressed that he had a low tolerance for the frustration that he felt while waiting for appointments that were even a little late in starting. The practitioner suggested that in the future he could keep his office waiting time to a minimum by calling the office ahead to see if she was on time or running behind. The client liked that suggestion and also agreed to consider a referral to a mental health professional.

A practitioner might also review the client's file and speak to the client to shed light on the client's behavior. Does the client have a history of violence and impulsive behavior? Against whom, under what circumstances, how recently? Does the client currently use alcohol or drugs? Does the client have a serious mental illness? Is the client verbally threatening violence or behaving in an angry and threatening manner?

Scenario 2

Deviations from usual practice (as demonstrated in this scenario) may be a warning signal to practitioners. After identifying such deviations, it is always useful for practitioners to review the treatment rationale and decision-making process by posing the following questions. Is this the best course of action? What is gained and what is lost by this treatment approach or intervention? Is this a one-time occurrence or an ongoing process? What review process is in place to evaluate the usefulness of this unusual practice? What are the risks to the client, the practitioner, the treatment? Is this practice negotiated openly or does the practitioner feel coerced?[13]

A male bodywork therapist had a VIP client, a nationally known cardiac surgeon, who had injured his foot while on vacation and was facing many months of rehabilitation. The surgeon requested that the therapist make house calls so that he wouldn't have to travel to receive treatments. The therapist obliged, even though he didn't usually make house calls, as he felt the client was a very important and busy man. However, the therapist found himself becoming annoyed as the surgeon regularly kept him waiting, causing him to fall behind in his scheduled office appointments. During the treatment sessions the surgeon peppered the therapist with intrusive personal questions. The therapist struggled to respond in a professional and cordial manner while protecting his privacy. After the sixth session the surgeon thanked him profusely for all his fine work and offered to let him and his family use his elegant vacation home. The therapist accepted his offer.

In supervision the therapist identified the multiple ways in which his treatment of this client was exceptional and deviated from customary practice. He saw that treating this man at home under these circumstances was probably not in his best interest. With discussion he became aware that deeply personal feelings and motives had shaped his clinical decision-making. His wish to be admired by an important man clouded his professional judgment. Envious of the surgeon's wealth and position, he wanted to share in the benefits of the wealth and status. This contributed to the therapist abandoning his professional standards and compromised the boundaries of his professional relationship with him. Additionally, he was angry with himself for his personal over-involvement and with the client for his unusual treatment requests that he was unable to handle appropriately.

The therapist became aware of how he had acquiesced to the surgeon's inappropriate behavior (keeping him waiting, taking calls during the treatment) to avoid disappointing him or provoking his disapproval. He wasn't afraid of the surgeon's anger or any possibility of violence, but fearful of his disapproval. The therapist's envy, unacknowledged longings and wish to win the client's approval contributed to his faulty decision-making. The supervisor modeled more appropriate responses to intrusive questions, such as, "I'm not comfortable answering personal questions. Let's concentrate on getting your foot back into working order." The therapist's wish to have his client's approval, admiration and material possessions was identified as an area for ongoing self-monitoring. The therapist focused his supervision sessions on self-monitoring and professional boundaries.

The therapist decided to decline the use of his client's vacation home. Thanking the client for the offer, he explained that he thought it was best to be clear about the professional nature of their relationship. He informed the surgeon that home visits and the late start of sessions didn't work in terms of his schedule and proposed that the surgeon receive treatments at the therapist's office. The client acknowledged the therapist's feedback, and together they came up with appropriate changes to their working agreement.

If the therapist had noticed his personal involvement earlier, he might have declined the client's invitation to treat him at home, saying he did not make house calls, instead recommending that he come to the office. In such instances the client may resist and try to convince the therapist to make an exception to his normal practice. If that should occur, the therapist may share his thinking and rationale with the client, offering what he believes is the best care. Setting such a limit, of course, involves the possibility that the client will go elsewhere for treatment.

Scenario 3

Clients routinely bring emotional personal dilemmas into the professional relationship, such as a low frustration tolerance, profound loneliness and deep longings to be special to someone. Health care professionals must be equipped to deal with the wide range of client behaviors and requests for treatment that may not be in the client's or the practitioner's best interest.[14] Clinical supervision is a valuable resource for assessing and monitoring the relationship aspects of care giving.

A 30-year-old male physical therapist had a 55-year-old unhappily married woman as a client. She had been seeking frequent contact with him for numerous minor physical complaints. During office visits the client repeatedly requested to be physically examined beyond what might be necessary to evaluate her complaints. In addition she came to the examination wearing bright red and black lace underwear. Frightened and disgusted by his client's provocative sexual behavior, the therapist felt unsure how to address the issue.

With clinical supervision the therapist identified his feelings of embarrassment and his anxiety about being vulnerable to an accusation of professional misconduct. The supervisor discussed the importance of clarifying the appropriate boundaries of the therapist/client relationship. Through discussion of the case the physical therapist hypothesized his client's seductive behavior to be an attempt to secure his emotional and physical attention or to repeat a history of sexual exploitation. He surmised that without seductive behavior and revealing attire, his client might believe she wasn't worthy of his care. Understanding that his client's behavior might be an attempt to express nonsexual needs in a sexualized manner, or that his client confused care-taking with sexuality, helped the therapist to regain a compassionate, caring, protective stance with her.

The physical therapist decided to inform his client that he would schedule monthly visits to discuss her status. Between these visits, if needed, he proposed to set her up with appointments with a physical therapy assistant. He explained that physical examinations would be deferred unless clearly necessary; instead, the visit would focus on her home therapy exercise program. The physical therapist chose not to comment directly upon his client's clothing as this would likely shame and humiliate her. By identifying his client's unsettling behavior and his own accompanying feelings through the supervisory process, the therapist formulated an approach that was both compassionate and protective of the client, her care and himself.

Sometimes clients are undeterred in pursuit of personal relationships with health care practitioners or are stuck in repeating, maladaptive, interpersonal dramas with their care providers. Clients are responsible for their behavior and may require professional assistance to understand the limits of the professional relationship and what's acceptable behavior. Professionals may have to set limits assertively in a non-punitive manner, and document repetitive, inappropriate behavior, or sexual advances in the client's record. Open, direct communication with clients, consultation from colleagues and documentation of the problem behavior and subsequent treatment approach protect the practitioner against litigation.

Scenario 4

See Sex, Touch and Intimacy, pages 125-127, for the **Intervention Model**.

Clients who have been sexually victimized as children may eroticize the professional relationship as they often confuse sexual contact with care taking.[15] Practitioners may on occasion be confronted with requests for sexual favors, sexualized verbal conduct and unwelcome overt sexual advances. While professionals may experience a range of intense feelings including annoyance or anxiety about such overtures from clients, it is their responsibility to re-establish professional boundaries and set safe limits. Often, this involves the use of professional authority educating the client about appropriate behavior and the limits of their relationship.[16]

After one month of weekly treatments with a female chiropractor, a male client began asking the practitioner to go to lunch with him. The chiropractor wished to be sensitive to her client's feelings and to educate him concerning her view of the professional relationship. She responded, "Thank you for the offer. I don't see clients outside the office. It is my policy not to mix professional and personal relationships." Despite her clear communication about the limits of the professional relationship, the client persisted in asking her to lunch. The chiropractor felt a need to further educate her client about his behavior and the professional relationship. She said, "I want you to stop asking me to go out to lunch. It concerns me that you don't seem to understand that our relationship is professionally based and won't expand outside the office. Your repeated requests for social contact distract from the professional care you deserve for your pain. If this continues, I may not feel comfortable treating you and will refer you to another practitioner."

Feeling upset and confused by his persistence; the chiropractor brought the situation to her supervision group. Through discussion she realized just how unsettling these overtures had been to her and how it affected her care of this man. The supervision group helped her sort through her feelings and needs while exploring many options. With the group's consultation, she experienced herself as once again in charge and developed clarity concerning a plan of action. Most of all, it was enormously comforting not to manage this challenging situation on her own.

To the chiropractor's surprise, the client didn't return for several weeks. She surmised that despite her best effort to be sensitive to his feelings while setting professional boundaries that her client might have felt injured, angry or humiliated. Additionally, she suspected that her client sensed her resolve and unambivalent stance about his overtures and that she would indeed refer him to another practitioner. When her client returned for an appointment several weeks later, he commented, "I hope you're not angry with me. I like you. I know your work is effective and don't want to start over with a new chiropractor." The chiropractor responded, "I know you like me and I would be happy to continue to treat you. I'm hopeful the treatments will continue to diminish your pain. It is important that we have an understanding about how we're going to work together including the limits of our relationship."

After this conversation, the chiropractor felt some relief as her client seemed to have realigned himself and she had a strong sense that he didn't want to jeopardize or lose their professional relationship. While she imagined her client would consciously try to behave differently, she wondered if he might have romantic or sexual feelings toward her. As she reflected on this possibility, she experienced a heightened sense of responsibility to behave in a manner that wouldn't further stimulate romantic or sexual feelings and fantasies. She was certain that she would use her supervision group to continue monitoring the unfolding of the professional relationship and manage her feelings.

When a practitioner senses or has confirmation of romantic or sexual feelings from a client, scrupulous attention to professional boundaries is crucial. If a practitioner feels attracted to a client, careful self-monitoring of interactions and the safeguarding of boundaries is in order. Be alert, sensitive and mindful of interactions with this client. By overly social or flirtatious conduct, a practitioner may signal that the professional boundaries are not secure or that the practitioner is personally or sexually interested in the client.[17] Supervision is usually recommended when sexual issues are involved.

Essential Elements of Helpful Supervision

While the fundamental role of supervision in clinical practice is generally acknowledged, there is little consensus about the theory and structure of useful supervision.[18, 19] Formal training or curricula for supervisors are nearly nonexistent and there is no one prevailing theory or model of clinical supervision. Most often supervisors rely upon imitating the valued aspects of their personal supervisory experiences while trying to avoid the painful or negative aspects. The decision and responsibility of assessing the right fit between practitioner/supervisor and the usefulness of the supervision lies with the supervisee. Some clear ideas defining useful supervision have emerged from research[20, 21] personal experiences and anecdotal accounts.

> *The trouble with most of us is that we would rather be ruined by praise than saved by criticism.*
>
> —Norman Vincent Peale

1. Useful supervision includes an interpersonal climate of reasonable safety including an atmosphere of warmth, respect, honesty and support that allows a trust-based relationship to develop. A collaborative approach with a sense of mutual empowerment and openness to new learning for both parties is valued. Definition and clarity about the supervisory contract including time, fees, issues of confidentiality, evaluation and learning goals are essential to establish a sense of safety and clear boundaries.

2. Supervision works best when the educational contract is as specific as possible and both parties communicate directly and clearly. The process of exposing and examining professional work and disclosing personal professional experiences commonly evokes feelings of anxiety or vulnerability. This is to be expected. Learning involves feeling like a beginner with a predictable sense of disruption as one transforms previous ways of understanding and integrates new material. These inevitable feelings of vulnerability, perhaps ineptness, diminish with time and are coupled with a sense of increasing

competence and self-confidence. Helpful supervisory experiences encourage the awareness that "mistakes" are an important part of the learning process. In a successful supervisory relationship the sense of comfort and self-disclosure deepens across time.

3. Supervisory approaches that foster the personal and professional development of the individual practitioner are preferable. Supervisors who encourage practitioners to creatively answer their own questions facilitate the development of a competent professional. Supervisors who communicate that they believe they ultimately know the best ways to understand and manage the clinical situation leave supervisees feeling incompetent, dependent and unprepared for the complexities of client care.

How to Find a Supervisor

Supervision Sources
• National Association of Social Workers (NASW)
750 First St NE, Suite 700
Washington, D.C. 20002
202-408-8600;
800-638-8799
http://www.naswdc.org

• Clinical Social Work Federation (CSWF)
PO Box 3740
Arlington, VA 22203
703-522-3866
http://www.cswf.org

• American Psychiatric Association (APA)
1400 K St NW
Washington, D.C. 20005
202-682-6000;
888-357-7924
http://www.psych.org

• American Psychological Association (APA)
750 First St NE
Washington, D.C. 20002
202-336-5510;
800-374-2721
http://www.apa.org

• American Nurses Association (ANA)
600 Marilyn Ave SW,
100 W
Washington, D.C. 20024
202-651-7000;
800-274-4262
http://www.nursingworld.org

A skillful supervisor is like a guide in unfamiliar territory, enhancing understanding and helping direct the practitioner toward constructive solutions, if necessary. A supervisor often helps by asking a variety of questions about what is needed and what the practitioner was thinking and feeling during the time he did not know what to do. In appropriate situations advice can be offered as to what to do with a client. The most important aspect of supervision, however, is the opportunity to explore and work through a problem.

Finding a supervisor is often not an easy task, particularly in small, out of the way places where there are few therapists familiar with somatic practices. Psychotherapy disciplines have the longest tradition of providing clinical supervision and thus psychotherapists are excellent sources. Psychiatrists, nurses, social workers, psychologists and counselors are likely to be experienced supervisors. Personal recommendations by a colleague or a valued teacher are also fine ways to secure names of potential supervisors. If a referral by a colleague or instructor is difficult to obtain, it is possible to contact state or national professional organizations to obtain names of professionals in good standing.

Interview Potential Supervisors

Practitioners should employ a consumer-oriented selection process in selecting and arranging clinical supervision. You are purchasing a professional service and should investigate and choose wisely. Supervisors are not equally talented, experienced, competent, or at the same developmental phase. Ann Alonso[22] explores the developmental process of supervisors, identifying issues for the novice, mid-career and late-career supervisor. Alonso notes that supervisors of clinical work change across time. An effective clinical supervisor has in-depth knowledge about human psychology and mind-body connections. A supervisor should teach what happens when clients become emotionally dependent upon practitioners, with particular attention to issues of transference and countertransference.

Remember, in essence you are selecting a teacher so you need to be sure that this person represents consonant values of care and ethical codes of conduct, and has the time and energy to support you. A good match in terms of compatible interpersonal and cognitive styles, methods of supervision, expertise and learning needs is important. These factors become increasingly important in the case of cross-discipline supervision where the supervisory dyad shares information about the unique features of practice in their respective professional cultures and develop a common language.

After an initial screening telephone call to assess if the supervisor has time, is affordable and sounds like a potential match, arrange an interview. During the face-to-face interview with the prospective supervisor you have an opportunity to experience how it feels to sit and speak with this person and gain an impression of how she thinks and works. Prepare in advance questions you would like answered in this meeting such as the following:

- What has been your experience as a supervisor? How long? For what disciplines?
- Have you ever worked with or supervised [name your discipline]?
- How do you describe your work as a supervisor?
- What is your fee for supervision? How long is the session?
- Are my discussions with you confidential? What are the limits, if any, of confidentiality?
- Can you give me the names of a few individuals you've supervised who would be willing to speak about their experiences?
- I would like to learn more about or want help with [list your professional or developmental concerns]. Is this something you can help me with?

These guidelines are designed to help you secure the best kind of supervisory assistance for your particular situation. If for any reason, even if it is difficult to articulate, you feel anxious, uncomfortable or threatened in the initial meeting with the prospective supervisor, trust your intuition and look elsewhere. Seriously consider any visceral discomfort and reservations. Remember there are other competent supervisors and you will find one that is a better match.

> "
> Those who bring sunshine to the lives of others cannot keep it from themselves.
> "
> —James Matthew Barre

Unhelpful Supervision

While one always hopes that supervisory experiences are helpful and useful, we know from research and anecdotal accounts that supervision may be a positive or a negative process and experience. Unfortunately, on occasion supervisors abuse the power inherent in their role and status. Because supervisors are professional role models and teachers, it is imperative that practitioners incorporate positive values and messages from the supervisor about the professional self and the care and treatment of clients. When supervisors use arrogant, inflexible and shaming techniques, and exploit the supervisee's vulnerability, the supervisee as well as client care is harmed.

Elements of negative supervisory relationships include supervisory relationships that evoke intense negative feelings and are burdened with disrespect and lack of honest self-disclosure.[23, 24] Supervisors who abandon the role of teacher and treat the supervisees as clients are not helpful. Supervisees who find themselves in a supervisory relationship characterized by these negative traits should seek other supervision. Remember, supervision should above all be helpful and enhance a sense of professional confidence, competence and mastery. It should also be very satisfying.

Peer Supervision

Peer group supervision is a valuable model of supervision for health care practitioners at any phase of professional life. Beginning practitioners may find it beneficial to engage in both individual and peer group supervision. Mid- and late-career practitioners often participate regularly in peer group supervision and seek individual consultations as required. Each practitioner designs a network of supervision that suits the demands and needs of his practice, phase of professional development and his personality.

Peer group supervision has easily identifiable advantages and some potential disadvantages. The strengths, limitations and success of peer groups rest with the composition of the individual members and the clarity of the peer group contract. Members must agree upon the time, location and frequency of meetings. The organizational structure and goals of the meeting and limits of confidentiality need to be defined and agreed upon. Vague, ambiguous, overly ambitious, or ambivalent goals and structure often lead to difficulties. As with individual or clinical group supervision, an interpersonal atmosphere of reasonable safety including respect, warmth, honesty and a collaborative openness is critical. Competitiveness, criticism, inconsistency of members, absence of support and warmth all diminish the effectiveness of the group and the pleasure for the members. Potential disadvantages of peer group supervision include the varying commitment and inconsistency of attendance of members.

Peer group supervision decreases professional isolation, increases professional support and networking, normalizes the stress and strain of professional life and offers multiple perspectives on any concern or problem. Intellectually stimulating and fun, peer supervision has the added benefit of being free of charge.

A brief, start-up consultation with a clinical supervisor or group specialist is helpful to define and establish the contract and framework for successful peer group supervision. When successful, peer group supervision far exceeds other forms of supervision and continuing education for individualized learning, intimacy, support, pleasure and a sense of belonging that anchors professional work. Many peer groups opt to have a clinical supervisor moderate meetings on a regular schedule, such as quarterly or twice a year. This supervisor might also be appropriate to meet with individually when additional support is desired.

> "
> *There are high spots in all of our lives, and most of them come about through encouragement from someone else.*
> "
>
> —George Adams

In Conclusion...

Clinical supervision is an excellent tool to enhance the professional development and satisfaction of the somatic practitioner. It provides practical help in the quest to maintain the highest ethical standards. Good supervision empowers the practitioner and supports the client's care, thereby improving the quality of the whole profession.

Chapter Highlights

- Ethical clinical practice for all somatic professionals includes self-awareness, self-monitoring and ongoing review of challenging or difficult cases with peers or a clinical supervisor.

- Effective supervision isn't about being told how to do your job, rather it's a venue in which you process your struggles, challenges and experiences with clients in order to do your best work.

- Practitioners need to be involved enough to care for clients, yet distant enough to decide objectively on and implement the best course of treatment.

- Particular clients may challenge the practitioner's capacity to manage his feelings, expose professional "blind spots," or touch on areas of personal vulnerability.

- Clinical supervision undertakes four functions: 1) addressing the relationship issues that arise between the client and practitioner; 2) functioning as a support group for the participants; 3) serving as a forum for didactic instruction on important psychological concepts (such as projection, transference, countertransference); and 4) training the participants in supervisory skills so they can continue this helpful type of coaching by themselves at a later date without the supervisor.

- Rather than offering advice and telling the practitioner what to do, a skilled supervisor helps the practitioner explore what is happening internally, define where the appropriate boundary might be for the practitioner and the client, and determine what action might correct the situation.

- Protecting and maintaining the boundaries of professional relationships is the responsibility of the professional even if the client requests or instructs the professional to behave otherwise.

- The following questions may facilitate self-supervision and assist practitioners in deciding when a consultation is needed: Does the care of this client deviate from the usual professional standards of care for this client's problem? Is the practitioner uncertain about the differentiation between professional and personal feelings and where to construct the clinical professional boundary?

- Practitioners should listen to their own anxiety as a reliable signal that a problem or client relationship deserves further attention and work.

- If a client presents threatening behaviors, the practitioner must assess whether the client presents a real, physical threat and danger to the practitioner by evaluating the client's capacity for violence. A consultation with a supervisor or mental health professional may be necessary.

- Clients who've been sexually victimized as children may eroticize the professional relationship as they often confuse sexual contact with care taking.

- The decision and responsibility of assessing the right fit between practitioner and supervisor and the usefulness of the supervision lies with the supervisee.

- Supervisors who encourage practitioners to creatively answer their own questions facilitate the development of a competent professional.

- Experienced supervisors are likely to be psychiatrists, psychologists, nurses, social workers and counselors.

- Obtain personal recommendations from a colleague or a valued teacher as a productive way to secure names of potential supervisors.

- Employ a consumer-oriented approach when "shopping" for a supervisor. Supervisors aren't equally talented, experienced or competent.

- Be sure your supervisor's values of care, ethical codes of conduct and attitudes resonate with your own. A good match includes compatible interpersonal styles, expertise and methods of supervision.
- When interviewing a potential supervisor, seriously consider any visceral discomfort and reservations. Trust your intuition and look elsewhere if negative feelings arise.
- Unhelpful supervision occurs when supervisors use arrogant, inflexible and shaming techniques and exploit the supervisee's vulnerability.
- If a supervisory relationship evokes intense negative feelings or is burdened with disrespect and lack of honest self-disclosure, the supervisee should work with a different supervisor.
- Peer group supervision is an alternative form of supervision. Its benefits include being free of charge, providing a network of professional support and offering multiple perspectives on any concern or problem. The potential disadvantages include the varying commitment and inconsistency of attendance by members.
- Peer supervision groups work best when an experienced supervisor trains the group how to conduct peer supervision and occasionally returns to lead the group.

Discussion Questions and Activities

- Create a detailed plan for finding a supervisor.
- What qualities and values would you look for in a supervisor?
- Identify several situations or issues that you have experienced that you might want to take to a supervisor.
- Set up guidelines for developing and running a peer supervision group.
- Brainstorm topics for discussion in a peer supervision group.
- Create a set of questions you would ask when interviewing a potential supervisor.
- Name several situations in which you would terminate using a particular supervisor.
- Develop a series of questions you would ask a participant in a peer supervision group who is presenting an issue.
- Recall an instance when talking to an individual or a small group was helpful in solving a problem.
- Identify any areas or issues that you might be reluctant to discuss in a supervision environment.
- Recall an ethical dilemma that would've been easier to resolve if you were in a supervision group.
- What are the advantages and disadvantages of clinical supervision over peer supervision?
- Identify the key elements of helpful supervision.

Appendix A

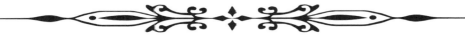

Forms

- Boundary Clarification Exercise Answer Key
- Client Bill of Rights
- Sample Oriental Medicine Office Policies
- Sample Massage Therapy Center Policies
- Sample School Clinic Informed Consent
- Sample Massage Therapy Informed Consent
- Trauma Survivor Handout: Feelings List

Boundary Clarification Exercise Answer Key

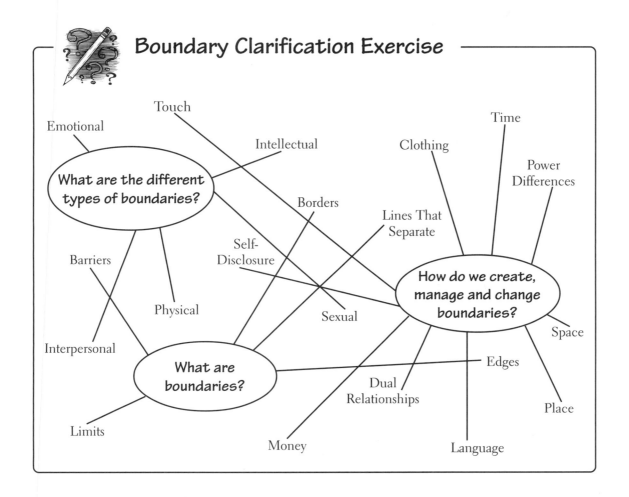

1. What are Boundaries?

> Lines That Separate, Limits, Barriers, Borders and Edges

2. What are the Different Types of Boundaries?

> Interpersonal, Physical, Emotional, Sexual and Intellectual

3. How Do We Create, Manage and Change Boundaries?

Power Differences	Time	Location	Language	Clothing
Space	Touch	Money	Dual Relationships	Self-Disclosure

Client Bill of Rights

An informational handout about sexual misconduct for consumers of health care services

This handout has been prepared to better inform you about sexual misconduct in the health care field. It will delineate your rights as a consumer and tell you how to protect yourself if your rights are violated.

In this brochure the client is defined as anyone who receives services for any therapy or health care. Sexual misconduct is defined as including sexual touching of the client by the practitioner and/or any activity or verbal behavior that is sexual in nature. Sexual contact includes a wide range of behaviors besides intercourse; it includes any behaviors that aim to arouse sexual feelings. They range from suggestive verbal remarks to erotic hugging and kissing in addition to direct sexual contact. The behavior does not have to be coercive to be inappropriate.

Broken Boundaries

Within the therapeutic relationship, it is always the responsibility of the therapist, doctor or health professional to set and maintain a professional boundary. It is not unusual or abnormal for a client to feel attracted to a health care practitioner who has treated them with kindness, care and attention. However, for a practitioner to take advantage of this special vulnerability and to move the relationship into a social or sexual one, even if the client wants it, is always inappropriate and unethical. At this point, we can say that a practitioner is abusing his/her power within the relationship and is no longer able to put the needs and rights of the client first.

All types of therapy and health care services can be of invaluable help to many people. The vast majority of therapists and health professionals practice in an ethical manner. Unfortunately, sometimes sexual misconduct does occur in treatment relationships. A sexually intimate relationship between a client/patient and a therapist, physician, or health care professional is never appropriate and is a violation of professional ethics.

Consumer Rights

You have a right:

1. to safe treatment, free from physical, sexual or emotional abuse.
2. to refuse treatment and not be pressured to continue.
3. to question any action that you experience as invasive or sexual
4. to terminate treatment if you feel threatened.
5. to discuss your therapy/health care with friends outside of the therapy relationship.
6. to professional consultation with other practitioners to discuss your situation.
7. to report unethical and illegal behavior.

Warning Signs of Sexual Inappropriateness

- The practitioner makes sexual jokes or references that are inappropriate to treatment.
- You have any concern that a treatment relationship is moving from the professional to the inappropriately personal.
- The practitioner tells you his or her intimate personal problems.
- You are asked to go outside the bounds of a professional relationship such as going on a dinner date or a social meeting outside the office.
- The practitioner tells you that having a sexual relationship with him or her is good treatment and/or the only way you can get well.
- The practitioner offers you recreational drugs or alcohol.
- The practitioner suggests that you be secretive about your relationship with him or her and that you do not discuss it with anyone.
- The practitioner suggests to you that forms of touching you consider to be intimate have been proven to be therapeutic for your condition.
- You feel that something is not right in the practitioner's behavior toward you, but you can't quite pinpoint what's happening.

If you experience any of these warning signs, trust your own feelings and intuition. Talk to a friend or neutral third party, or talk directly to the practitioner if you feel comfortable doing so. Otherwise, talk to his or her supervisor, consult a different practitioner, or if you get no satisfactory response, call the appropriate licensing board or professional association to check on and report the practitioner's behavior.

Common Experiences

If sexual behavior occurs with a health professional, a client might experience feelings that may include but are not limited to:

- Confusion about the experience that sometimes encompasses protective, loving and angry feelings about the abuser, and/or feelings that the client's mind is being controlled.
- Fear, isolation and distrust because the client believes that there is no one to tell, that no one will believe what happened, and/or that he/she is the only one to whom this has happened.
- Indecision and/or a temporary inability to make decisions, to work at a job, or to tend to personal needs.
- Guilt, shame and feelings of responsibility (a sexual relationship with a practitioner is always the health professional's responsibility, not the client's).
- Depression, feeling out of control or suicidal because the client's trust has been betrayed.
- Recurrent nightmares, fears or images of intrusion and/or flashbacks about the experience, and difficulty concentrating in other areas of life.

Options for Recovery

Talk to someone you trust about your experience. There are other clients who have been survivors of sexual misconduct in every state. Many of these individuals have sought and received help from therapy and support groups.

Therapy: Subsequent psychotherapy or body therapy is difficult for many victims to consider, yet it is often vital in providing the necessary support for someone who has been through the trauma of sexual misconduct. Choose a therapist carefully by finding someone who is appropriately outraged by what has happened, someone who has experience in this type of case, someone who can help think through an effective course for recovery and/or recourse.

Networking: Contacting other individuals who have experienced sexual abuse or misconduct—individually or through support groups—can be extremely helpful. Breaking the silence can be liberating and may help prevent the victimization of others.

Therapist Responsibility: Accept that the therapist is responsible for what has occurred. Understand that most people who have experienced sexual abuse feel that they are at fault or should have behaved differently in some way. These feelings are natural but do not change the fact that the therapist is responsible for his/her misconduct.

Reporting Misconduct: It is important to report abusive therapists. Most people who abuse others do so with many of their clients. Stopping them is essential whether it takes psychological help, professional censure, revocation of a license, education or action by the courts.

Possible Actions

The first step, if the situation was not overtly abusive or dangerous, is to speak directly to the therapist and tell him/her what you are feeling. If this is not possible or unsuccessful try to talk with the offending practitioner about what happened in the presence of a neutral third party.

This kind of session can be very helpful. If the practitioner fears a lawsuit, he/she is less likely to be willing to do this with you, since the neutral third party could become a witness in a trial. The practitioner that realizes that he/she has made a big mistake and wants an opportunity to apologize may consent to meet with you in the hopes of avoiding legal action. You can often find psychotherapists willing to serve as the third party through a professional therapy association or local advocacy group, such as a Rape Crisis Center. If you choose this option make sure you are very comfortable with the person you find to be the third party.

If the offending practitioner is willing to meet with a third party you might want an additional fourth person to be present. Choose someone close to you who is level-headed and could support you and help you talk about this confrontation afterward.

If you choose to approach the practitioner or the organization where you were treated directly, and are satisfied with the response, you may wish to leave it at that. For example, a satisfactory response, depending on the violation, might be that you are given a sincere apology by the practitioner, have your money refunded, and feel assured that appropriate educational measures and psychotherapy for the practitioner will occur or that disciplinary action by the place of employment is being taken. If you are not satisfied with the response you get you might consider registering a complaint or taking legal action.

Registering Complaints

When ready, and with appropriate support, filing a complaint can be an important phase of the healing process. There are local and state government agencies called Licensing Boards that receive and investigate complaints. Licensing Boards have the authority to discipline an individual (for example, revoke a license) if that person violates the law. No matter how serious your complaint may be, the Boards have no legal authority to award money damages or to criminally prosecute someone.

Professional organizations also receive complaints about members of their societies. The ethical codes of most professional organizations specifically prohibit sexual contact between therapists/ health professionals and their clients/patients.

Legal Recourse

Another course of action is through the legal system. Be aware that there are time limitations for civil and criminal actions.

Civil Action: A civil lawsuit may be a way to derive some monetary compensation for losses incurred and damages suffered. Attorneys specializing in these cases may be located through victim advocacy groups.

Criminal Action: Criminal prosecution may be pursued through the Office of the District Attorney in the abuser's county. The District Attorney's Office may also have a victim advocate who can assist you and answer questions.

Remember, if you feel that you have been sexually abused in a therapy or health care relationship, you can get help. We encourage you to seek help as an important part of your healing process. Please feel free to photocopy, adapt and distribute this handout. It is important that this information be available to all consumers of health care services.

*This handout was prepared and edited by Ben Benjamin with materials obtained from: The Education Subcommittee of the Massachusetts Committee on Sexual Misconduct by Physicians, Therapists and Other Health Professionals; and materials provided by Estelle Disch, clinical sociologist.

Sample Oriental Medicine Office Policies

The purpose of these policies is to assure that your care is as effective and efficient as possible. We have found that patients who adhere to these policies get the best results.

Timeliness

It is important that you are on time for all appointments. A certain amount of time is allotted for each patient visit. If you are late, your remaining time may not be sufficient for your full treatment. We will do our best to make accommodations, nevertheless, the full session fee is charged.

During your first visit, you may agree to a course of treatment, designed specifically for you. If a certain number of treatments in a set period is required to get the results we both desire and you need to change the time of an appointment, please plan to come at another time that same day. If the same day is not possible, please be sure to make it up within one week.

24 Hours Advance Notice Is Required for All Cancellations.
(True emergencies are excepted.)

We request 24-hour notice for cancellations. If we do not receive this, we will have to charge you $35 for the reserved time.

Payment

Payment for all services is due at the time of your visit. Many insurance carriers now cover acupuncture, including Workers' Compensation, auto accident policies and other private carriers. If you have insurance, you must still pay for your visits. We will provide you with a receipt that you can submit to your insurance company for reimbursement. We highly recommend that you call your insurance company to find out if Oriental Medicine services are covered and if there are any restrictions such as needing a prescription from your primary care physician.

We accept Mastercard and Visa.

Patient Signature: _____

Date: _____

Sample Massage Therapy Center Policies

Background and Training

I have been practicing massage therapy since 1985. I was trained at the Montana School of Massage Therapy in a 750-hour program. The style of bodywork that I practice incorporates Swedish massage, Shiatsu, and a therapy called deep frictioning, which reduces scar tissue caused by injuries. I specialize in working with people of all ages who are athletic and suffer from various types of tension and pain problems. My style of bodywork focuses in two directions:

1. Stress reduction and relaxation
2. Work with pain and injury problems

Massage therapy is useful for a variety of pain, injury and tension problems, but does not address serious medical conditions. After assessing a client, I may refer you to an osteopath, chiropractor, nutritionist, orthopedic surgeon, or an Alexander teacher, among other possibilities.

Who Can Benefit

Massage therapy is successful in working with problems related to excess tension build up, chronic pain and musculoskeletal injuries. In addition to working with pain and tension problems in the neck, back, ankle, knee, shoulder and so forth, massage therapy is very effective with people who suffer from chronic headaches, insomnia and problems of fatigue. These are the areas in which I feel I have competency.

Massage therapy is also beneficial for pregnant women, and is often used as an adjunct to certain medical conditions on the recommendation of a physician, (e.g., high blood pressure, anxiety or stress).

Others who may benefit greatly from massage are people in psychotherapy who would like to be more in touch with their bodies.

Client/Practitioner Expectations

The first session begins with an interview and health history. You are asked a series of questions and an assessment is performed. Keep in mind that privacy and confidentiality are maintained at all times. Clients may wear a smock and may leave on their underwear if they wish. During the session, clients are covered and draped with sheets and towels, uncovering only the body part to be worked on. The genitals are never exposed or massaged.

Massage sessions may start with the client lying face up or face down, depending on the purpose of the session. If the session focuses on a particular injury, that body part is generally worked on first. For a regular stress-reduction session, the back and neck are worked on first, followed by the legs, feet and arms. Clients can ask for different parts of the body to be worked on, or not worked on, and are encouraged to discuss this with me at the beginning of the session.

Some kinds of massage sessions use oil or lotion, and others do not. When Swedish massage is employed, oil/lotion is used. When Shiatsu or friction therapy is performed to eliminate scar tissue, oil/lotion isn't used. When oil/lotion is used, clients may request that it be cleaned off with alcohol to keep their clothes clean, as I do not have shower, sauna or whirlpool facilities at the office.

During the session, clients are encouraged to relax, and inform me if anything makes them uncomfortable, either physically or psychologically. Talking may occur during the session, but often I will ask you to talk with me before or after, as the massage session may take a good deal of concentration. If something feels uncomfortable during the session, please speak up immediately. I want to know as soon as possible.

The sessions don't vary much in length. They last between 50 and 60 minutes. You might be sore after an injury massage session for one to two days. Be sure to tell me if this occurs. If you are sore for longer than two days, the massage needs to be adjusted to be gentler.

- I reserve the right to refrain from working on a person who is under the influence of alcohol or drugs.
- Sexual harassment is not tolerated. If the practitioner's safety feels compromised, the session is stopped immediately.

Appointment Policies

- Each session is 60 minutes long.
- The first appointment, which includes a history and an assessment, lasts approximately 90 minutes.
- If a client is late for a treatment session, the session still falls within the 60-minute allotted time slot.
- If I am late, the session lasts the full 60 minutes or the treatment rate is discounted.
- If you wish to cancel an appointment, you must do so 24 hours in advance, or you are charged for the full amount of the session unless the appointment can be filled. Someone answers the telephone from 9 A.M. until 6 P.M., but if you get an answering machine, please leave a message on the machine, including the date and time of the call. Emergency cancellations aren't charged for at the practitioner's discretion. If I need to cancel an appointment, I do so within 24 hours whenever possible. If I can't do so, your next session is at no charge.
- All of the appointments occur at 122 Mellon St.
- I don't do house calls.
- I see clients Monday through Friday from 10 A.M. to 6 P.M. I also hold extended hours on Thursday evening until 9 P.M.
- I return calls within 24 hours unless I'm out of town.

Fees

- If during my assessment I determine with reasonable certainty that my work won't help you, we end the session at that time and you aren't charged for the initial appointment.
- Massage therapy sessions are $55.
- If you would like a double session, the charge is $100.
- Payment is due at the time of service unless other arrangements have been made prior to treatment. I accept cash, checks and credit cards. I do not bill clients nor provide direct billing for insurance.
- Individuals who have financial constraints are welcome to discuss this with me to see what can be worked out, such as a sliding fee scale, referral to a practitioner with a fee you can afford, or referral to a student clinic at a nearby massage school.
- Sometimes private insurance companies reimburse clients for my services. It is best to get a prescription from a doctor if you wish to submit to your insurance company. I provide you with a receipt but can't guarantee that your visits will be covered by insurance. In many cases they will be covered, but that is at the discretion of the insurance company.
- Fees are generally not raised more than once per year.

Professionalism

- Our profession ascribes to a code of ethical behavior, which is available upon request. I follow all of the statements in this ethical code and have strong beliefs that practitioners and their clients shouldn't engage in intimate social relationships.
- Personal and professional boundaries are respected at all times.
- I perform services for which I'm qualified (professionally, physically and emotionally) and able to do, and refer to appropriate specialists when work is not within my scope of practice or not in the client's best interest.
- I customize my treatment to meet the client's needs.
- I keep accurate records and review charts before each session.
- I respect all clients regardless of their age, gender, race, national origin, sexual orientation, religion, socio-economic status, body type, political affiliation, state of health, and personal habits.

Recourse Policy

- If you are dissatisfied with the massage session, you receive a full refund for that session or a complimentary treatment.
- You may return for refund any unused products (in salable condition) within 10 days of purchase.

Sample School Clinic Informed Consent

I, _____ HEREBY voluntarily request to receive clinical services from the Acupuncture Clinic of the Arizona School of Acupuncture and Oriental Medicine. I consent that these services may include acupuncture, moxabustion, nutritional/dietary counseling, herbology, Bach flower essences, TuiNa therapeutic massage, and lifestyle counseling, among other related services. I acknowledge that no guarantees have been made to me as to the effect of such care.

I further acknowledge that none of the above services is meant to be construed by me as the diagnosis or treatment of disease, but rather as an aid to balancing my energy and to improving my general wellness.

I understand that the acupuncture clinic holds traditional Oriental medicine to be complementary to orthodox medical treatment, unless contrary medical advice is given. I am advised that if I am sick, I should consult my doctor.

I understand that prior to the beginning of any procedure, I will receive an explanation of its nature and purpose and any probable risks involved. I understand that I may refuse any and all services at any time.

I understand that the clinic is part of the acupuncture school and that, as such, its main purpose is the training of acupuncture interns. Interns are supervised by a faculty member who is a Board Certified Acupuncturist. Interns do not receive compensation.

I recognize that I am responsible for my health and well-being, and that it is my duty to myself to be an informed partner in the care I receive at the clinic. To this end, I will secure the self-knowledge that I need in order fully to work with my intern.

In the event that I am not able to keep my appointment, I will try to give at least 48 hours notice so that someone else can use the time. For any cancellation that is made within 24 hours from the appointment time, I will pay the fee of $20. Or, if I don't show up for the appointment, as scheduled, then I will pay the fee of $20.

I understand that payment by cash, check or credit card is due at the time of service. Should I have a complaint or grievance regarding services, I will speak with the clinic coordinator.

Finally, I understand that all records will be kept confidential.

Witness: _____   Date: _____

Patient's Signature: _____

We are a fragrance-free facility.

Sample Massage Therapy Informed Consent

I, _____[client's name]_____, understand that massage therapy provided by, _____[therapist's name]_____, is intended to enhance relaxation, reduce pain caused by muscle tension, increase range of motion, improve circulation and offer a positive experience of touch. Any other intended purposes for massage therapy are specified below:

The general benefits of massage, possible massage contraindications and the treatment procedure have been explained to me. I understand that massage therapy is not a substitute for medical treatment or medications, and that it is recommended that I concurrently work with my Primary Caregiver for any condition I may have. I am aware that the massage therapist does not diagnose illness or disease, does not prescribe medications, and that spinal manipulations are not part of massage therapy.

I have informed the massage therapist of all my known physical conditions, medical conditions and medications, and I will keep the massage therapist updated on any changes. I understand that there shall be no liability on the practitioner's part due to my forgetting to relay any pertinent information.

If I experience any pain or discomfort during the session, I will immediately communicate that to the therapist so the treatment can be adjusted.

I have received a copy of the therapist's policies, I understand them and agree to abide by them.

Client Signature: _____ Date: _____

Trauma Survivor Handout

Feelings List

There is no "right" way to feel after a treatment. Listen to your body. Feel your own experience; that is what is right for you.

1. A sense of aliveness or pleasure in your body or a feeling of physical well-being. This may include a sense of connectedness in your whole body, awareness of sexual energy or feelings, and a sense of deep relaxation. You may find that you sleep more restfully that evening.

2. Less numbness in specific areas of your body. You may experience a sense of "letting go," "thawing" or "melting" in those areas that felt "frozen." Those areas may actually become warmer to the touch. On the other hand, you may experience trembling or shakiness. Keep warm by covering yourself with a blanket, applying a heating pad or wearing additional layers of clothing.

3. Awareness of more tension in parts of your body. You may notice tension in areas that you were previously unaware that held stress. If this occurs think of things that helped you reduce tension in the past. Some people find it helpful to imagine breathing into those areas to relax them and give attention to any feelings that have been held in those muscles and are now more accessible.

4. Increased emotional awareness. Being more in touch with your body brings awareness of new and different emotions. You may start to feel things that you knew about before but were disconnected from emotionally. Unexpected memories may surface, you might feel fear or sadness or a sense of emptiness. For instance, you may experience feelings of deprivation, stimulated by the nurturing touch that you did not get enough of as a child. Grieving for the nurturing touch you never received, or never received enough of, is appropriate. Feelings of anger about your deprivation may also be part of your experience.

5. Apprehension about returning. It is common to feel apprehensive about returning for another session. This reluctance stems from feelings of exposure and vulnerability with the practitioner. Realize that this experience is different from your past experiences with touch. If the session feels good, you do not need to feel guilty for wanting, even longing, for safe nurturing touch. It is what you always deserved—even when you did not get it. Let yourself take it in now.

6. Shutting down. Another natural reaction to experiencing increased sensation in your body is for your body to contract and shut down temporarily. If this happens, be patient with yourself and ask your therapist to go slower with you. Everyone needs to move at their own pace. Respect your own body's rhythm.

Adapted with permission from a client handout developed by Krishnabai.

Appendix B

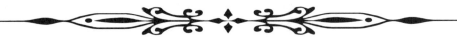

Specialized Protocols

- ✦ Specific Techniques for Working with
  Self-Disclosed Survivors of
  Trauma and Abuse
- ✦ BITE Model of Cult Mind Control

Specific Techniques for Working with Self-Disclosed Survivors of Trauma and Abuse

We have discussed the nature of abuse, critical psychological concepts and a number of prerequisites for working with survivors. The ethical practitioner attends not only to his treatment skills but his relational interactions and business practices as well. Nowhere is this more important than in working with a survivor of abuse or trauma.

A practitioner begins working with a survivor in a number of ways: a client is referred by her psychotherapist as part of the psychotherapy process; the practitioner is contacted by a survivor who has heard about the practitioner through a friend, or who has read about the benefits of hands-on therapy; and a current client discloses his status of previous abuse.

Initial Contact—The Phone Interview

The first contact begins when a practitioner talks with a client who has disclosed during a telephone call that he is a survivor of abuse. After asking for the caller's name and the name of the referring person or psychotherapist, an opportunity exists to create an appropriate context. The therapeutic relationship starts here by establishing boundaries, structure and an initial sense of safety. Advance knowledge of the practitioner's approach to the initial and subsequent sessions benefits potential clients. Ask the person if she would like a brief description of an initial session. You might say something like:

> "My first session is an hour and a half long. For the first half of the session I will ask you for some information and give you a chance to ask me any questions. I see the first session as an exploration of whether we would like to work together. After 30-40 minutes of conversation you decide if you would like a short hands-on session."

Let the client know from the start that she is in charge. You might also say:

> "If you aren't sure, or if you want to think about it for a week or if the match doesn't feel right to you, we can stop to give you time to decide."

Note: We recommend not charging anything if the session stops at this point. The client should not pay a practitioner to determine if the practitioner instills a sense of safety. At this point you could say something like, "My fee for the first hour and a half session is $100 and for subsequent hour-long sessions it's $75. If you decide not to continue the session I don't charge anything for the initial 40 minutes. If we do decide to work together and continue, I charge you for the full session." Always establish financial arrangements on the telephone to minimize the possibility of misunderstanding.

Many practitioners also include additional information on the telephone such as clarifying that the client is in charge of where on the body the practitioner works and the amount of clothing the client removes for the treatment. The initial telephone call is a good time to mention if you have a sliding fee scale and how it is negotiated.

During the telephone conversation also ask the client if there's anything she would like to ask you before the appointment. This invitation opens the door if the client feels hesitant. What you have done during this initial telephone conversation is begin the relationship. The client knows that she is free to interview you and shares control of the process.

Everything you discuss on the phone is to be repeated at the beginning of the first session. It is also best to put everything in writing for clarity, especially if the person's primary mode of processing information is visual. Sometimes the client is experiencing fear and anxiety just making the telephone call, and most of what is discussed will be forgotten. Conducting telephone interviews along these lines gives a feeling of mutuality and respect, regardless of the specific arrangements.

The Physical Environment

The physical environment of the practitioner's office should create a sense of safety and comfort. Some suggest making the office colors soft and neutral. If the practitioner works in a medical clinic, he might make it look less sterile by adding a few personal effects and some plants in the office. If the practitioner works in a home office, keep the treatment room separate from living space (if at all possible) and decorate it in a way that makes it feel professional. Minimize clutter in the waiting area and office. Be sure the windows are covered and there is a smock or a sheet laid out for the client. If possible have a separate bathroom that's free of personal belongings. Before the client enters the office or treatment room, draw the curtains or blinds to ensure privacy.

Be sure the office is reasonably soundproof. Use a sleep sound machine or quiet music, if the soundproofing is not up to par. Choose music carefully; avoid songs with sexual lyrics, seductive instrumental music or indistinct sounds. For instance, chants easily trigger flashbacks of cult abuse. Place literature (e.g., books, brochures and articles that deal with abuse) in the waiting room. The practitioner might put a statement of policies in a small binder for clients to read (this statement can also be sent to the client prior to the first session). Exercise restraint with scents as they can be powerful flashback triggers, particularly flowery fragrances and incense.

First Session Preliminaries

As the client enters the treatment room or waiting area, greet the client in a friendly yet professional way. Shake hands only if the client extends a hand toward you first. If the client has to wait before you begin together, give him relevant literature to read or the written history form to fill out.

The Pre-Treatment Mutual Interview

After a client is settled in a chair, restate what was discussed on the telephone. As previously noted, it is very likely that the client was anxious during the initial phone conversation and does not remember everything that was said. Let the client know that the first half of the session is spent in conversation during which the client has an opportunity to ask questions.

Review Policies

After reviewing the structure of the first session, outline the policies for the client. Make sure that everything is understood. Have a written set of standard policies as well as a statement about survivors available for the client and go over those documents together. The following section highlights additional policy considerations for working with abuse survivors. Give the client opportunities to ask questions about your policies so that mutuality can be established. She has the right to ask questions about your approach, the ethical dimensions of the work and any other questions about the treatment.

- Cancellation Policy. When working with a survivor, as with any client, be clear about the cancellation policy. Some practitioners have a two-, five-, or 24-hour cancellation policy. Whatever your policy is, make the boundary clear and stick to it, allowing for the same flexibility you would give to any client if a situation arises where there is unusual distress or extraordinary circumstances.
- Supervision. Inform the client of the kind of professional supervision you receive on all your clients and its function.
- Code of Ethics. Tell the client that you follow a professional code of ethics developed by your profession or yourself and offer to give him a copy. Clearly state that you do not engage in social, intimate, sexual or business relationships with your clients.
- Confidentiality. Speak about the confidential nature of the therapeutic relationship. Let the client know that you will not ask for any details about her abuse history, and are interested in hearing anything that she feels is helpful to your work together.
- Collaborative Nature of Your Work. Stress the importance of a collaborative relationship with the client and his psychotherapist or counselor. If the client is not currently in psychotherapy, explain the benefits to consider it while receiving bodywork. Describe the possibility of opening up areas of memory, experience and feelings,

and the necessity of having a place to share and explore those experiences. It is assumed here that the treatment you undertake is specifically aimed at helping the client reconnect with her body—focused on dealing with the physical ramifications of the abuse.

- Delayed Discovery of Sexual Abuse. Sometimes a person comes for hands-on therapy and does not know he is a survivor, but figures it out after a period of treatment (this occurs with some frequency). If the client is not in psychotherapy or his counselor is not specifically trained to work with survivors, it is wise to delay treatment until the person settles into a supportive psychotherapy situation. Keep a list of referrals for such situations.
- Level of Therapy. After establishing that the client is in psychotherapy, ask the client if his psychotherapist agrees that he is in an appropriate stage of recovery for body therapy. When the client is referred by a psychotherapist, the appropriateness of treatment has probably been previously established.
- Informed Consent. As an addendum to the confidentiality agreement, inform the client that the only other persons who know about your work together are your supervisor, (who will not know the client's name and identity) and the client's psychotherapist.
- Disrobing. If the type of treatment you provide normally involves removal of clothing, a clear statement about disrobing is critical when working with survivors. Stress the importance of comfort for the client. Let the client know she dresses and undresses in private. Make it clear that the client decides what she feels comfortable wearing: she can wear some or all of her clothing; take off shoes and socks only; or wear a smock. Let the client know it is not at all unusual to leave clothes on for some time. It is recommended that a survivor not completely disrobe, even if completely covered under a sheet. Leaving underwear on helps create a safe boundary for the genital area.

Tell the client that she is always covered with a sheet or towel except for the area you are working on. Give instructions such as, "I leave the room for you to change in private. Once you have had time to change, get on the table and cover yourself, I'll knock on the door before entering and ask if you are ready."

Taking the Client History

After the mutual interview and policy discussion, review the client's history to build further rapport and gain valuable knowledge about the client's situation. Establish the survivor's strengths in creating strategies for his survival. Practitioners need to identify and build on the capacities and skills that helped the survivor get to where she is now. The history also assists the practitioner in finding out whether it is appropriate for the client to undertake bodywork at this time. When the client comes in, some practitioners have the client fill out a brief history form in the outer office before entering the treatment room, while others just ask the questions verbally. The history form, in addition to the normal details, should cover these questions:

- Are you seeing any other health care practitioners (e.g. medical doctor, psychotherapist) regularly?
- Have you had any type of body therapy before?
  If yes, was it a positive, negative, or neutral experience?
- What strategies help you manage some of the symptoms and stresses you have worked through?
- How are you feeling now in anticipation of this session?
- What would you like to accomplish from of our work together?

At the end of the history form or on a separate form include the following statement:

I hereby give permission to (practitioner's name) and my psychotherapist (the psychotherapist's name) to exchange relevant information to help me in my healing process.

_____   _____
Signature   Date

At the bottom of the history form you might add, "Please feel free to add additional comments below that might be helpful in our working together."

Follow-Up Questions

When reviewing the history you have the opportunity to build a connection in addition to gaining some relevant new information. Ask the client about:

- Pains, injuries or medical conditions. This lets you know where to exercise caution. You do not want to cause the client any pain in the treatment.
- Medications and drugs. Certain medications, like Thorazine, Elavil and Zoloft affect the client's ability to feel sensations in the skin. Ask about the use of alcohol, recreational drugs and smoking. These questions give you some idea if substance dependency is an issue for the client.
- Personal care. This indicates how much the client takes care of himself physically, (e.g., exercise, diet and health care). Answers to these questions tell you the degree to which the client takes care of or abuses his body.
- Body Awareness. Obtain an idea of the degree to which the client is in touch with her body by asking where she carries stress and tension. Compare the client's assessment with your own after working on the client. If the client is fairly unaware, you may approach working with this client somewhat differently than if the client were more aware. For example, if a client thinks that her body is relaxed but in fact is quite tense, move gently and slowly in bringing that awareness to the client. Do not say, "Your back is really tense like a rock." On the other hand, you can speak more directly with a client who demonstrates keen awareness when telling you where she feels tension or deadness.
- Previous Bodywork. If the client has had a bad experience or has never had bodywork before, you know what to be careful of or what needs more preparation. If the previous bodywork was a good experience, ask why the client did not go back to that practitioner. This gives you information as to what the client is hoping to get from working with a new practitioner.

Ask a few open-ended questions after the history and follow-up to give the client an opportunity to offer additional information. At this time, it might be appropriate to ask if the client has ever experienced flashbacks. If so, ask what has been helpful in those experiences. You may ask, "Is there anything else you would like me to know?" but not "Have you had any particular abuse experiences that might impact our work?" In the second instance the client might experience the question as intrusive—putting pressure on the client to reveal more than he initially wants to share.

Asking questions in a neutral manner shows care and interest. When clients feel comfortable and need to tell the practitioner about some aspect of their experience, they will. During one such open-ended conversation a client described being sexually molested and tortured around her face and neck. She had let the practitioner know when she was ready. The practitioner then knew to take care when working near or on her face and neck. Another client revealed that a therapist had sexually abused him and that he was very anxious about the session. Others simply respond to this question by saying "No." Never push to elicit information from clients. When a client is ready, she will tell you what she wants you to know.

Let the client know that sometimes survivors experience difficult emotional feelings or bodily sensations during or after a bodywork session, like a tingling feeling in the hands or feet, intense heat, or momentary dizziness. Give them the Trauma Survivor Handout found in Appendix A, page 265. You might also say, "If that happens, I will do my best to help you understand what's happening and refer you to additional sources of support if that appears necessary or appropriate."

Transition to Bodywork

In the first session the mutual interview and history-taking requires about 30-40 minutes. After this phase is complete it is time to ask the client, "Would you like to continue the session and have a hands-on treatment today, or would you prefer to stop now and think about whether you would like to work with me?" If the client is not sure, suggest that he think about it and call to schedule a hands-on session, if it feels right. Do not let anxiety or the desire to work with a particular client allow you to apply any pressure on the client to continue. Allowing the client to be in charge makes the treatment more effective.

If the client decides that he wants to continue the session and try the hands-on work, move to the next phase which involves the specific work that the client and practitioner undertake together.

Set Goals Together

Ask the client what goals and expectations she has for the treatment. Discuss long-term goals and set short-term goals for the first session together. If the client has difficulty with this, give some examples of realistic goals such as: This treatment process helps me reduce the tension in my body so I feel positive and enjoyable sensations when touched; I remain present when being touched; I am not afraid when being touched; I feel connected with my body; I become more aware of how my body feels.

A short-term goal for the session might be to see if touch therapy is something he wants to do. Other short-term goals could be specific such as: "I remain present while having my feet touched," or "I learn how to relax when touched on the foot," or "I allow my lower legs to be worked on." Having the client establish a goal that the practitioner agrees can be accomplished in a session or two places a manageable limit or boundary on the session and puts the client in charge of the treatment options.

Empower the Client

Emphasize that you work as a team and that the client knows more about what he needs than the practitioner does. Consider saying something like, "I may make certain suggestions which you can decide to accept or reject." Invite the client to make suggestions. If you are uncertain about the appropriateness of the requests, discuss these with a supervisor or psychotherapist.

Tell the client, "You determine where on your body I work, how deeply I work and how long I work in certain areas." Some clients like to use a body chart to identify zones where it is okay to be touched and zones where it is not okay to be touched. The client is free to stop the session at any point. A technique that might make the client comfortable is citing examples of statements other clients made that relate to this situation such as: "One client asked me to work on her head and neck the first three months, and added the feet during the next two months," or "One client asked me to only insert acupuncture needles on the front of her body for the first few sessions," or "One client requested that I refrain from any direct manipulations to his neck for the first two months." It is reassuring for a client to know that it took someone else a bit of time to receive a standard treatment. The examples given must be real and truthful. To safeguard confidentiality when discussing another client's experience, be careful to change details to protect the person's identity.

Sometimes survivors see practitioners to receive the physical benefits of the work while others utilize the practitioner's work as a means to reconnect the survivor with her body and to gain control of that process. When the body is touched, many abuse survivors dissociate and a major part of treatment is working with the client to stay with her body sensations while being touched. Other survivors become hypervigilant, or overfocus on the specifics of what is being done and consequently are unable to relax. For these clients the task is to defuse the narrowed concentration and to learn to focus on a wide area or on the entire body at once.

Create Emotional Safety

Ascertain what degree of safety has been established so far by asking how the client feels in anticipation of the physical part of the session. You might ask, "How would you like me to respond if you become upset—for instance, if you feel sad and begin to cry?" One client might request that you leave the room for a few minutes, while another may ask you to just sit quietly for a moment and wait for him to finish. Remember that even though a client has expressed a preference beforehand, it is vital to check when feelings come up as the client may have a need that wasn't previously expressed.

During the initial discussion a client may ask you to induce memories. If this happens, explain that memories come when the person feels safe enough to remember and that forcing memories to surface is not useful. In fact this can often be detrimental or harmful to the process and can derail your work together. Perhaps share examples from this book and say something like, "Many clients experience emotional difficulty when trying to induce memories. Several clients related stories of being overwhelmed by memories that were forcefully induced in this way. One had to go to bed for weeks, another started a cycle of frequent uncontrollable flashbacks that took months of therapy to stabilize."[1]

Ask if the client has ever had a flashback or experienced being regressed to a frightening situation. Ask if this has ever occurred during a touch therapy session. Inquire as to what would be useful if a flashback occurred in a session. For instance, some clients might want the practitioner to immediately take her hands off the body and make eye contact; others would feel more comfortable if the practitioner's hand was placed on the client's arm or shoulder, or held the client's hand; and yet other clients might recommend that the practitioner cover them with a blanket and ask them to sit up or stand up to bring them back from the flashback.

The following exercise[2] assists to create safety, determine where to work and to support the client in taking control of the bodywork. Some clients find the exercise helpful and others do not. After describing it ask the client if he would be willing to try the exercise.

 First Touch Exercise

1. **Tell the client**, "You have control of the treatment process with regard to the parts of the body I work on, the amount of pressure used, the types of work performed and so forth. I would like to try something if you are willing." Then explain 2, 3 and 4.

2. **With the client clothed and sitting in a chair say**, "Tell me a part of your body where it would be comfortable to be touched while sitting here, for example your shoulder, hand or back."

3. **Say to the client**, "Tell me when it's okay to touch you." When the client signals it is okay, touch firmly but gently.

4. **Now tell the client**, "Let me know when you would like me to remove my hand with a nod or a few words."

The Hands-On Treatment

When beginning the hands-on work, the practitioner demonstrates to the client that she intends to allow the client to take the lead in the process and starts the treatment on the area that the client requests.

Structure

Treatment structures create safety. It does not matter what the structure is as long as it is clear and establishes a routine that the client can count on. Do certain things the same way each week at each session. Pay special attention to being on time for the appointment. Whenever possible, schedule the appointment for the same time each week. Always ask the same one or two questions at the beginning of each treatment, for instance, "Is there anything about the last session or how you felt afterward that you want to tell me?" Then ask the client what he would like you to do today and where he would like you to work. Refrain from altering the routine unless the client is included in the process of making the change.

---

[1] Judith Herman, M.D., lecture, Bunting Institute of Radcliffe College, Harvard, Cambridge, MA, May 1994.
[2] Clyde Ford, D.C., adapted from a seminar, 1991.

Set goals for each session and encourage the client to talk about the goals at the beginning of the session. *The Handbook on Sensitive Practice for Health Professionals* states, "Consent must be an ongoing, interactive process. Do not assume that consent given today applies to all successive days: ask for consent on each successive day of treatment." At the beginning of each session also repeat the statement that the client undress to her level of comfort. Do not allow interruptions during the session, including answering the telephone. Distractions interrupt attention and focus. Maintain clear touch boundaries; be careful not to touch the client's body casually when she is not on the table.[3]

Pace and Predictability of Touch

Move slowly from one part of the body to another. Before moving to the next part of the body to be touched, tell the client what will be done there, especially if it is different from the kinds of touch done just previously. For instance, when moving from the hand to the upper arm, or from the neck to the lower back, tell the client this is about to happen. Then ask if it feels okay to proceed.

Create a kind of shorthand communication. If what you are is doing is fine with the client, it may be suggested that the client say "okay" when asked. If not, he might say "no," which signals you to move on. This again puts direct control in the hands of the client. Every time the client says "okay" or "no," he is setting the boundaries. At first, you may ask rather frequently, "How's this?" "Is this movement all right?" As the work on a particular body part progresses over time, the frequency with which you ask questions may diminish. But as the work moves to another body part, the questioning process starts over again. If it becomes obvious that all the moves are okay, ask the client if he wants less "checking in" or for you to stop asking. The responses to this technique vary. Some find it very empowering, but after a while, it might become annoying.

Voice Quality

The tone of voice carries emotional messages such as warmth, kindness, professional distance, boredom, impatience and condescension. Be conscious of the messages created through your voice. The quality and presence of voice is important. When a practitioner feels empathic, accepting and positively disposed toward the client, she is gentle, genuine, concerned and present in the feeling tone of the voice. When this is not occurring (it is not easy to recognize in oneself), the practitioner may want to work with a teacher, supervisor or colleague to get some feedback on empathic abilities and what is coming through in the quality of her voice.

Be aware that some clients may react to a hypnotic voice by going into a trance state that encourages dissociation. Check out how your voice is being received by the client.

Language

Practitioners must have a feel for appropriate language when working with trauma survivors. Language should be warm and professional, not intimate, yet not so formal as to be distancing. Practitioners who use language that is too familiar, too critical, or contains a sexual overtone inevitably violate a client's boundary. For instance, making unsolicited comments about the person's body (i.e., not in the treatment contract) is a violation of a client's boundary if the client hasn't asked for this feedback. Comments like, "Boy, your spine is kind of twisted, it needs work!" or "Was it hard for you to lose weight?" are inappropriate boundary crossings even if these issues were part of the reason the client came to see the practitioner.

---

[3] Candice Schachter, Carol Stalker and Eli Teram, Handbook on Sensitive Practice for Health Professionals: Lessons from Women Survivors of Childhood Sexual Abuse (Ottowa, Canada: Health Canada, 2001) 20.

Being Present

Being present is the most important factor in treating survivors. This means that the practitioner needs to be attentive moment by moment to where the client is in relation to the work being done. Because it is common for survivors to dissociate or become hypervigilant, the practitioner needs to find ways to frequently check in to see if the client is present, and if not, bring the client more into contact with himself. The practitioner can explore creative ways to help the client remain present to his experience of touch as it occurs. If the client is dissociating, one helpful technique is to instruct the client to focus attention on the point being worked on, or to imagine breathing into that part of the body. If the person becomes hypervigilant and overfocused, suggest releasing that focus onto a broader, more general area. If this is a problem, try frequently switching the area of the body being worked on.

Suggest visual images, or request that the client brings a favorite piece of music to listen to during the session. Sometimes having the eyes open allows the client to feel more present, while others prefer their eyes closed. Actively working together to find what assists the client continues to build trust and a sense of safety. The more present the practitioner is, the more possible it is for the client to be present as well.

Continuous Communications

Working with survivors of abuse requires a special type of communication during the treatment. Actively track the client as the session proceeds to prevent disassociation. For instance, it is helpful to regularly ask, "How are you doing?" or "Where are you?" This brings the client's attention and awareness into the body. Another possibility is to say something like, "I am focusing on your foot," and then begin to make positive affirming statements from time to time, like, "Are you experiencing your foot relaxing?" or "I think your foot is letting go, but I'm not sure. Tell me what you feel."

Clients frequently withdraw or lose connection to their experience and have no idea how or why this happened. By exploring these reactions together, over time an awareness develops that helps a client begin to understand her own behavior. These kinds of interactions encourage the client's collaboration with the practitioner in the exploration of her body.

Closure

As you move toward the last two or three minutes of the hands-on portion of the session, tell the client that the hands-on part of the session is close to finishing. As this segment ends always fully redrape the client or re-adjust the clothing (this may seem obvious, but many practitioners forget this simple act). Tell the client that the bodywork portion of the session is over and then leave the room. After you leave, the client dresses (or rests awhile before dressing). Knock before returning or instruct the client to indicate he is ready by opening the door.

Leave time to talk with the client at the end of the session. After returning to the room ask how the client is feeling and how the session went. Ask if the client wants to talk about anything specific that happened during the session and see if anything could've been done differently which would be helpful in the future. Encourage the client to tell you if any boundaries were inadvertently crossed. Because this is usually difficult for the client, consider an opening like: "Did I work too hard on any part of your body?" or "Did I move too quickly?" Use your judgment as to when such questions are appropriate. Often, the first or second session is too soon.

Feelings

Feelings often surface after touch therapy. Discuss this with your client at the end of the first session. The Trauma Survivor Handout: Feelings List found in Appendix A, page 265 briefly describes common after-effects that may be experienced after the session. Supplying the client with this information, either verbally or in writing (or both), is quite useful to the survivor, especially given that in the first few weeks of bodywork many of these sensations and feelings occur. Knowledge of these possible responses helps create client safety and comfort. You have permission to copy the Feelings List (simply white-out the "Trauma Survivor Handout" title) and give it to your clients.

BITE Model of Cult Mind Control

Extensive trauma and abuse can take place within mind control cults. There are 5,000 destructive cults in North America with approximately 15 million members.[1] The likelihood is high that some of your clients, client's loved ones, or colleagues are involved in this type of group. This information is useful in identifying whether the group's intent is honest and ethical. Feel free to make copies of the model and refer people to the web site.

Many people think of mind control as an ambiguous, mystical process that can't be defined in concrete terms. In reality, mind control refers to a specific set of methods and techniques, such as hypnosis or thought stopping, that influence how a person thinks, feels and acts. Like many bodies of knowledge, it isn't inherently good or evil. Mind control techniques can be beneficial if they are used to empower an individual to have more choice, and authority for his life remains within himself. For example, benevolent mind control can be used to help people quit smoking without affecting any other behavior. Mind control becomes destructive when the locus of control is external and it's used to undermine a person's ability to think and act independently.

As employed by the most destructive cults, mind control seeks nothing less than to disrupt an individual's authentic identity and reconstruct it in the image of the cult leader. The BITE model helps people determine whether a group is practicing destructive mind control and assists people to understand how cults suppress individual member's uniqueness and creativity. BITE stands for the cult's control of an individual's **Behavior**, **Intellect**, **Thoughts** and **Emotions**.

Destructive mind control can be determined when the overall effect of these four components promotes dependency and obedience to some leader or cause. It isn't necessary for every single item on the list to be present. Mind-controlled cult members often live in their own apartments, have nine-to-five jobs, are married with children, and still are unable to think for themselves and act independently.

The BITE Model

I Behavior Control

1. Regulation of individual's physical reality
    a. Where, how and with whom the member lives and associates
    b. What clothes, colors, hairstyles the person wears
    c. What food the person eats, drinks, adopts and rejects
    d. How much sleep the person is able to have
    e. Financial dependence
    f. Little or no time spent on leisure, entertainment, vacations
2. Major time commitment required for indoctrination sessions and group rituals
3. Need to ask permission for major decisions
4. Need to report thoughts, feelings and activities to superiors
5. Rewards and punishments (behavior modification techniques—positive and negative)
6. Individualism discouraged; "group think" prevails
7. Rigid rules and regulations

II Information Control

1. Use of deception
    a. Deliberately holding back information
    b. Distorting information to make it more "acceptable"
    c. Outright lying
2. Access to non-cult sources of information minimized or discouraged

---

[1] www.wellspringretreat.org

   a. Books, articles, newspapers, magazines, TV, radio

   b. Critical information

   c. Former members

   d. Keep members so busy they don't have time to think and check things out

3. Compartmentalization of information; Outsider vs. Insider doctrines

   a. Information is not freely accessible

   b. Information varies at different levels and missions within pyramid.

4. Spying on other members is encouraged

   a. Pairing up with "buddy" system to monitor and control

   b. Reporting deviant thoughts, feelings and actions to leadership

   c. Individual behavior monitored by whole group.

   d. Leadership decides who "needs to know" what and when

5. Extensive use of cult-generated information and propaganda

   a. Newsletters, magazines, journals, audiotapes, videotapes and other media

   b. Misquotations, statements taken out of context from non-cult sources

6. Unethical use of confession

   a. Information about "sins" used to abolish identity boundaries

   b. Past "sins" used to manipulate and control; no forgiveness or absolution

7. Need for obedience and dependency

III Thought Control

1. Need to internalize the group's doctrine as "Truth"

   a. Adopting the group's map of reality as "Reality" (Map = Reality)

   b. Black-and-White thinking

   c. Good vs. Evil

   d. Us vs. Them (inside vs. outside)

2. Use of "loaded" language (for example, "thought-terminating clichés"). Words are the tools we use to think with. These "special" words constrict rather than expand understanding and can even stop thoughts altogether. They function to reduce complexities of experience into trite, platitudinous "buzz words."

3. Only "good" and "proper" thoughts are encouraged.

4. Use of hypnotic techniques to induce altered mental states

5. Manipulation of memories and implantation of false memories

6. Use of thought-stopping techniques, which shut down "reality testing" by stopping "negative" thoughts and allowing only "good" thoughts

   a. Denial, rationalization, justification, wishful thinking

   b. Chanting

   c. Meditating

   d. Praying

   e. Speaking in "tongues"

   f. Singing or humming

7. Rejection of rational analysis, critical thinking, constructive criticism. No critical questions about leader, doctrine, or policy seen as legitimate

8. No alternative belief systems viewed as legitimate, good or useful

IV Emotional Control

1. Manipulate and narrow the range of a person's feelings
2. Make the person feel that if there are ever any problems, it is always his fault, never the leader's or the group's
3. Excessive use of guilt
   a. Identity guilt
      1.) Who you are (not living up to your potential)
      2.) Your family
      3.) Your past
      4.) Your affiliations
      5.) Your thoughts, feelings, actions
         a.) Social guilt
         b.) Historical guilt
4. Excessive use of fear
   a. Fear of thinking independently
   b. Fear of the "outside" world
   c. Fear of enemies
   d. Fear of losing one's "salvation"
   e. Fear of leaving the group or being shunned by group
   f. Fear of disapproval
5. Extremes of emotional highs and lows
6. Ritual and often public confession of "sins"
7. Phobia indoctrination: inculcating irrational fears about ever leaving the group or even questioning the leader's authority. The person under mind control cannot visualize a positive, fulfilled future without being in the group.
   a. No happiness or fulfillment outside of the group
   b. Terrible consequences will take place if you leave: hell, demon possession, incurable diseases, accidents, suicide, insanity, 10,000 reincarnations, etc.
   c. Shunning of leave takers; fear of being rejected by friends, peers and family
   d. Never a legitimate reason to leave. From the group's perspective, people who leave are: weak; undisciplined; unspiritual; worldly; brainwashed by family or counselor; or seduced by money, sex and rock music

Steven Hassan is one of America's leading cult mind abuse counselors. He has been involved in educating the public about destructive cults in America for more than twenty-six years. He is a licensed mental health counselor and holds a Master's degree in counseling psychology from Cambridge College. He is the author of *Combatting Cult Mind Control: The #1 Best-selling Guide to Protection, Rescue and Recovery from Destructive Cults* and *Releasing The Bonds: Empowering People to Think for Themselves.*

www.freedomofmind.com   617-628-9918

Appendix C

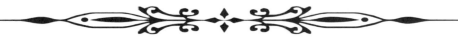

Codes of Ethics

- American Chiropractic Association
- American Massage Therapy Association
- American Organization for Bodywork Therapies of Asia™
- American Physical Therapy Association
- American Polarity Therapy Association
- Associated Bodywork & Massage Professionals
- Feldenkrais Guild® of North America
- International Massage Association Group
- Kripalu Yoga Teachers Association
- Nat'l Certification Board for Therapeutic Massage & Bodywork
- Nat'l Certification Commission for Acupuncture & Oriental Medicine
- Ontario Massage Therapist Association
- Trager International

American Chiropractic Association (ACA)
Code of Ethics

Preamble

This Code of Ethics is based upon the fundamental principle that the ultimate end and object of the chiropractor's professional services and effort should be: "The greatest good for the patient."

This Code of Ethics is for the guidance of the profession with respect to responsibilities to patients, the public and to fellow practitioners and for such consideration as may be given to them by state legislatures, state administrative agencies and also by state chiropractic associations to the extent that they are authorized under state law to exercise enforcement or disciplinary functions.

A. Responsibility to the Patient

A (1) Doctors of chiropractic should hold themselves ready at all times to respond to the call of those needing their professional services, although they are free to accept or reject a particular patient except in an emergency.

A (2) Doctors of chiropractic should attend their patients as often as they consider necessary to ensure the well-being of their patients.

A (3) Having once undertaken to serve a patient, doctors of chiropractic should not neglect the patient. Doctors of chiropractic should take reasonable steps to protect their patients prior to with-drawing their professional services; such steps shall include: due notice to them allowing a reasonable time for obtaining professional services of others and delivering to their patients all papers and documents in compliance with A (5) of this Code of Ethics.

A (4) Doctors of chiropractic should be honest and endeavor to practice with the highest degree of professional competency and honesty in the proper care of their patients.

A (5) Doctors of chiropractic should comply with a patient's authorization to provide records, or copies of such records, to those whom the patient designates as authorized to inspect or receive all or part of such records. A reasonable charge may be made for the cost of duplicating records.

A (6) Subject to the foregoing Section A (5), doctors of chiropractic should preserve and protect the patient's confidences and records, except as the patient directs or consents or the law requires otherwise. They should not discuss a patient's history, symptoms, diagnosis, or treatment with any third party until they have received the written consent of the patient or the patient's personal representative. They should not exploit the trust and dependency of their patients.

A (7) Doctors of chiropractic owe loyalty, compassion and respect to their patients. Their clinical judgment and practice should be objective and exercised solely for the patient's benefit.

A (8) Doctors of chiropractic should recognize and respect the right of every person to free choice of chiropractors or other health care providers and to the right to change such choice at will.

A (9) Doctors of chiropractic are entitled to receive proper and reasonable compensation for their professional services commensurate with the value of the services they have rendered taking into consideration their experience, time required, reputation and the nature of the condition involved. Doctors of chiropractic should terminate a professional relationship when it becomes reasonably clear that the patient is not benefiting from it. Doctors of chiropractic should support and participate in proper activities designed to enable access to necessary chiropractic care on the part of persons unable to pay such reasonable fees.

A (10) Doctors of chiropractic should maintain the highest standards of professional and personal conduct, and should refrain from all illegal conduct.

A (11) Doctors of chiropractic should be ready to consult and seek the talents of other health care professionals when such consultation would benefit their patients or when their patients express a desire for such consultation.

A (12) Doctors of chiropractic should employ their best good faith efforts that the patient possesses enough information to enable an intelligent choice in regard to proposed chiropractic treatment. The patient should make his or her own determination on such treatment.

A (13) Doctors of chiropractic should utilize only those laboratory and X-ray procedures, and such devices or nutritional products that are in the best interest of the patient and not in conflict with state statute or administrative rulings.

B. Responsibility to the Public

B (1) Doctors of chiropractic should act as members of a learned profession dedicated to the promotion of health, the prevention of illness and the alleviation of suffering.

B (2) Doctors of chiropractic should observe and comply with all laws, decisions and regulations of state governmental agencies and cooperate with the pertinent activities and policies of associations legally authorized to regulate or assist in the regulation of the chiropractic profession.

B (3) Doctors of chiropractic should comport themselves as responsible citizens in the public affairs of their local community, state and nation in order to improve law, administrative procedures and public policies that pertain to chiropractic and the system of health care delivery. Doctors of chiropractic should stand ready to take the initiative in the proposal and development of measures to benefit the general public health and well-being, and should cooperate in the administration and enforcement of such measures and programs to the extent consistent with law.

B (4) Doctors of chiropractic may advertise but should exercise utmost care that such advertising is relevant to health awareness, is accurate, truthful, not misleading or false or deceptive, and scrupulously accurate in representing the chiropractor's professional status and area of special competence. Communications to the public should not appeal primarily to an individual's anxiety or create unjustified expectations of results. Doctors of chiropractic should conform to all applicable state laws, regulations and judicial decisions in connection with professional advertising.

B (5) Doctors of chiropractic should continually strive to improve their skill and competency by keeping abreast of current developments contained in the health and scientific literature, and by participating in continuing chiropractic educational programs and utilizing other appropriate means.

B (6) Doctors of chiropractic may testify either as experts or when their patients are involved in court cases, worker's compensation proceedings or in other similar administrative proceedings in personal injury or related cases.

B (7) The chiropractic profession should address itself to improvements in licensing procedures consistent with the development of the profession and of relevant advances in science.

B (8) Doctors of chiropractic who are public officers should not engage in activities which are, or may be reasonably perceived to be in conflict with their official duties.

B (9) Doctors of chiropractic should protect the public and reputation of the chiropractic profession by bringing to the attention of the appropriate public or private organizations the actions of chiropractors who engage in deception, fraud or dishonesty, or otherwise engage in conduct inconsistent with this Code of Ethics or relevant provisions of applicable law or regulations within their states.

C. Responsibility to the Profession

C (1) Doctors of chiropractic should assist in maintaining the integrity, competency and highest standards of the chiropractic profession.

C (2) Doctors of chiropractic should by their behavior, avoid even the appearance of professional impropriety and should recognize that their public behavior may have an impact on the ability of the profession to serve the public. Doctors of chiropractic should promote public confidence in the chiropractic profession.

C (3) As teachers, doctors of chiropractic should recognize their obligation to help others acquire knowledge and skill in the practice of the profession. They should maintain high standards of scholarship, education, training and objectivity in the accurate and full dissemination of information and ideas.

C (4) Doctors of chiropractic should attempt to promote and maintain cordial relationships with other members of the chiropractic profession and other professions in an effort to promote information advantageous to the public's health and well-being.

D. Administrative Procedures [Please refer to web site for this extensive section]

Addendum
Rental Arrangements and Clinic or Laboratory Referrals

It is unethical for a doctor of chiropractic to receive a fee, rebate, rental payment or any other form of remuneration for the referral of a patient to a clinic, laboratory or other health service entity.

The ACA Code of Ethics mandates, as primary obligation of the doctor of chiropractic, the exercise of clinical judgement and practice "solely for the patient's benefit." In the view of this association, the receipt of any form of remuneration for a patient referral runs directly counter to this primary obligation and tends to adversely impact upon the relationship between chiropractor and patient.

Arrangements in which "rental fees," "rebates," or free gifts are received in return for patient referrals are, in the ACA's view, unethical and unacceptable in the professional practice of chiropractic.

The ACA recognizes that there are some forms of rental agreements for space or equipment which are legitimate arm-length business transactions not conditioned on patient referrals. However, some forms of rental agreements may be designed to conceal the real nature of the payment, that is, to induce referrals. The ACA also recognizes that the federal government has developed guidelines which outline those circumstances in which space or equipment rentals would not constitute an illegal or improper form of remuneration in return for Medicare or Medicaid referrals.

The ACA feels these federal guidelines provide an excellent basis by which a doctor of chiropractic can ethically evaluate and engage in space or equipment rental agreements. These guidelines appear in Title 40 of the Code of Federal Regulations, Part 1001 and may be summarized and adapted for the purposes of our ethical standards as follows:

A lease agreement for space or equipment in which a doctor of chiropractic refers a patient to an entity which either leases to or from the doctor space or equipment, will not constitute an unethical practice where:

1. The lease agreement is in writing and signed by the parties.
2. The lease specifies the space or equipment covered by the lease.
3. If the lease is intended to provide the lessee with access to the premises or equipment for periodic intervals of time, rather than on a full-time basis for the term of the lease, the lease specifies exactly the schedule of such intervals, their precise length, their periodicity, and the exact rent for such intervals.
4. The term of the lease is for not less than one year.
5. The rental charge is consistent with fair market value in arms-length transactions and is not determined in a manner that takes into account the volume or value of any referrals of business between the parties.

Doctors of chiropractic are advised to consult with their local examining board or other regulatory agencies for specific requirements which may relate to clinic or laboratory referrals. (Approved 1989)

Sexual Intimacies with a Patient

The ACA Ethics Committee ("Committee") has received numerous requests for clarification relative to the ethical implications of sexual intimacies between a doctor of chiropractic and a patient he or she is treating. This advisory opinion is intended to resolve any misunderstanding and to state that it is the opinion of the Committee that sexual intimacies with a patient is unprofessional and unethical based on the existing ethical provisions in the aca Code of Ethics: A(6), A(7), A(10) and C(2).

The physician/patient relationship requires the doctor of chiropractic to exercise utmost care that he or she will do nothing to "exploit the trust and dependency of the patient." Doctors of chiropractic should make every effort to avoid dual relationships that could impair their professional judgement or risk the possibility of exploiting the confidence placed in them by the patient. (Approved 1991)

Printed with permission

American Massage Therapy Association (AMTA)
Code of Ethics

This Code of Ethics is a summary statement of the standards by which massage therapists agree to conduct their practices and is a declaration of the general principles of acceptable, ethical, professional behavior.

Massage therapists shall:

1. Demonstrate commitment to provide the highest quality massage therapy/bodywork to those who seek their professional service.
2. Acknowledge the inherent worth and individuality of each person by not discriminating or behaving in any prejudicial manner with clients and/or colleagues.
3. Demonstrate professional excellence through regular self-assessment of strengths, limitations and effectiveness by continued education and training.
4. Acknowledge the confidential nature of the professional relationship with clients and respect each client's right to privacy.
5. Conduct all business and professional activities within their scope of practice, the law of the land, and project a professional image.
6. Refrain from engaging in any sexual conduct or sexual activities involving their clients.
7. Accept responsibility to do no harm to the physical, mental and emotional well-being of self, clients and associates.

Printed with permission

American Organization for
Bodywork Therapies of Asia™ (AOBTA)
Code of Ethics

AOBTA Members pledge to honor the ethical and professional requirements set forth in the AOBTA Code of Ethics

1. Social/Ecological Concern

Members recognize their intrinsic involvement in the total community of life on the planet Earth.

2. Professional Conduct

AOBTA members conduct themselves in a professional and ethical manner, performing only those services for which they are qualified, and represent their education, certification, professional affiliations and other qualifications honestly. They do not in any way profess to practice medicine or psychotherapy, unless licensed by their State or Country to do so.

3. Health History and Referrals

AOBTA members keep accurate client records, including profiles of the body/mind health history. They discuss any problem areas that may contraindicate use of Asian Bodywork techniques, and refer clients to appropriate medical professionals when indicated.

4. Professional Appearance

AOBTA members pay close attention to cleanliness and professional appearance of self and clothing, of linens and equipment, and of the office environment in general. They endeavor to provide a relaxing atmosphere, giving attention to reasonable scheduling and clarity about fees.

5. Communication and Confidentiality

AOBTA members maintain clear and honest communications with their clients, and keep all information, whether medical or personal, strictly confidential. They clearly disclose techniques used, appropriately identifying each in the scope of their professional practice.

6. Intention and Trust

AOBTA members are encouraged to establish and maintain trust in the client relationship and to establish clear boundaries and an atmosphere of safety.

7. Respect of Clients

AOBTA members respect the client's physical/emotional state and do not abuse clients through actions, words or silence, nor take advantage of the therapeutic relationship. They, in no way, participate in sexual activity with a client. They consider the client's comfort zone for touch and for degree of pressure, and honor the client's requests as much as possible within personal, professional and ethical limits. They acknowledge the inherent worth and individuality of each person and therefore do not unjustly discriminate against clients or colleagues.

8. Professional Integrity

AOBTA members present Asian Bodywork in a professional and compassionate manner representing themselves and their practice accurately and ethically. They do not give fraudulent information, nor misrepresent AOBTA or themselves to students or clients, nor act in a manner derogatory to the nature and positive intention of AOBTA. They conduct their business honestly.

9. Professional Courtesy

AOBTA members respect the standards set by the various AOBTA modalities, and they respect service marks, trademarks and copyright laws. Professional courtesy includes respecting all ethical professionals in speech, writing, or otherwise, and communicating clearly with others.

10. Professional Excellence

AOBTA members strive for professional excellence through regular assessment of personal and professional strengths and weaknesses, and by continued education and training.

Printed with permission

American Physical Therapy Association (APTA) Code of Ethics

Preamble

This Code of Ethics of the American Physical Therapy Association sets forth Principles for the ethical practice of physical therapy. All physical therapists are responsible for maintaining and promoting ethical practice. To this end, the physical therapist shall act in the best interest of the patient/client. This Code of Ethics shall be binding on all physical therapists.

Principle 1

A physical therapist shall respect the rights and dignity of all individuals and shall provide compassionate care.

Principle 2

A physical therapist shall act in a trustworthy manner toward patients/clients, and in all other aspects of physical therapy practice.

Principle 3

A physical therapist shall comply with laws and regulations governing physical therapy and shall strive to effect changes that benefit patients/clients.

Principle 4

A physical therapist shall exercise sound professional judgment.

Principle 5

A physical therapist shall achieve and maintain professional competence.

Principle 6

A physical therapist shall maintain and promote high standards for physical therapy practice, education and research.

Principle 7

A physical therapist shall seek only such remuneration as is deserved and reasonable for physical therapy services.

Principle 8

A physical therapist shall provide and make available accurate and relevant information to patients/clients about their care and to the public about physical therapy services.

Principle 9

A physical therapist shall protect the public and the profession from unethical, incompetent and illegal acts.

Principle 10

A physical therapist shall endeavor to address the health needs of society.

Principle 11

A physical therapist shall respect the rights, knowledge and skills of colleagues and other health care professionals.

Printed with permission

American Polarity Therapy Association (APTA) Foundations of Professionalism in Polarity Therapy Practice Code of Ethics

APTA acknowledges the American Psychological Association (APA) for permission to use portions of content and elements of format of the Ethical Principles for Psychologists to develop the American Polarity Therapy Association Code of Professional Ethics; permission was granted by the APA Administrative Officer for Ethics.

This Code of Professional Ethics (Code) is intended to serve polarity practitioners and instructors who are members of the American Polarity Therapy Association (APTA) in matters of professional conduct. It provides these practitioners and instructors, as well as the general public, a guide for determining the propriety of these professionals' conduct. The Code applies to all APTA members regardless of their form of practice as administrators, clinical practitioners, student and general members, instructors, or researchers (hereinafter referred to as practitioners). While the statements of ethical principles apply to all APTA members, specific circumstances determine their appropriate application.

The interpretations expressed in this Code are not to be considered all-inclusive of situations that could develop under a specific principle of the Code. This Code also is subject to change as the dynamics of professional practice change and as new patterns of educational and therapeutic health care delivery are developed and accepted by the professional community and the public at large. Input related to current interpretations, or situations requiring interpretation, is encouraged from APTA members.

Membership in the APTA commits the member to abide by these principles. Polarity practitioners cooperate with the Committee on Professional Ethics and Conduct and the Board of Directors of the APTA by responding to inquiries concerning alleged ethical violations in a prompt and thorough manner.

Preamble

Polarity practitioners respect the dignity and the worth of all individuals and endeavor to promote human rights. They are committed to furthering knowledge of human behavior, to fostering people's understanding of themselves and others, and to using this knowledge to promote human well-being. While striving for these goals, they conscientiously protect the welfare of their clients, students and research participants (hereinafter referred to as consumers). They use professional skills only for purposes consistent with these values, and do not knowingly allow their misuse by others. While establishing for themselves freedom of inquiry and communication, polarity practitioners and instructors accept the responsibility engendered by this freedom: competence, diligent and nonprejudicial application of skills, and concern for the best interests of consumers, colleagues, and society at large. To uphold these ideals, polarity practitioners pledge themselves to the following ethical principles: Responsibility; Competence; Confidentiality; Consumer Welfare; Moral and Legal Standards; Professional Relationships; Public Statements.

Principle 1: Responsibility

In providing services, polarity practitioners maintain the highest standards of their profession. They accept responsibility for the consequences of their actions and make every effort to ensure that services are used appropriately.

a. Polarity practitioners recognize and accept a profound social responsibility because their suggestions and professional actions may have a significant impact on the lives of others. They recognize personal, social, organizational, economic, or political circumstances that may contribute to an inequality in power between themselves and consumers, or other circumstances that might result in misuse of their influence.

b. Polarity practitioners recognize a primary obligation to assist others to acquire knowledge and skill. They maintain high standards of scholarship by presenting information accurately, thoroughly, and objectively while attempting to prevent misuse, suppression, or distortion of research findings and the body of polarity knowledge.

c. Polarity practitioners participate in activities which contribute to the improvement of their community and address the health and well-being of the public. They strive to promote cooperation among providers of physical, mental, emotional, social, spiritual and legal services relevant to health and well-being.

Principle 2: Competence

In the best interests of the public and the profession, it is the responsibility of all polarity practitioners to maintain high standards of competence. Polarity practitioners recognize the limitations of polarity, and therefore do not diagnose, prescribe, or treat physical or mental conditions. They also acknowledge the limitations of their competence as well as of their techniques. They only provide services and techniques for which they are qualified by training and experience. In addition, they keep abreast of current scientific, social, and professional information relevant to the services they provide.

a. Polarity practitioners accurately represent their level of competence, education, training, and experience. Only those polarity credentials conferred under authorization of the APTA Bylaws and Standards for Practice are used as evidence of APTA-approved qualifications. Polarity practitioners do not represent general membership in APTA as evidence of polarity competence, education, training, or experience.

b. Polarity practitioners carefully prepare the instruction that they give to consumers to reflect current and accurate information based on the body of polarity knowledge.

c. Polarity practitioners recognize the need for and obtain continuing education and remain open to the development and use of new procedures, to changes in values, and to changes in the interpretation of the body of polarity knowledge. Practitioners comply with all applicable APTA requirement for continuing education.

d. Polarity practitioners recognize and respect differences among people, such as those which may be associated with health condition, age, gender, sexual orientation, religious or spiritual beliefs, socioeconomic, racial, and ethnic variables. They acquire training, experience, or consultation as necessary to ensure competent and affirming service to such persons or refer such persons for competent services elsewhere.

e. Polarity practitioners recognize that their own personal problems may interfere with their professional effectiveness. Therefore, they refrain from initiating any professional activity, which, due to their personal problems, is likely to result in inadequate performance or harm to a consumer or colleague. Should practitioners become aware of their personal problem while engaged in such activity, they obtain competent professional consultation to determine whether they should suspend, terminate, or limit the scope of their professional activities.

Principle 3: Confidentiality

Polarity practitioners have a primary obligation to respect the confidentiality of information obtained from persons in the course of their work. They reveal such information to others only with the consent of the person or the person's legal representative, except in those unusual circumstances in which not to do so would result in clear danger to the person or to others. Where appropriate, practitioners inform consumers of the legal limits of confidentiality.

a. Information obtained in clinical or consulting relationships, or evaluative data concerning consumers, employees, and others, is discussed only for professional consultation or supervision purposes and only with persons providing such consultation or supervision services or those approved by the client. Written and oral reports present only data pertinent to the purpose of the evaluation, and every effort is made to avoid invasion of privacy.

b. Practitioners who present personal information obtained during the course of professional work in writings, lectures, or other public forums either obtain adequate prior consent to do so or disguise all identifying information.

c. Practitioners make provisions for maintaining confidentiality in the storage and disposal of records.

d. When working with minors or other persons who are unable to give voluntary, informed consent, practitioners take special care to protect these persons' best interests.

Principle 4: Consumer Welfare

Polarity practitioners respect the integrity and protect the welfare of the people and groups with whom they work. When conflicts of interest arise between practitioners and consumers or employers, practitioners clarify the nature and direction of their loyalties and responsibilities and keep all parties informed of their commitments. Practitioners fully inform consumers of the purpose and nature of an evaluative, educational, therapeutic, or training procedure. They also freely acknowledge that consumers have freedom of choice with regard to participation.

a. Practitioners are continually aware of their own needs and of their potentially influential position in relation to persons such as consumers and subordinates. They avoid exploiting the trust and dependency of such persons. Practitioners make every effort to avoid dual relationships of any kind that could impair their professional judgement or increase the risk of exploitation. Practitioners are aware that the intensity of a therapeutic relationship may activate sexual and other needs and desires on the part of both the consumer and the practitioner while weakening the objectivity necessary for control. Sexual activity with a client is unethical.

b. When a practitioner agrees to provide services to a client, the practitioner assumes the responsibility of clarifying the nature of the relationships of all parties involved, including any third party involved.

c. Where the demands of any other organization require practitioners to violate the Code, the practitioners clarify the nature of the conflict between the demands and the Code, inform all parties of practitioners' ethical responsibilities, and take appropriate action in keeping with the Code.

d. Practitioners make financial arrangements in advance that safeguard the best interests of and are clearly understood by the consumers of their services. Practitioners are encouraged to contribute a portion of their services to work for which they receive little or no financial return.

e. Practitioners formulate a plan for achieving evaluative, educations, and therapeutic goals which they communicate to the consumers of their services. They carry out this plan with diligence, modify it as necessary, and make every effort to accomplish the goals which have been agreed upon by consumers of their services.

f. Practitioners terminate a clinical, educational, or consulting relationship when it is reasonably clear that the consumer is not benefiting from it. They offer to help the consumer locate alternative sources of assistance.

Principle 5: Moral and Legal Standards

Practitioners' moral standards of behavior are a personal matter to the same degree they are for any other citizen, except as these may compromise the fulfillment of their professional responsibilities or reduce the public trust in polarity and polarity practitioners. Practitioners also are aware of the possible impact of their public behavior upon the professional practice of their colleagues. Practitioners comply with the laws and regulations which govern the practice or instruction of polarity, as well as the limits of confidentiality.

a. Polarity practitioners are aware of the fact that their personal values may affect the selection and presentation of instructional material. They recognize and respect the diverse attitudes that consumers may have toward various topics.

b. As employers and employees, practitioners do not engage in behavior or condone practices that are abusive or that result in illegal or discriminatory actions. Such practices include but are not limited to those based on considerations of race, handicap, age, gender, sexual preference, religion, or national origin in hiring, promotion, or training.

c. In their professional roles, practitioners avoid any action that will violate or diminish the legal rights of consumers or of others who may be affected by their actions.

d. Practitioners act in accord with APTA standards and guidelines related to practice, instruction, and the conduct of research.

e. In the ordinary course of events, practitioners adhere to relevant governmental laws and institutional regulations. When federal, state, provincial, organizational, or institutional laws, regulations, or practices are in conflict with the APTA Code and Standards, practitioners make known their commitment to the APTA Code and Standards and, wherever possible, work toward a resolution of the conflict. Practitioners are concerned with the development of such legal and quasi-legal regulations as best serve the public interest, and they work toward changing existing regulations that are not beneficial to the public interest.

Principle 6: Professional Relationships

Practitioners act with due regard for the needs, special competencies, and obligations of their colleagues in polarity and other professions. They respect the prerogatives and obligations of the institutions and organizations with which these other colleagues are associated.

a. Practitioners understand the areas of competence of related professions. They make full use of all the professional, technical, and administrative resources that serve the best interests of consumers. The absence of formal relationships with other professional workers does not relieve practitioners of the responsibility of securing for consumers of their services the best possible professional service, nor does it relieve them of the obligation to exercise foresight, diligence, and tact in obtaining the complementary or alternative assistance needed by consumers.

b. Practitioners take into account the traditions and practices of other professional groups with whom they work, and cooperate respectfully with such groups. If a practitioner is contacted by a person who is already receiving similar services from another professional, the practitioner carefully considers that professional relationship and proceeds with caution and sensitivity to the therapeutic issues as well as the consumer's welfare. The practitioner discusses these issues with the consumer so as to minimize the risk of confusion and conflict.

c. Practitioners who employ or supervise other professional or professionals-in-training accept the obligation to facilitate the further professional development of these individuals. They provide appropriate working conditions, timely evaluations, constructive consultation, and experience opportunities.

d. Practitioners do not exploit their professional relationships with consumers, supervisees, or employees, sexually or otherwise. Practitioners do not condone or engage in sexual harassment.

e. When conducting research in institutions or organizations, practitioners secure appropriate authorization to conduct such research. They are aware of their obligations to future researchers and ensure that host institutions receive adequate information about the research and proper acknowledgment of their contributions.

f. Publication credit is assigned to those who have contributed to a publication in proportion to their professional contributions. Major contributions of a professional nature made by several persons to a common project are recognized by joint authorship, with the individual who made the principal contribution listed first. Minor contributions of a professional nature and extensive clerical or similar nonprofessional assistance may be acknowledged in footnotes or in an introductory statement. Acknowledgment through specific citations is made for unpublished as well as published material that has directly influenced the research or writing. Practitioners and instructors who compile and edit material of others for publication publish the material in the name of the originating group, if appropriate, with their own name appearing as chairperson or editor. All contributors are to be acknowledged and named.

g. In some circumstances, when practitioners know of an ethical violation by another polarity practitioner they may personally attempt to resolve the issue by bringing the behavior to the direct attention of the individual. If the misconduct is of a minor nature that appears to be due to lack of sensitivity, knowledge, or experience, such a personally derived solution may be appropriate. Such direct, personal corrective efforts are made with sensitivity to any rights of confidentiality involved. If the violation does not seem amenable to or is not resolved by a direct, personally derived solution, or is of a more serious nature, practitioners must bring it to the attention of the Committee on Professional Ethics and Conduct.

Principle 7: Public Statements

Public statements, announcements of services, advertisements, and promotional activities of polarity practitioners serve the purpose of helping the public make informed judgments and choices. Practitioners represent accurately and objectively their professional qualifications, affiliations, and functions, as well as those of the schools or organizations with which they or the statements may be associated. In public statements providing health information or professional opinions or providing information about the availability of polarity products, publications, and services, practitioners base their statements on the body of professionally accepted polarity knowledge and techniques, with full recognition of the limits and uncertainties of such evidence.

a. When announcing or advertising professional services, practitioners may list the following information to describe the provider and services provided: name, professional education and training, relevant academic degrees, date, type, and level of competence, certification, or licensure, diplomate status, APTA general membership status, address, telephone number, office hours, a brief listing of the type of services offered, and an appropriate presentation of fee information. Additional relevant or important consumer information may be included if not prohibited by other sections of the Code.

b. In announcing or advertising the availability of polarity products, publications, or services, practitioners do not present their affiliation with any organization in a manner that falsely implies sponsorship or certification by that organization. In particular and for example, practitioners do not state APTA general membership status in a way to suggest that such status implies specialized professional competence or qualifications, Public statements include, but are not limited to, communication by means of periodical, book, list, directory, television, radio, or motion picture. They do not contain any false, fraudulent, misleading, deceptive, or unfair statement; any misinterpretation of fact or statement likely to mislead or deceive because in context it makes only a partial disclosure of relevant facts; a statement intended or likely to create false or unjustified expectations of favorable results.

c. Practitioners do not compensate or give anything of value to a representative of the press, radio, television, or other communication medium in anticipation of or in return for professional publicity in a news item. A paid advertisement must be identified as such, unless it is apparent from the context that it is a paid advertisement. If communicated to the public by use of radio or television, an advertisement is prerecorded and approved for broadcast by the practitioner, and a recording of the actual transmission is retained by the practitioner.

d. Announcements or advertisements of individual, family, and group services or instruction, schools, and agencies give a clear statement of purpose and a clear description of the experiences provided. The education, training, and experience of the state members are appropriately specified.

e. Practitioners associated with the development or promotion of polarity and/or health building devices, books, or other products offered for commercial sale make reasonable efforts to ensure that announcements and advertisements are presented in a professional and factually informative manner.

f. Practitioners present the art and science of polarity and offer their services, products, and publications fairly and accurately, avoiding misrepresentation through sensationalism, exaggeration, or superficiality. Practitioners are guided by the primary obligation to aid the public in developing informed judgements, opinions, and choices.

g. Practitioners ensure that workshop, seminar, and class descriptions and course outlines are accurate and not misleading, particularly in terms of subject matter to be covered, bases for evaluating progress, and the nature of course experiences. Announcements, brochures, or advertisements describing educational programs accurately describe the audience for which the program is intended as well as eligibility requirements, educational objectives, and nature of the materials to be covered. These announcements also accurately represent the education, training, and experience of the instructors presenting the programs and any fees involved.

h. Public announcements or advertisements soliciting research participants in which clinical services or other professional services are offered as an inducement make clear the nature of the services as well as the costs and other obligations to be accepted by the participants in the research.

i. Practitioners accept the obligation to correct others who represent a practitioner's professional qualifications, or associations with products or services, in a manner incompatible with the Code.

j. Individual evaluative and therapeutic services are provided only in the context of a professional relationship. When personal advice is given by means of public lectures or demonstrations, newspaper or magazine articles, radio or television programs, mail, or similar media, the practitioner uses the most current relevant data and exercises the highest level of professional judgement.

Printed with permission

Associated Bodywork & Massage Professionals (ABMP)
Professional Code of Ethics

As a member of Associated Bodywork & Massage Professionals, I hereby pledge to abide by the ABMP Code of Ethics as outlined below.

Client Relationships

- I shall endeavor to serve the best interests of my clients at all times and to provide the highest quality service possible.
- I shall maintain clear and honest communications with my clients and shall keep client communications confidential.
- I shall acknowledge the limitations of my skills and, when necessary, refer clients to the appropriate qualified health care professional.
- I shall in no way instigate or tolerate any kind of sexual advance while acting in the capacity of a massage, bodywork, somatic therapy or esthetic practitioner.

Professionalism

- I shall maintain the highest standards of professional conduct, providing services in an ethical and professional manner in relation to my clientele, business associates, health care professionals, and the general public.
- I shall respect the rights of all ethical practitioners and will cooperate with all health care professionals in a friendly and professional manner.
- I shall refrain from the use of any mind-altering drugs, alcohol, or intoxicants prior to or during professional sessions.
- I shall always dress in a professional manner, proper dress being defined as attire suitable and consistent with accepted business and professional practice.
- I shall not be affiliated with or employed by any business that utilizes any form of sexual suggestiveness or explicit sexuality in its advertising or promotion of services, or in the actual practice of its services.

Scope of Practice / Appropriate Techniques

- I shall provide services within the scope of the ABMP definition of massage, bodywork, somatic therapies and skin care, and the limits of my training. I will not employ those massage, bodywork or skin care techniques for which I have not had adequate training and shall represent my education, training, qualifications and abilities honestly.
- I shall be conscious of the intent of the services that I am providing and shall be aware of and practice good judgment regarding the application of massage, bodywork or somatic techniques utilized.
- I shall not perform manipulations or adjustments of the human skeletal structure, diagnose, prescribe or provide any other service, procedure or therapy which requires a license to practice chiropractic, osteopathy, physical therapy, podiatry, orthopedics, psychotherapy, acupuncture, dermatology, cosmetology, or any other profession or branch of medicine unless specifically licensed to do so.
- I shall be thoroughly educated and understand the physiological effects of the specific massage, bodywork, somatic or skin care techniques utilized in order to determine whether such application is contraindicated and/or to determine the most beneficial techniques to apply to a given individual. I shall not apply massage, bodywork, somatic or skin care techniques in those cases where they may be contraindicated without a written referral from the client's primary care provider.

Image / Advertising Claims

- I shall strive to project a professional image for myself, my business or place of employment, and the profession in general.
- I shall actively participate in educating the public regarding the actual benefits of massage, bodywork, somatic therapies and skin care.
- I shall practice honesty in advertising, promote my services ethically and in good taste, and practice and/or advertise only those techniques for which I have received adequate training and/or certification. I shall not make false claims regarding the potential benefits of the techniques rendered.

Printed with permission

Feldenkrais Guild® of North America
Code of Ethics

This Code of Professional Conduct describes how we, as *Feldenkrais* Practitioners/Teachers, relate to our clientele and students, our peers, and other professional people. We agree to:

1. Keep the welfare and needs of the client/student foremost in our minds in our professional practice.
2. Create a safe environment:
    a. do no injury or harm to any individual.
    b. do not create an unreasonable risk of any individual being harmed.
3. Protect confidentiality of any conversation between us and the client/student.
4. Do no physical insult or sexual misuse of any person who may be considered as under our professional influence:
    a. neither *Functional Integration* nor *Awareness Through Movement* involves the client/student's disrobing.
    b. The practitioner guides the individual's awareness through hands-on movement, touching the head, neck, shoulder girdle, rib cage, pelvis, legs, arms, hands, and feet, in the context of the professional relationship in the lesson.
5. Respect the legal and civil rights of any person.
6. Refer clients/students to physicians and other professionals as needed and/or indicated.
7. Represent ourselves clearly, objectively, and honestly with regard to training and experience:
    a. inform clients/students as to fees and conditions of work, expected duration, and results.
    b. describe ourselves as teachers of movement and awareness using the *Feldenkrais Method*® and clearly state when we are teaching by this Method and when we are not.
8. Be honest in all dealings, professional and otherwise.
9. Do no fraud or misrepresentation in any business or professional activity.
10. Do no practice under the influence of alcohol or any controlled substance.
11. Cooperate fully in the event of any grievance, whether or not we are directly involved:
    a. reasonably respond to inquiries, furnishing papers and explanations as requested.
    b. follow the result of a grievance procedure, as agreed.
    c. Do not interfere with investigation of any grievance proceeding by misrepresenting facts or by threatening or harassing any one involved.
12. Establish cooperative professional relationships with other practitioners and other professions.

Adopted October 1997

Printed with permission

International Massage Association (IMA) Group
Code of Ethics

As an IMA Group member, you agree to abide by the following standards of professional and ethical behavior in your field:

- To put my clients well being first and foremost.
- To conduct myself professionally and responsibly.
- To uphold the integrity of my profession.
- To acknowledge, respect and cooperate with my colleagues and peers in order to advance our profession and ensure that the highest level of excellence is available to the consuming public.
- I shall promote myself, The IMA Group, and my profession honestly, tactfully, and with the aim of educating both my peers and the public, so that they may be empowered to demand and receive all the benefits that my profession provides.
- To acknowledge the limitations of my skills and scope of practice and refer clients, when necessary, to other health professionals to provide the most appropriate care.
- To maintain a safe and comfortable working environment, paying particular attention to avoidable hazards and respecting personal boundaries.
- To ascertain and comply with the requirements of all governing laws and abide by them to the best of my ability. Where laws are unjust, I will labor with my association to change them.
- To communicate responsibly, truthfully and respectfully with clients, and to hold their communications in strict confidence.
- Any member failing to abide by the Code of Ethics shall be answerable to the board of directors for peer review.

Printed with permission

Kripalu Yoga Teachers Association (KYTA)
Code of Ethics

Kripalu offers experiential programs within a safe environment. The nature of yoga (union of the body, mind and spirit)-on or off the mat-is to induce non-ordinary states of consciousness in the process of opening the body and psyche, through which profound transformation can occur. As a teacher or other program staff member of any program presented at Kripalu, we are stewards of the trust the guests place in us. It is our responsibility to uphold and foster this sacred, safe environment in which to allow this work to happen. It is essential that anyone teaching or assisting in any program at Kripalu Center possesses a high degree of personal integrity and maintains clear boundaries in the role of serving the guests. Holding ourselves as teachers or program staff member places us in a position of power to the guests, however subtle or obvious. We become their mentors, facilitators, and helper. Some guests may idealize us or project that we are wiser or more evolved than they are.

As professionals, we must remain aware of this power dynamic and never exploit the vulnerability of a guest for our personal gain or gratification. Professional organizations (such as Insight Meditation Center, The American Psychological Association, etc.) require waiting periods of 6 months to 2 years before acting on an attraction that began in a care-giving or mentor-student context.In addition to awareness of the power dynamic, we ask our program staff to uphold the environment of inner focus. Over the years many guests have expressed their gratitude to have a place to come where they can safely open their hearts, observe their own deeper dynamics and be free from romantic, sexual distractions and conditioned behaviors. This is what makes the Kripalu experience unique. Because of this, we ask that all our program staff refrain from sexual, romantic involvement with all guests at Kripalu, no matter what program they are in.

Note: Kripalu guests include those in all General Group Programs, Retreat & Renewal, Spiritual Lifestyle Program, Karma Yoga Lifestyle Program, and Seva Program.Our intention is not to be punitive or repressive. Although our first commitment is to practice restraint with romantic involvements, we do recognize that an attraction between a guest and staff member could develop, with care and sensitivity, into a healthy, conscious relationship. Our Ethics Development Team provides caring, non-judgmental support for clarity in these matters.

Agreement

Specifically, I agree to the following code of ethics within the time frame that my programs are promoted in The Kripalu Program Guide, or while I am in relationship with Kripalu Center as a program staff member:

- I agree to hold myself as steward of safe and sacred space by restraining from romantic or sexual relationship with any guest at Kripalu Center. I understand that any sexual or romantic relationship is potentially distracting and possibly even harmful for the guest who has come here to do inner work. I will not invite, act on, respond to or allow sexual, romantic contact with a Kripalu guest during the guest's stay at Kripalu—even if the guest is the initiator.
- If a romantic attraction does develop with a guest while they are at Kripalu, I agree to seek support and clarity from a member of Kripalu's Ethics Development Team (see list below) before involving the guest or acting on the attraction. I understand that the purpose of the Ethics Team and this agreement is to protect the environment of sanctuary for the guests and to support the clarity, consciousness and self-responsibility of individuals. I understand that the Ethics Team develops an individual approach to each situation in a dialogue between the individual(s) and a team member or members.
- I recognize that the aforementioned issues of power dynamic and upholding sanctuary apply to teacher/assistant and I agree to the same ethical behavior as stated in points 1 and 2.
- I agree that my purpose in a program held at Kripalu Center is to serve the guests' personal exploration. I agree that I will avoid any activity or influence that is in conflict with the best interests of the guests or is solely for my own personal gain or gratification.
- I agree to represent my qualifications honestly and to provide only the services I am qualified and contracted by Kripalu to perform. I agree to refrain from recommending treatment, diagnosing a condition or suggesting a guest go against a physician's advice.

I understand that all actions that breach the principles of this code will be fairly investigated by the Ethics Development Team. I understand that if the situation warrants, my future involvement as a teacher or program staff at Kripalu may be revoked. I have read and understand this document in its entirety and agree to honor this code of ethics.

Printed with permission

The National Certification Board for Therapeutic Massage and Bodywork (NCBTMB) Code of Ethics

The Code of Ethics of the National Certification Board for Therapeutic Massage and Bodywork (NCBTMB) requires certificants to uphold professional standards that allow for the proper discharge of their responsibilities to those served, that protect the integrity of the profession, and that safeguard the interest of individual clients. Those practitioners who have been awarded national certification by the NCBTMB will:

- Have a sincere commitment to provide the highest quality of care to those that seek their professional services.
- Represent their qualifications honestly, including their educational achievements and professional affiliations, and will provide only those services which they are qualified to perform.
- Accurately inform clients, other health care practitioners, and the public of the scope and limitations of their discipline. Acknowledge the limitations of and contraindications for massage and bodywork and refer clients to appropriate health professionals.
- Provide treatment only where there is reasonable expectation that it will be advantageous to the client.
- Consistently maintain and improve professional knowledge and competence, striving for professional excellence through regular assessment of personal and professional strengths and weaknesses and through continued education training.
- Conduct their business and professional activities with honesty and integrity, and respect the inherent worth of all persons.
- Refuse to unjustly discriminate against clients or other health professionals.
- Safeguard the confidentiality of all client information, unless disclosure is required by law, court order, or is absolutely necessary for the protection of the public.
- Respect the client's right to treatment with informed and voluntary consent. The NCBTMB practitioner will obtain and record the informed consent of the client, or client's advocate, before providing treatment. This consent may be written or verbal.
- Respect the client's right to refuse, modify, or terminate treatment regardless of prior consent given.
- Provide draping and treatment in a way that ensures the safety, comfort and privacy of the client.
- Exercise the right to refuse to treat any person or part of the body for just and reasonable cause.
- Refrain, under all circumstances, from initiating or engaging in any sexual conduct, sexual activities, or sexualizing behavior involving a client, even if the client attempts to sexualize the relationship.
- Avoid any interest, activity or influence which might be in conflict with the practitioner's obligation to act in the best interests of the client or the profession.
- Respect the client's boundaries with regard to privacy, disclosure, exposure, emotional expression, beliefs, and the client's reasonable expectations of professional behavior. Practitioners will respect the client's autonomy.
- Refuse any gifts or benefits which are intended to influence a referral, decision or treatment that are purely for personal gain and not for the good of the client.
- Follow all policies, procedures, guidelines, regulations, codes, and requirements promulgated by the National Certification Board for Therapeutic Massage and Bodywork.

Printed with permission

National Certification Commission
for Acupuncture and Oriental Medicine (NCCAOM)
Code of Ethics

Practitioners certified by the National Certification Commission for Acupuncture and Oriental Medicine are committed to responsible and ethical practice, to the growth of the profession s role in the broad spectrum of American health care, and to their own professional growth. Candidates seeking certification agree to be bound by the NCCAOM Code of Ethics.

Commitment to the Patient
I will:
1. Respect the rights, dignity, and person of each patient.
2. Render to each patient the highest quality of care and make timely referrals to other Oriental medicine providers or health care professionals as may be appropriate.
3. Avoid treating patients when my judgment or competence is impaired by untreated chemical dependency or physical or mental incapacity reasonably believed to be hazardous to the safety of the patient.
4. Accept and treat all those seeking my services in a nondiscriminatory manner.
5. Keep accurate records of history and treatment and respect the confidentiality of those records or any other personal information imparted by the patient in accordance with law.
6. Keep the patient informed by explaining treatments and outcomes and avoid making promises with regard to outcomes that will create inappropriate expectations.
7. Follow the U.S. Department of Health and Human Services regulations regarding the protection of human subjects in research studies and clinical trials (45 CFR Part 46).
8. Follow U.S. Public Health Service Policy on Humane Care and Use of Laboratory Animals (Office for Protection from Research Risks, National Institutes of Health, Revised September 1986).

Commitment to the Profession
I will:
1. Continue to work to raise the standards of the profession.
2. Use appropriate professional mechanisms to report ethical and professional practice violations.
3. Maintain the highest standard of ethical and professional practice to the benefit of my patients and the profession.

Commitment to the Public
I will:
1. Provide accurate information regarding my education, training, experience, professional affiliations, and certification status.
2. Refrain from making public statements on the efficacy of Oriental medicine that are not supported by the generally accepted experience of the profession.
3. Respect the integrity of other forms of health care and other medical traditions and seek to develop collaborative relationships to achieve the highest quality of care for individual patients.
4. Refrain from any representation that nccaom certification implies licensure or a right to practice unless so designated by the laws in the jurisdiction in which I practice.
5. Use only the appropriate professional designations for my credentials.

(Revised May 2001)

Printed with permission

Ontario Massage Therapist Association
Code of Ethics

Preamble

The ethical foundation of the practice of Massage Therapy consists of moral obligations which ensure the dignity and integrity of the profession.

The aim of the Code is to define clearly those obligations and those professional duties which must be observed by every practitioner and also to define some of the major and minor abuses which must be avoided.

Study of the Code should develop in every student and every practitioner a highly sensitive professional conscience. It is the imperative duty of every Massage Therapist to adhere strictly not only to the regulations prescribed by the Code of Ethics, but equally to its moral precepts.

In addition to the items covered in the Code of Ethics, every Massage Therapist should be cognizant of and must abide by the regulations in the Regulated Health Professions Act and the Massage Therapy Act as they pertain to Massage Therapy.

Section 1 Service to the Public

1. The Massage Therapist's first duty is to the public.
2. The Therapist should inform the patient of fees, and the type of treatment recommended prior to such treatment.
3. When it is necessary in the interests of the patient, the Therapist should recommend that the patient seek expert medical advice.
4. A Therapist must respect the confidence of the patient, not discussing the patient by name without his or her consent.
5. A Therapist's establishment must be clean and neat.
6. Linens and towels must be laundered before use with another patient.
7. On the patient's request, the Therapist must render a receipt for all monies paid.
8. A Therapist must not make unreasonable or unsubstantiated claims regarding massage generally or his or her technique specifically.

Section 2 Service to the Profession

A Therapist must not make disparaging remarks concerning the practices, abilities or competence of other Massage Therapists or about practitioners in other health disciplines.

Notwithstanding the above, where a member of this Association is aware and has proof of the misconduct of, breach of trust or other violation or transgression of this Code of Ethics by any member of this Association, it is his or her duty to bring such knowledge and proof to the attention of the Board of Directors of this Association.

Section 3 Records

The Therapist must maintain accurate and up-to-date records of the dates and types of treatment given each patient, and fees charged.

Printed with permission

Trager International
Code of Ethics and Conduct

I. Preamble

The Code of Ethics and Conduct describes the level of behavior, which *Trager* Practitioners maintain in order to protect *Trager* International, national Associations, the public, and themselves. All Students and Practitioners of the *Trager* Approach are expected to follow these principles.

The guidelines for following Code of Ethics and Conduct are taught within the training program. Detailed instruction of the principles of the Code of Ethics and Conduct is included in the Level I and all subsequent levels of training and continuing education. Support materials in this process include the Standards of Practice, The *Trager* Handbook, the Code of Ethics and Conduct itself, all signed agreements, and other printed materials as needed.

Students' and Practitioners' compliance with the principles outlined in the Code is evaluated through trainings, tutorials, feedback from the public and peers, and other programs or communications as needed.

This ongoing process of evaluation is done in interaction with a combination of Instructors, Tutors and the Board of the National Association.

Matters involving possible violation of the principles of this Code, if not resolved according to the process mentioned above, are brought to the attention of the Board of Directors for action. Principles of basic fairness are followed in all these procedures. Only the authorized distributor of the license has the power to refuse to grant or renew the individual's service mark license and right to use the *Trager* service marks.

II. Precepts

A. Use of the *Trager* name
1. Only authorized *Trager* Students and Practitioners may do the tablework or demonstrate *Mentastics* or *Trager* psychophysical integration and *Mentastics* (The *Trager* Approach).
2. Authorization requirements are specified in "The *Trager* Handbook."

B. Instruction
1. Only Instructors and/or Workshop Leaders designated by *Trager* International may conduct trainings—required or elective—in The *Trager* Approach.
2. Authorization requirements for these functions are listed on page 8-2 of this handbook.

C. *Trager* Practitioners provide accurate information to the public about The *Trager* Approach.
1. The *Trager* Approach is always described in terms of an educational model rather than a medical one.
2. Practitioners do not diagnose, prescribe, or claim to treat any condition unless otherwise licensed to do so.
3. Within the context of a session or demonstration, any approach other than *Trager* shall not be represented as The *Trager* Approach.
4. Practitioners refer clients to colleagues and health professionals with care, stating the reason for referral and their knowledge of the practitioner or methods recommended.

D. *Trager* Practitioners are responsible for complying with state and local laws and regulations governing their practice.

III. Professional Integrity

A. *Trager* Practitioners uphold *Trager* International standards for professional practice.
1. References for the standards of practice are including the standards of practice supported by The *Trager* Handbook, the Practice Guides, the Tutor Manual, the Code of Ethics and Conduct, and all signed agreements.
2. Practitioners fulfill all ongoing continuing education requirements.
3. Practitioners abide by the Code of Ethics and Conduct and all signed agreements.

B. Each *Trager* Practitioner is responsible for the quality of her or his work and for the exercise of sound judgment.
1. Practitioners assess their own state, skills and knowledge so as to avoid misleading or harming a client physically, emotionally, mentally, socially, financially, or in any regard.
2. Practitioners do not work when alcohol, drugs, strong attitudes, motivations or emotional states so impair their ability to do.
3. Practitioners bear in mind that their own actions may reflect on other Practitioners.
C. *Trager* Practitioners respect the rights and dignity of all individuals and protect the welfare of their clients.
1. Practitioners respect the client's authority about his or her own experience.
2. Practitioners hold as confidential all personal information about others learned in a professional capacity.
   a. Information learned in a professional context is not divulged in any way that lets the client's identity be known, except with the client's permission.
   b. Confidentiality and anonymity are maintained when discussing professional issues with teachers and colleagues.
   c. In the event that a client or colleague presents a personal or public danger, Practitioners are encouraged to refer that person to the proper service directly.
3. Practitioners respect the reputation of colleagues. When discussion of problems about colleagues is necessary, it is done in terms of principles, not personalities.
4. When possible, Practitioners communicate directly with the individuals involved to resolve issues; when necessary they use the resources of Tutors and the National Organization for assistance.
5. Practitioners do not use the professional relationship to further their own personal or sexual interests or to promote their own political or religious beliefs.
6. Practitioners do not place their own financial interests above the welfare of their clients.
   a. Fees reflect the customary range for the experience of the Practitioner, the setting, and the region in which the services are provided.
   b. Practitioners do not conduct or recommend sessions for the sole reason of receiving payment.
D. Trager Practitioners maintain clear and honest professional relationships with clients and colleagues.
1. Fees, appointments, length of session, location and other business arrangements are agreed upon between client and Practitioner.
2. Practitioners are responsible for keeping professional agreements they make.
E. Trager Practitioners show sensible regard for the social codes and moral expectations of the community in which they practice.

January 1999/rev. August 2001

Printed with permission

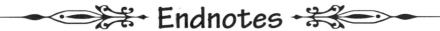

Endnotes

Chapter 1: Ethical Principles

1. Thomas J. Peters and Robert H. Waterman, Jr., *In Search of Excellence* (New York: Harper & Row 1982).
2. Thomas J. Peters, "Ethics is everyday, lifetime endeavor," <u>The Arizona Daily Star</u>, 26 September 1989.
3. Norman Vincent Peale & Kenneth Blanchard, *The Power of Ethical Management* (New York: William Morrow and Company, Inc., 1988) 30-31.
4. Mark Annett, *The Scruples Methodology*, June 16, 2002 http://www.scruplestore.com/ TheScruplesMethodology/thebook.html.
5. Marianne Corey, Gerald Corey and Patrick Callanan, *Issues and Ethics In the Helping Professions* (Pacific Grove, CA: International Thomson Publishing Inc., 1998) 16-17.
6. Frank J. Navran, *Crossing the Spectrum: Steps for Making Ethical Decisions*, Ethics Resource Center, www.ethics.org.
7. Phyllis K. Davis, PH.D., *The Power of Touch* (Carlsbad, CA: Hay House, Inc. 1999) 173-174.
8. Daphne Chellos, *Creating Boundaries Handbook*, 1992.
9. Carol D. Tamparo, B.S., PH.D., C.M.A.-A., and Wilburta Q. Lindh, C.M.A., *Therapeutic Communications for Health Professionals* (Clifton Park, NY: Delmar Thomson Learning, 2000) 70.
10. Tamparo and Lindh 69-76.
11. Ronan M. Kisch, PH.D., *Beyond Technique: The Hidden Dimensions of Bodywork* (Dayton, OH: BLHY Growth Publications, Inc., 1998) 325.
12. Jean L. McKechnie, ed., *Webster's New Universal Unabridged Dictionary* (New York: Simon and Schuster, 1979) 1536.
13. Kisch 325.

Chapter 2: Boundaries

1. Jane Bluestein, PH.D., *Parents, Teens and Boundaries* (Deerfield, FL: Health Communications, Inc., 1993).
2. Ronan M. Kisch, *Beyond Technique: The Hidden Dimensions of Bodywork* (Dayton, OH: BLHY Growth Publications, Inc., 1998) 331-332.
3. Salvador Minuchin, *Families and Family Therapy* (Cambridge, MA: Harvard University Press, 1974).
4. Sonia Nevis, personal interview, 1995.
5. Ernst Hartmann, M.D., Boundaries in the Mind: a New Phychology of Personality New York, NY: Basic Books, 1991) 4-9.
6. Charles Whitfield, M.D., *Boundaries and Relationships: Knowing, Protecting and Enjoying the Self* (Deerfield, FL: Health Communications, Inc., 1993).
7. Hartmann 113.
8. Thomas Guthiel, M.D., and Glen Gabbard, M.D., "The Concept of Boundaries in Clinical Practice: Theoretical and Risk-Management Dimensions," *American Journal of Psychiatry*, Feb. 1993.
9. Kisch 325.
10. Estelle Disch, PH.D., "Are You in Trouble with a Client," *Massage Therapy Journal*, Volume 31, Number 3 (Summer 1992).

Chapter 3: Dynamics of Effective Communication

1. Robert Bolton, PH.D., *People Skills: How to Assert Yourself, Listen to Others and Resolve Conflicts* (New York: Simon & Schuster, Inc., 1979).
2. Stuart Simon, personal interview, 1997.
3. Richard Bandler, *Using Your Brain—for a Change* (Moab, UT: Real People Press, 1985).
4. Howard Gardner, *Multiple Intelligences: The Theory in Practice* (New York: Basic Books, 1993).
5. Kylea Taylor, *The Ethics of Caring* (Santa Cruz, CA: Handford Mead Publishers, 1995). 6.
6. Bolton 50-76, 87-113.
7. Bolton 87.
8. Bolton 92.

9. Bolton 93-94.
10. Bolton 80.
11. Sheldon Kopp, *Back to One: A Practical Guide for Psychotherapists* (Palo Alto, CA: Science of Behavior Books, 1977).
12. Martin Seldman, PH.D., and David Hermes, *Personal Growth Thru Groups: A Collection of Methods* (San Diego, CA: The We Care Foundation, Inc., 1975).
13. Bolton 144.
14. Bolton 137-176.
15. Bolton 218-225.

Chapter 4: Dual Relationships

1. Mary Jo Bennett and Katy Butler, "Can We Tell the Truth: Let's End Our Conspiracy of Silence about our Ambiguous Boundaries," *Psychotherapy Networker*, March/April 2002: 32-77.
2. Daphne Chellos and Ben Benjamin, "Dual Roles and Other Ethical Considerations," *Massage Therapy Journal*, Spring 1992: 23.
3. Nanette Gartrell et al., "Psychiatrist-Patient Sexual Contact: Results of a National Survey, I: Prevalence," *American Journal of Psychiatry*, 143 (1986): 1126. (See also: Judith Herman et al., "Psychiatrist-Patient Sexual Contact: Results of a National Survey, II: Psychiatrists' Attitudes," *American Journal of Psychiatry*, 44 (1987): 164.).
4. Jean. C. Holroyd and Annette M. Brodsky, "Psychologists' Attitudes and Practices Regarding Erotic and Nonerotic Physical Contact with Patients," *American Psychologist*, 32 (1977): 843.
5. Chellos and Benjamin 22.
6. Chellos and Benjamin, 22.

Chapter 5: Sex, Touch and Intimacy

1. William Greenburg of the AMTA Grievance Board, personal interview, 11 October 1995.
2. June M. Reinisch and Ruth Beasley, *The Kinsey Institute New Report on Sex: What You Must Know to be Sexually Literate* (New York: St. Martin's Press, 1990) xviii.
3. A. P. Stern, "The feeling we can't do without," *McCall's*, November 1992: 84, 86.
4. Tiffany Field, *touch* (Cambridge, MA: A Bradford book, MIT Press, 2001) 59.
5. Phyllis Davis, PH.D., *The Power of Touch* (Carlsbad, CA: Hay House, Inc., 1999) 6.
6. Ashley Montagu, *Touching* (New York: Harper & Row Publishers, 1971) 34, 46.
7. Montagu 198-203.
8. Montagu 198-203.
9. Montagu 237-392.
10. Laurel Catherine Bentsen, "Women and Touch Deprivation," *Massage Therapy Journal*, Volume 33, Number 4 (Fall 1994): 54-106, 60.
11. Stern 84, 90.
12. T. Field, M. Hernandez-Reif, O. Quintino, et. al., *Journal of Applied Gerontology*, Volume 17 (1998) 229-239.
13. Grant Jewell Rich, ed., Ruth Remington, "Hand massage in the agitated elderly," *Massage Therapy: The Evidence for Practice* (New York: Mosby, Harcourt Publishers Limited, 2002) 165-185).
14. Jeffrey D. Fisher et al., "Hands Touching Hands: Affective and Evaluative Effects of an Interpersonal Touch." *Sociometry*, Volume 39, Number 4 (1976): 417.
15. Richard Heslin and Tari Alper, "Nonverbal Communication," *Sage Annual Reviews of Communications Research*, Volume 11 (1982).
16. Helen Colton, *Touch Therapy* (New York: Kenshington Publishing Corp., 1983) 159.
17. *Webster's New Universal Unabridged Dictionary*, 2nd ed., (New York: Simon and Schuster, 1981).
18. Stephen Thayer, "Close Encounters," *Psychology Today* (March 1988).
19. Susan Forward and Craig Buck, *Betrayal of Innocence: Incest and Its Devastation* (New York: St. Martin's Press, 1978).
20. *Sexual Health Magazine*, http://www.sexualhealth.com, 1.
21. Ruth Brecher and Edward Brecher, *An Analysis of Human Sexual Response* (New York: New American Library, 1966).
22. *Sexual Health Magazine*.

23. William H. Gotwald Jr. and Gale Holtz Golden, *Sexuality: The Human Experience* (New York: Macmillan Publishing, 1981) 295.

24. Gotwald and Golden, 297-298.

25. *Sexual Health Magazine.*

26. Alfred C. Kinsey et al., *Sexual Behavior in the Human Male* (Philadelphia, PN: W. B. Saunders, 1948).

27. Kinsey et al.

28. The American Association of Sex Educators, Counselors and Therapists, *Contemporary Sexuality*, Volume 33 (March 1999).

29. Miriam Ehrenberg and Otto Ehrenberg, *The Intimate Circle: The Sexual Dynamics of Family Life* (New York: Simon and Schuster, 1988).

30. *Fowler's Modern English Usage*, 2nd Ed. (New York: Oxford University Press, 1985).

31. Carol D. Tamparo, B.S., PH.D., C.M.A.-A., and Wilburta Q. Lindh, C.M.A., *Therapeutic Communications for Health Professionals* (Clifton Park, NY: Delmar Thomson Learning, 2000) 72.

32. Daphne Chellos, "Creating Boundaries Handbook," Boulder, CO, 1993.

33. Steven B. Bisbing, Linda Mabus Jorgenson, and Pamela K. Sutherland, *Sexual Abuse by Professionals: A Legal Guide* (Charlottesville, VA: Michie, 1995).

34. Department of Health, Board of Massage Therapy, Petitioner, vs. Miodrag Visacki, L.M.T., Respondent. Case No. 01-2257PL
State of Florida Division of Administrative Hearings
2001 Fla. Div. Adm. Hear. LEXIS 3131
September 18, 2001, Recommended Order.

35. Dr. Melvin Mashner v. W. Pennington, Jr., 1970738
Sumpreme Court of Alabama
729 So. 2D 262; 1998 Ala. LEXIS 301
November 20, 1998; Released.

36. From "The Hippocratic Oath," a translation by Ludwig Edelstein, *Supplements to the Bulletins of the History of Medicine*, no.1 (Baltimore, MD: John Hopkins University Press, 1943).

37. John C. Gonsiorek, *Breach of Trust: Sexual Exploitation by Health Care Professionals and Clergy* (Thousand Oaks, CA: Sage Publications 1995).

38. From the schedule of conference events published by organizers of "It's Never O.K., The Third International Conference on Sexual Exploitation by Health Professionals, Psychotherapists and Clergy," held in Toronto, Ontario, Canada, Oct. 13-15, 1994.

39. Angelica Redleaf, D.C., *Behind Closed Doors: Gender, Sexuality & Touch in the Doctor/Patient Relationship.* (Westport, CT: Auburn House, 1998). 129-133.

40. Linda Greenhouse, "Same-Sex Harassment Ruled Illegal," *The Providence Journal-Bulletin* sec. A-1, 11 (Tuesday, 5 March 1998).

41. Pamela R. Fletcher and Martha Roth, eds., *Transforming a Rape Culture* (Minneapolis, MN: Milkweed Editions, 1995) 130.

42. Redleaf, 119.

Chapter 6: Ethical Practice Management

1. Noah Webster, *Webster's New Universal Unabridged Dictionary*, (Cleveland, OH: Dorset & Baber, 1983) 1436-1437.

2. Jerry Buley, PH.D., "What Is a Professional?," Arizona Communication Association, The Hugh Downs School of Human Communication, 2000, http://com.pp.asu.edu/ACA/Professional.html.

3. Noah Webster, Webster's New Universal Unabridged Dictionary, (Cleveland, OH: Dorset & Baber, 1983) 953.

4. George F. Sheldon, M.D., F.A.C.S., *Bulletin of the American College of Surgeons*, Volume 83, Number 12 (Chicago, IL, 1998) 16.

5. Sandy Fritz, *Mosby's Fundamentals of Therapeutic Massage* (St. Louis, MO: Van Hoffmann Press, 1995) 435.

6. Whitney Lowe, L.M.T., "Exploring Orthopedic Assessment," Massage Today Volume 1, Number 1 (January 2001) 7.

7. Donald Veres, M.D., M.S.J., ed., *Taber's Cyclopedic Medical Dictionary* (Philadelphia, PN: F.A. Davis Company, 1997).

8. Sandy Fritz, James M. Grosenbach, and Kathy Paholsky, "Ethics and Professionalism: Scope of Practice," *Massage Magazine*, March/April 1997.

9. Patricia J. Benjamin, "Paper Tiger Credentials," *Massage Therapy Journal*, Volume 29, Number 3 (Summer 1990) 9.

10. Nina McIntosh, *The Educated Heart: Professional Guidelines for Massage Therapists, Bodyworkers, and Movement Teachers* (Memphis, Tennessee: Decatur Bainbridge Press, 1999) 97.

11. M. Corey, G. Corey and P. Callanan, *Issues and Ethics in the Helping Professions*, 5th ed., (Pacific Grove, CA: International Thomson Publishing Inc., 1998) 16-17.

12. Cherie M. Sohnen-Moe, *Business Mastery* (Tucson, AZ: Sohnen-Moe Associates, Inc., 1997) 157-162.

13. Sohnen-Moe 163-167.

13. Case Management Society of America, *Standards of Practice for Case Management* (Little Rock, AR: Case Management Society of America, 1995).

15. Cindy Ling, *Why and What you Should Know about Case Management*, www.NurseWeek.com.

16. Sohnen-Moe 167-172.

Chapter 7: Business Ethics

1. Kenneth Blanchard and Norman Vincent Peale, *The Power of Ethical Management* (New York: William Morrow and Company, Inc., 1988).

2. 1 Timothy 6:10.

3. Lu Bauer, "Clean Up Your Money Operating System," *Massage Therapy Journal*, Volume 39, Number 1 (Spring 2000).

4. Suze Orman, *9 Steps to Financial Freedom: Practical and Spiritual Steps So You Can Stop Worrying* (New York: Three Rivers Press, 2001).

5. Cherie M. Sohnen-Moe, *Business Mastery* (Tucson, AZ: Sohnen-Moe Associates, Inc., 1997) 99.

6. Sohnen-Moe 99-100.

7. Sohnen-Moe 190-194.

8. Sohnen-Moe 181.

9. The California Codes, Civil Code Section 1749.5 states:

    1749.5. (a) On or after January 1, 1997, it is unlawful for any person or entity to sell a gift certificate to a purchaser containing an expiration date. Any gift certificate sold after that date shall be redeemable in cash for its cash value, or subject to replacement with a new gift certificate at no cost to the purchaser or holder.

    (b) A gift certificate sold without an expiration date is valid until redeemed or replaced.

10. Sohnen-Moe 195-196.

11. Sohnen-Moe 197.

12. Gary Wolf, personal interview, June 2001.

13. Cherie Sohnen-Moe, "Copyright," *Massage Therapy Journal*, Volume 40, Number 4 (Winter 2002).

14. Sohnen-Moe 140-141.

15. Stewart Levine, *Getting to Resolution: Turning Conflict into Collaboration* (San Francisco, California: Berrett-Koehler Publishers, Inc., 1998).

16. Joan C. Calcagno, "Mediation is the Best Way to End a Dispute," *Massage Therapy Journal*, Volume 38, Number 4 (Winter 2000).

17. Massachusetts Continuing Legal Education, Inc., *Jury Instructions for Civil Trials* (MA: Massachusetts Continuing Legal Education, Inc., 1995) 36 (95-05.34);

18. Brine v. Belinkoff, 235 N.E.2d 23, 26 (Wis. 1987).

19. Sohnen-Moe 136-140.

20. Internal Revenue Service, *Employer's Tax Guide* (Publication 15, Circular E).

Chapter 8: Special Considerations In Cases of Trauma

1. Melissa Soalt, personal interview, 1994.
2. Stephanie Mines, "Secrets: Healing Triumphs over Domestic Violence," *Massage and Bodywork* Oct/Nov 2001: 18.
3. Karrie Mowen, "Trauma Touch Therapy: An Interdisciplinary Approach to Trauma," *Massage and Bodywork*, Oct/Nov 2001: 28-36.
4. Janet Yassen, personal interview, 1994.
5. Janet Yassen, personal interview, 1991.
6. Maryanna Eckberg, PH.D., *Victims of Cruelty: Somatic Psychotherapy in the Treatment of Posttraumatic Stress Disorder* (Berkeley, CA. North Atlantic Books, 2000) 3.
7. Eckberg 45.
8. Tiffany Field, *touch* (Cambridge, MA: A Bradford book, MIT Press, 2001) 136.
9. Patricia Tjaden and Nancy Thoennes, "Prevalence, Incidence and Consequences of Violence Against Women: Findings From the National Violence Against Women Survey," *NCJ* (Washington DC: U.S. Department of Justice, Bureau of Justice Statistics, November 1998): 172837.
10. Howard N. Snyder, "Sexual Assault of Young Children as Reported to Law Enforcement: Victim, Incident, and Offender Characteristics," *NCJ* (Washington DC: U.S. Department of Justice, Bureau of Justice Statistics, July 2000): 182990.
11. R. Badgley, *Report of the federal committee on sexual offenses against children and youth*, Canadian Government Publishing Centre (Ottowa) 1984.
12. Judith Herman, *Trauma and Recovery* (New York: Harper Collins Publishers, 1992) 6-32.
13. Mines 22.
14. Herman 6-32.
15. Steven Hassan, *Releasing the Bonds: Empowering People to Think for Themselves* (Somerville, MA: Freedom of Mind Press, 2000).
16. American Psychiatric Association, *Diagnostic and Statistical Manual of Mental Disorders*, 4th ed. (Washington DC: American Psychiatric Association, 1994).
17. Herman 6-32.
18. Eckberg.
19. Herman 6-32.
20. *Incest: The Victim No One Believes*, film, Motorola Teleprogram Information (MTI), Deerfield IL, 1978.
21. Herman 121.
22. Herman 121.
23. Herman 168.
24. Herman 195.
25. Herman 207.
26. Leslie Lebowitz, M.R. Harvey, and J.L. Herman, "A Stage-by-Dimension Model of Recovery From Sexual Trauma," *Journal of Interpersonal Violence*, Volume 8 (September 1993).
27. Lebowitz et al.
28. Soalt.
29. Eckberg 41-48.
30. Eckberg 48-58.
31. *Survivor Interviews*, videotape, Ben Benjamin, Boston, MA, 1992.
32. Eckberg 58-61.
33. *Survivor Interviews*.
34. Robert Timms and Patrick Connors, *Embodying Healing* (Brandon, VT: The Safer Society Press, 1992) 24.
35. Timms and Connors 38.
36. Soalt.
37. Mines 24.
38. Eckberg 63.
39. Mowen 32.
40. Yassen 1994.
41. Eckberg 216-218.

42. Herman 196-213.

43. Herman 175-195.

44. Yassen 1991.

45. Soalt.

46. *Incest: The Victim No One Believes.*

47. Kirtland C. Peterson, Maurice F. Prout, and Robert A. Schwartz, *Post Traumatic Stress Disorder: A Clinician's Guide* (New York: Plenum Press, 1992).

48. Candace Pert, "Neuropeptides: The Emotions and Bodymind," *Massage Therapy Journal*, Volume 26, Number 4 (Fall 1987): 39.

49. Wilhelm Reich, *Character Analysis* (London, England Vision Press, 1950) 55, 357-365.

50. *Incest: The Victim No One Believes.*

51. Mines 24.

Chapter 9: Supervision

1. Nancy Bridges, "Psychodynamic perspective on therapeutic boundaries: Creative clinical possibilities," *Psychotherapy Practice and Research*, Volume 8, Number 4 (1999): 1-9.

2. Ann Alonso, *The Quiet Profession* (New York: Macmillan Publishing Company, 1985).

3. Nancy Bridges, "The role of supervision in managing intense affect and constructing boundaries in therapeutic relationships," *Journal of Sex Education and Therapy*, Volume 24, Number 4 (2000): 218-225.

4. Nancy Bridges, "Meaning and management of attraction: Neglected areas of psychotherapy training and practice," *Psychotherapy*, Volume 31, Number 3 (1994): 424-433.

5. Bridges, "The role of supervision."

6. Bridges, "Psychodynamic perspective on therapeutic boundaries."

7. Alonso.

8. Les Kertay, "Ethical considerations for bodyworkers who counsel," *Massage Magazine*, July/August 1998.

9. Bridges, "Meaning and management of attraction."

10. Bridges, "Psychodynamic perspective on therapeutic boundaries."

11. Jeannette Milgrom, *Boundaries in Professional Relationships* (Minneapolis, MN: Walk-In Counseling Center, 1992).

12. Angelica Redleaf and Susan Baird, *Behind Closed Doors: Gender, Sexuality, & Touch in the Doctor/ Patient Relationship* (Westport, CT: Auburn House, 1998).

13. Milgrom.

14. Glen O. Gabbard, "Can patients sexually harass their physicians?" *Archives of Family Medicine*, Volume 4 (1995): 261-265.

15. Redleaf and Baird.

16. Redleaf and Baird.

17. Redleaf and Baird.

18. George J. Allen, Sandor J. Szollos, and Bronwen E. Williams, "Doctoral students comparative evaluations of best and worst psychotherapy supervision," *Professional Psychology: Research and Practice*, Volume 17, Number 2 (1986): 91-99.

19. Christine H. Hutt, Judith Scott, and Mark King, "A phenomenological study of supervisees' positive and negative experiences in supervision," *Psychotherapy: Theory, Research and Practice*, Volume 20, Number 1 (1983): 118-122.

20. Allen, Szollos, and Bronwen.

21. Hutt, Scott, and King.

22. Alonso.

23. Allen, Szollos, and Bronwen.

24. Hutt, Scott, and King

Index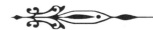

A

Abuse 21, 59, 62, 107, 111, 114, 115, 122–124, 128, 131, 134, 158, 216–239, 256–259, 268–275. *See also* Trauma

Child 9, 115, 163, 218

Cult 220, 269, 276–278

Emotional 218–220, 236, 257

Mental 218

Neglect 158, 220

Physical 218–221, 224

Sexual 21, 22, 114, 122–124, 127, 218–222, 248, 249

Accountability 4, 23, 87, 90, 93, 99, 145, 149, 150, 151, 160, 184, 185. *See also* Self-Accountability

Advertising 157, 172, 281, 289, 290. *See also* Marketing

Alliance 62, 144, 171

Anger 18, 19, 21, 35, 38, 57, 64, 75, 82, 123, 125, 227, 245, 246, 265

Annoyance 64, 248

Anxiety 20, 38, 62, 63, 69, 108, 139, 218, 222, 244, 245, 247–249, 253, 261, 268, 271

Appearance 28, 49, 52, 135, 141, 150, 151, 171, 281, 284

Arbitration 199

Arousal 115, 116, 120–126, 134, 137, 140, 141, 236, 239

Arouse 135, 257

Assertion Sequence 75–80, 83, 84

Assertive 75, 76, 79, 83, 84, 125, 140

Assessment 61, 65, 73, 147, 152, 166, 173, 177, 261, 262, 271

Self-Assessment 7, 8, 10

Associations 92, 151, 152, 280–298

Attitude 2, 3, 6, 8, 23, 26, 36, 37, 51, 87, 109, 110, 114, 118, 131, 144, 155, 168, 177, 182, 183, 261, 288, 298

Authenticity 93

Authority 15, 17, 18, 86, 92, 163, 165, 191, 209, 244, 245, 248, 276, 278, 298

Autonomy 10, 11, 23, 163, 164, 294

Awareness 7, 19, 20–23, 26, 29, 30, 37–45, 51–53, 56–58, 69–74, 86, 87, 98, 119, 121, 131, 133, 136–139, 149, 162, 164, 165, 177, 216, 221–228, 233, 237, 253, 261, 265, 271, 275, 281, 291

B

Babies 107

Barter 48, 89, 95, 96, 99, 101, 130, 184, 188, 189, 191, 211, 213

Benevolence 15

Bill of Rights 137, 257–259

Bite Model 220, 276, 278

Body Language 56–58, 66, 69–71, 74, 76, 79, 82–84, 125

Body Memory 231–234

Boundaries 8, 16, 18, 19, 26–53, 58–62, 65, 67, 69–73, 75–78, 80–84, 86, 93, 94, 97, 112–115, 118–121, 124, 125, 128, 131, 135–138, 140, 141, 151–153, 156, 157, 177, 184, 186, 189, 200, 211, 212, 217, 222, 224–228, 230, 231, 235–239, 242–249, 253, 256, 257, 262, 268, 274, 275, 277, 284, 292, 294

Boundary Crossing 32, 39–43, 51–53, 76, 80, 113, 227, 274

Boundary Indicator Exercise 33

Boundary Models 30–32

Permeable boundary 30, 33, 51

Rigid boundary 31, 33, 51

Semi-permeable boundary 33, 51

Boundary Violation 39–43, 51, 71, 75, 76, 83, 104, 129, 131, 132, 200, 203, 205, 206, 242

Burnout 71, 242

Business 8, 88, 90, 92, 151–155, 171, 172, 176–178, 182–213

C

Cancellation 78, 153, 154, 187, 260, 262, 263, 269

Case Management 173–175, 178, 179

Certification 145, 146, 149, 177, 179

Change Agents 49, 50

Cheating 5, 6, 23

Child 9, 15, 17, 18, 20, 21, 23, 27, 105–107, 114, 115, 118, 139, 140, 158, 162–164, 177, 216–222, 232, 233, 248, 253

Civil Lawsuits 196, 201–204, 211

Client Custody 206, 207, 211

Client Files 158, 162, 207. *See also* Documentation

Client–centered 14, 15, 23, 61, 113

Codes of Ethics 3, 4, 7, 10, 24, 92, 196, 197, 279–297

Collaboration 173, 175, 199, 226, 227, 229

Communication Barriers 56, 57, 84

Compassion 30, 36, 138, 247, 282, 283, 288

Competency 145, 149, 150, 177, 179

Confidentiality 7–9, 24, 127, 157–162, 177, 179,
203, 209, 210, 249, 251, 252, 261, 269, 270, 272,
284, 286–288, 291, 294, 295, 298

Continuing Education ix, 242, 287, 297

Continuum 30, 31, 114, 117, 121, 127, 129

Contract 14, 23, 100, 126, 154, 168, 172, 174, 176,
178, 187, 199, 200, 205–208, 211, 213

Copyright 197, 198, 211, 284

Core Psychological Concepts 14–22

Core Values Assessment 7, 8

Countertransference 14, 17, 19, 20, 23, 24, 62, 92,
93, 122, 167–169, 227, 229, 237, 239, 250

Credentials 149, 194, 211, 287, 295

Credit 154, 184, 187, 198

Cults 218, 220, 276–278

Culture 3, 6, 35–39, 51, 53, 105–107, 110, 114–123,
139, 141

D

Dating 7, 41, 42, 97, 99, 109, 122, 123, 126, 127, 132,
140

Defense Mechanism 20–24

Denial 22–24, 277

Diagnosis 147, 160, 165, 177

Discriminate 8, 208, 209, 284, 294

Dispute Resolution 199, 200

Documentation 207, 209, 256. *See also* Client
Files

Draping 15, 119, 124, 129, 136, 155

Dual Relationships 38, 41, 42, 44, 85–101, 135, 156,
237, 239, 256, 282, 287

Duty 9–12, 23, 160, 200, 201–203

E

Emotions 27–29, 36, 51, 62–67, 71, 74, 83, 112, 139,
218–220, 229, 231, 233, 236, 237, 239, 242, 265,
276

  Emotional Release 62, 83, 233

Empathy 30, 45, 49, 66, 81, 82, 229

Employee 88, 132–134, 152, 171, 172, 174, 189, 196,
203–207, 211

Energy 6, 29, 30, 42–45, 51, 52, 120, 121, 135, 183

Erections 123–126

Ethical Congruency 13, 14

Ethical Dilemmas 9–12, 23, 73, 83, 142, 184, 185,
212

Etiquette 156

F

Fair Use Factor 197, 198

Family 4, 5, 6, 8, 24, 36, 37, 51, 53, 87, 89, 99, 101,
104, 110, 111, 112, 116–119, 139, 142, 156, 163, 182,
213, 218–220, 228, 230, 234

Fear 16, 17, 28, 38, 63, 64, 66, 91, 106, 109, 110, 120,
121, 139, 218, 220, 221, 228, 231, 237, 265, 268,
278

Fee Structure 154, 184–187, 206, 211

Feedback 44, 57, 82, 108, 111, 227, 274, 275

Fiduciary Relationship 14, 15, 23

Finances 144, 152, 154, 171, 172, 177, 178, 182–191

First Touch Exercise 273

Flashback 34, 62, 64, 216, 217, 221, 227, 230–239,
258, 269, 271, 273

Fraud 160, 190, 199, 281, 284, 289, 291

Friend 48, 86, 90, 91, 94, 96, 101, 157, 185, 186,
193, 213

Friendship 41, 42, 71

G

Gender 108–110, 114, 115, 117, 120, 134, 137, 139, 141,
286–288

Gestalt Theory 32

Gift Certificate 188, 190, 211, 213

Goodwill 190, 192

Grief 95, 222, 236

Group Practice 132, 171–173, 178, 179, 205

Guarantee 7, 194, 195

H

Harassment 131–134, 141, 142, 288

HIPAA 159–162

Hippocrates 127, 145

Honesty 6, 8, 12, 144, 201, 249, 252, 280, 281, 290,
294

I

Image 3, 23, 37, 38, 171, 176, 178, 194, 195, 211, 276, 283, 290

Independent Contractor 172, 205, 206, 211

Informed Consent 68, 69, 83, 84, 111, 129, 136, 141, 147, 159, 164–166, 178, 179, 230, 263, 264, 270, 287, 294

Insurance
  Coverage 184, 196, 197, 204, 207, 208, 211
  Issues 207–210

Integrity 6, 8, 10, 113, 114, 144, 151, 163, 176, 177, 190, 201, 218, 281, 284, 287, 292–297

Interactive Speaking 67–71, 82, 84

Internet 159, 160, 197

Intervention 46, 72, 119, 228, 245

Intervention Model 125–127, 140

Intimacy 28–30, 42, 89, 92, 93, 99, 100, 104, 105, 108, 109, 112, 113, 119, 120, 139, 141

L

Laws 3, 4, 6–13, 15, 23, 24, 51, 104, 132, 133, 145–152, 156, 158–162, 171, 177, 179, 191, 193, 196–198, 211, 212, 258, 259, 280, 281, 283–285, 288, 292–297

Lawsuit 87, 97, 131, 171, 196, 200–204, 207, 211, 259

Learning Styles 57, 58, 82, 84. *See also* Multiple Intelligences

Libel 196, 197, 211

Licensure 145, 147, 148, 153, 177, 179, 196

Limbic System 115, 116, 140

Location 49, 52, 119, 130, 155, 171, 206, 207

M

Malpractice 129, 131, 196, 200–205, 211

Marketing 171, 172, 176, 178, 190, 191, 194, 195, 199, 206, 207, 211, 213
  Marketing Materials 194, 195, 211, 213

Maturity 93, 95, 99, 100

Media 37, 38, 51, 106, 118, 139, 195, 277, 289

Memory 21, 24, 62, 64, 199, 217, 221–226, 230–232, 234, 237, 239, 269

Minor 9, 162–164, 177, 179

Money 12, 24, 26, 48, 50, 52, 89, 96, 97, 101, 132, 141, 154, 162, 182–191, 193, 196, 198, 203–207, 211, 213, 256, 259

Morals 2–4, 23, 24, 196

Multiple Intelligences 58, 82, 83. *See also* Learning Styles

N

Network 150, 151, 174, 189, 193, 258

Nutritional Supplements 192, 193

P

Parasympathetic Nervous System 108, 115, 116, 139, 140

Partnership 88, 92, 171, 172, 174, 179

Perception 16, 56, 105, 116, 123, 223

Policy/Policies 11, 13, 49, 59, 61, 72, 75–78, 80, 82, 97, 100, 101, 137, 152–162, 166, 172, 176, 177, 179, 185–187, 238, 260–262, 264, 269, 270
  Sample Policy Statements 260–262

Post Traumatic Stress Disorder 221, 222, 236

Power Differential/Power Dynamic 14–18, 20, 23, 24, 39, 45, 49, 52, 59, 64, 69, 83, 86, 88, 89, 92, 93, 99, 100, 111, 162, 191–193, 213, 227, 237, 239

Prejudice 31, 57

Privacy 15, 36, 51, 129, 136, 141, 155, 157–161, 196, 246, 261, 269, 283, 287, 294

Pro bono 183, 186

Proactive Principle 71–73

Process Recording 73–75, 83, 84

Product Sales 172, 191–193, 211

Professional Conduct 151, 177, 284, 286, 290, 291

Professionalism 3, 4, 8, 23, 49, 127, 134–136, 144, 151, 152, 155, 177, 179, 195, 211, 262

Projection 20, 21, 23, 71, 121, 253

Psychosocial 104–106

Punctuality 153, 154

R

Record Keeping 145, 177, 191, 207

Recourse Policy 162, 177, 262

Recovery 110, 216, 217, 221–223, 225, 229, 230, 235–237, 239, 258, 270

Referrals 12, 41, 91, 94, 149, 172, 174, 185, 193, 281, 282, 284, 295

Reflective Listening 65–67, 82, 84

Registration 145, 177, 179

Rejection 18, 132

Religion 7–9, 23, 37, 38, 51, 104, 118, 262, 288

Repression 14, 20–23, 115, 235

Rights 9–11, 137, 141, 151, 157, 159, 161, 165, 171, 257–259, 285, 286, 288, 290, 291, 295, 298

S

Sadness 30, 38, 63, 265
Salon Issues 176
Schools 5, 6, 37, 51, 87, 88, 97, 98, 145
Scope of Practice 2, 3, 18, 62, 82, 144–152, 172, 174,
    177, 192, 195, 227, 262, 283, 290, 292
Secondary Traumatization 19, 227–229, 237,
    239. *See also* Vicarious Traumatization
Self-Accountability 47, 150, 151, 184, 185
Self-Awareness 74, 98, 226, 237, 242, 253
Self-Disclosure 6, 42, 48–50, 52, 61, 82, 84, 155,
    250, 251, 256
Self-Esteem 75, 182, 183, 220, 223
Sensual 121, 135, 224
Sex 86–142
    Continuum 114, 117, 127
    Cultural Values 104, 114
    Erections 123–126
    Family Sex Types 118, 139
        Sex Avoidant 118, 139
        Sex Expressive 118, 140
        Sex Obsessive 118, 139
        Sex Repressive 118, 139
    Sex and Touch Therapy 103, 119
    Sexual Response Cycle 115, 116, 140
Sexual Enterprise 146, 148
Sexual Feelings 104, 114, 116, 119, 120–123, 140, 257
    Attraction to Clients 19, 121–123
Sexual Misconduct 41, 42, 87, 127–134, 137, 140,
    142, 156, 197, 203, 204, 257–259
    Harassment 131–134, 141, 142, 288
    Lawsuit 87, 97
    Prevention 133–136, 151, 207
    Risk Factors 130, 131
Sexuality 29, 37, 38, 104, 105, 109, 114–121, 133, 134,
    139–142, 226, 228, 237, 290
    Sexual Behavior 29, 51, 114–118, 120, 121, 127,
    139, 258
    Sexual Identity 117, 139
    Sexual Orientation 109, 117, 139, 142, 262, 287
Six-Step Resolution Model 11
Slander 196, 197, 211
Sliding Fee 186, 213, 262, 268
Socializing 18, 130
Society 3, 11, 23, 24, 104, 106, 110, 114–116, 131, 139,
    183, 196
Standards of Practice 151, 152, 171, 177, 179
Students 5–7, 86–90, 97–101, 128, 213

Sublimation 20
Sympathetic Nervous System 108, 125, 139

T

Taxes 145, 191, 205, 206
Teenagers 37, 162–165
Termination 76, 80, 83, 94, 167–170, 179
Therapeutic Constellation 162, 163, 177
Tips 7, 56, 75, 101, 174, 182, 187, 188, 211, 213
Titles 145, 146, 149, 177
Transference 14, 17–20, 23, 24, 43, 61, 62, 64, 82,
    92, 93, 97, 169, 187, 229, 231, 237, 239, 250
Trauma 21, 62, 110, 111, 215–239, 258, 268–275. *See
    also* Abuse
    Flashbacks 216, 217, 221, 227, 230–239
    Statistics 107, 127, 139, 219
    Working with Self-Disclosed Survivors 268–275

V

Values 2–4, 7, 8, 10, 11, 13, 23, 24, 36, 37, 104, 114–
    116, 139, 173, 182, 196, 211
Vicarious Traumatization 229, 237
Victim 131, 133, 200–204, 218, 221–223, 259
Virtues 3